LABORATORY MATHEMATICS

Medical and Biological Applications

Joe Bill Campbell, Ph.D.

Shorter College
Rome, Georgia

June Mundy Campbell, M.Ed., MT(ASCP)

FIFTH EDITION

with 50 illustrations

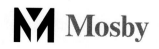 Mosby

St. Louis Baltimore Boston Carlsbad Chicago Naples New York Philadelphia Portland
London Madrid Mexico City Singapore Sydney Tokyo Toronto Wiesbaden

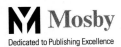

Mosby
Dedicated to Publishing Excellence

A Times Mirror
Company

Vice President and Publisher: Don Ladig
Editor: Jennifer Roche
Developmental Editor: Sandra J. Parker
Project Manager: Deborah L. Vogel
Production Editor: Karen L. Allman
Designer: Elizabeth Rohne Rudder
Manufacturing Manager: Theresa Fuchs
Cover Designer: Elizabeth Rohne Rudder

FIFTH EDITION

Copyright © 1997 by Mosby-Year Book, Inc.

Previous editions copyrighted 1976, 1980, 1984, 1990

Printed in the United States of America
Composition by The Clarinda Company
Printing/binding by R. R. Donnelly & Sons Company

Mosby-Year Book, Inc.
11830 Westline Industrial Drive
St. Louis, Missouri 63146

Library of Congress Cataloging in Publication Data

Campbell, Joe Bill, 1941-
    Laboratory mathematics : medical and biological applications / Joe
Bill Campbell, June Mundy Campbell. -- 5th ed.
        p.   cm.
    Includes bibliographical references and index.
    Previous edition has main entry under Campbell, June.
    ISBN 0-8151-1397-8 (alk. paper)
    1. Medical laboratory technology--Mathematics.   I. Campbell, June
Mundy, 1933-   . II. Title.
    RB38.3.C36   1996
    616.07′5′0151--dc20
                                                96-26753
                                                CIP

96 97 98 99 00 / 9 8 7 6 5 4 3 2 1

Preface

Mathematics is a science, a set of concepts, a way of thinking, a tool, and a mystery. It can be all of these things to anyone. However, each has its own importance to any individual. To most people who work in laboratories, the tool and the mystery are usually the most important.

Laboratory Mathematics provides simplified explanations of the calculations used in clinical and biological laboratories. It is primarily meant to help the student who has an inadequate background in mathematics develop the essential skills necessary to meet the standards for competent laboratory work. Also, it provides a source of review for the experienced worker in specific areas of laboratory mathematics.

Explanations are presented in a way to allow the reader to understand each step of the calculations. The chemical and physical principles are explained as they relate to the calculations. This book is meant to be a beginning for the study of the mathematics needed in laboratory work. It is not meant to be an end. It is not a reference on the theory of mathematics, nor is it complete in its scope. It is a beginning; it should not be an end. But is this not the way of most things in life?

The changes in the fifth edition include the addition of educational objectives. These will help the instructor in the planning of a course. Also, they will be a guide to the student in the study of each chapter. The book has changed to reflect changes in the way mathematics is currently being done in laboratories. Computers and the machines they are connected to now carry out the repetitive calculations of laboratory work. However, it is still important that the student know the way mathematics is used to produce a result. Also, the worker must know what is reasonable for a particular result. We can let machines do our work, but we cannot let the machines do our thinking, at least not yet.

As always, we solicit, encourage, and appreciate any and all suggestions for improvement of this work. Please send these to the authors at the address below.

Joe Bill Campbell
June Mundy Campbell
P.O. Box 115
Cave Spring, GA 30124

Contents

8 IONIC SOLUTIONS, 188

9 COLORIMETRY, 208

10 GRAPHS & STANDARD CURVES, 217

11 HEMATOLOGY MATH, 253

LABORATORY MATHEMATICS

Medical and Biological Applications

1

Basic Mathematics

EDUCATIONAL OBJECTIVES

To have successfully learned the material in this chapter, the student should be able to do the following properly:

- ◆ Describe the organization of the number systems using Arabic numerals and Roman numerals and the major uses of these two systems in the clinical laboratory.
- ◆ Manipulate signed numbers during addition, subtraction, multiplication, and division.
- ◆ Manipulate signed common and decimal fractional numbers during addition, subtraction, multiplication, and division.
- ◆ Convert common fractions to decimal fractions and vice versa.
- ◆ Manipulate percent values using addition, subtraction, multiplication, and division.
- ◆ Complete chain calculations using the proper order of calculations.
- ◆ Calculate values using simple algebra.
- ◆ Identify the significant figures in values and use proper techniques of rounding off results.
- ◆ Carry out algebraic manipulation of exponential numbers.
- ◆ Manipulate values expressed in scientific notation and convert values to and from scientific notation.

SECTION 1.1 GENERAL CONCEPTS

Students of laboratory technology have varying degrees of expertise in mathematics. This chapter considers some basic concepts of mathematics that anyone completing 12 years of public education should know. However, we realize that in many schools the goal is not that of disseminating useful knowledge but rather of sheltering incompetent personnel and frustrating competent teachers. This book cannot cover every aspect of mathematics and still remain within its designed scope. This chapter provides a review of the major concepts of mathematics needed for the technical aspects of most medical and biological laboratories. If the student does not understand these concepts after studying the review in this chapter, further sources of study should be sought to learn enough about the science and application of mathematics to use this book.

As far as possible, the student should not only understand how to do mathematical calculations but *why* the manipulations of the figures work as they do. When a formula is presented as a method of solution to a problem, the student should attempt to understand the principle on which the formula is based. Understanding the basis of a formula often allows one to modify the formula to better suit a particular situation.

In doing mathematical calculations, there are several general considerations to make when determining the most efficient method of solving a problem and reducing error. Some of these are included in the following list:

1. Read the problem carefully. Be sure the entire problem has been read *and understood.*
2. Determine what principles and relationships are involved.
3. Determine exactly what results are to be produced by the calculations.
4. Think about the possible methods to use in solving the problem.
5. Write the intermediate stages of the calculations clearly. Avoid writing one number on top of another as a method of correction. Make each digit legible.
6. Recognize different forms of the same value, such as $\frac{1}{2}$, ½, 1 ÷ 2, 0.5, 50%, and 0.50.
7. Be extremely careful when positioning the decimal point.
8. Where possible, mentally estimate an answer before working the problem; compare the calculated result with the estimated answer. If the two figures disagree drastically, determine which one is wrong.

SECTION 1.2 NUMBER SYSTEMS

Two major number systems are used today. These are referred to as Arabic and Roman numerals. The most useful are the Arabic numerals.

Arabic Numerals

The Arabic system is the most widely used system of expressing values and in calculations. This is a base-10 system with 10 digits: 0, 1, 2, 3, 4, 5, 6, 7, 8, and 9. These digits express values when used alone or in combination. The system is positional in nature. This means that the value of any digit is affected by the position it occupies in the number. Each digit in a number has a place value beginning from a point called a **decimal.** Digits to the left of the decimal point indicate values greater than 1. Digits other than zero to the right of the decimal point indicate values greater than zero but less than 1. A zero between the decimal point and a nonzero digit serves to determine the place value of the nonzero digit. Every place is 10 times the next closest place to the right. Consider the number 245.609. The 5 is in the units place, expressing 5 × 1; the 4 is in the tens place, expressing 4 × 10; and the 2 is in the hundreds place, expressing 2 × 100. Successive digits occupy a place value 10 times the preceding place value. Digits to the right of the decimal point follow the same pattern, except that these indicate values less than 1. In the above number, the 6 is in the tenths place, expressing a value of 6 × ¹⁄₁₀; the 0 expresses 0 × ¹⁄₁₀₀, and the 9 expresses 9 × ¹⁄₁,₀₀₀. The zero digit in the ¹⁄₁₀₀ place is used to indicate that the value of the number is greater than 245.6 but less than 245.61. The next digit, 9, indicates how near to 245.61 the number is. The chart at the top of p. 3 may help you understand this system.

This system allows for relatively simple manipulation of numbers for the four basic computational processes: addition, subtraction, multiplication, and division. These processes are discussed in detail later in this chapter.

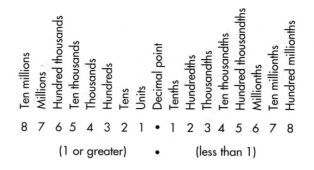

8 7 6 5 4 3 2 1 • 1 2 3 4 5 6 7 8

(1 or greater)   •   (less than 1)

At the present time there are two methods used to separate digits in a number into groups of three (thousands, millions, billions, etc.) In English documents, it is common practice to use a period (a point or dot) *on* the line for the decimal point and a comma to separate the groups of three. However, the International Union of Pure and Applied Chemistry (IUPAC) and the International Federation of Clinical Chemistry (IFCC) recommend that the comma be used for the decimal point and that numbers with many digits be written with a small space separating the groups of three, counting from the decimal point both to the left and the right. A period or comma should not be used for separation.

The two systems are illustrated below. Use whichever seems more logical to you. In this book the English system is used.

IUPAC	English
0,02	0.02
1 962,7	1,962.7
1 928 760,178 48	1,928,760.17848

Roman Numerals

The Roman numeral system uses letters to represent numbers. It does not have a constant base system and hence makes calculations difficult or impossible. This system is used only to identify values. Roman numerals are used sporadically in writing. For example, Roman numerals are used in medicine to indicate dosages of drugs that are written in apothecary units. Hence one needs to understand the current system of Roman numerals even though the Arabic numerals are much more common and useful.

Roman numerals are expressed as seven capital or lowercase letters.

Roman Numerals	Arabic Equivalent
I, i	1
V, v	5
X, x	10
L, l	50
C, c	100
D, d	500
M, m	1,000

A capital letter with a bar over it indicates 1,000 times the simple letter.

$\overline{V}$	$(5 \times 1{,}000)$	5,000
$\overline{C}$	$(100 \times 1{,}000)$	100,000
$\overline{D}$	$(500 \times 1{,}000)$	500,000
$\overline{M}$	$(1{,}000 \times 1{,}000)$	1,000,000

These letters are combined in specific ways to indicate the magnitude of a value. There are some general rules for the combining of Roman numerals.

1. When a numeral of lesser value follows one of greater value, add the two values.

$$VI = 5 + 1 = 6$$

$$LX = 50 + 10 = 60$$

$$MDC = 1{,}000 + 500 + 100 = 1{,}600$$

2. When numerals of the same value are repeated in sequence, add the values.

$$XX = 10 + 10 = 20$$

$$III = 1 + 1 + 1 = 3$$

3. When a numeral of lesser value precedes one of greater value, the value of the first is subtracted from the value of the second. The numerals V, L, and D are never used as a subtracted number.

$$IV = 5 - 1 = 4$$

$$XL = 50 - 10 = 40$$

$$XLV = 50 - 10 + 5 = 45 \text{ (not VL)}$$

4. When a numeral of lesser value is placed between two numerals of greater value, the numeral of lesser value is subtracted from the numeral following it.

$$XIV = 10 + 5 - 1 = 14$$

$$XXIX = 10 + 10 + 10 - 1 = 29$$

5. Numerals are never repeated more than three times in sequence.

$$XXX = 30$$

$$XL = 40 \text{ (not XXXX)}$$

6. Arrange the letters in order of decreasing value from left to right except for letters having values to be subtracted from the next letter.

$$MDCLXVI = 1{,}666$$

$$MCM = 1{,}900$$

$$MCMXLIV = 1{,}944$$

SECTION 1.3 ARITHMETIC

The fundamental area of mathematics is arithmetic. This is the manipulation of real numbers by use of the four basic operations of mathematics: addition, subtraction, multiplication, and division. Nearly everyone can carry out these operations with simple problems. However, most people have some difficulty with specific parts of arithmetic. This section provides a general review of the major concepts of this area of mathematics.

Terminology of the Basic Operations

The following terms are used to describe the four basic operations of arithmetic.

ADDITION. Addition is the combination of numbers to obtain an equivalent single quantity. A number added to others is called an **addend.** When two or more addends are combined the result is called a **sum.**

SUBTRACTION. Subtraction is the operation of deducting one number from another. The number from which another is deducted is called the **minuend.** The number that is deducted from the minuend is called the **subtrahend.** The result of a subtraction is called the **difference.**

MULTIPLICATION. Multiplication is the adding of a number to itself a specified number of times. The **multiplicand** is the number that is multiplied. The **multiplier** is the number of times the multiplicand is added to itself. The result of a multiplication operation is called the **product.**

DIVISION. Division is the operation of finding how many times one number or quantity is contained in another. The **dividend** is the number that is to be divided. The **divisor** is the number that is divided into the dividend. The result of a division operation is called the **quotient.**

Use of Plus and Minus Signs

The plus (+) and minus (−) signs have two uses in mathematics: (1) to indicate the addition and subtraction operations, and (2) to determine the direction of progression of a number from zero. The first use is the generally known use. The second use is often not well understood. The following is an explanation of this use.

Numbers are used to denote a progression of values from a beginning point. The beginning point is zero. The progression of values moves away from zero in two directions.

Infinity .... −7 −6 −5 −4 −3 −2 −1   0 +1 +2 +3 +4 +5 +6 +7 .... Infinity

Customarily, numbers to the right of the zero point are spoken of as **positive numbers,** whereas numbers to the left of zero are spoken of as **negative numbers.** A **signed number** is one written with a plus or minus sign. Positive numbers have a plus sign; negative numbers a minus sign. Unless otherwise indicated, a number without a specific sign can be assumed to be positive.

Addition of Signed Numbers

The addition of signed numbers involves either simple arithmetic addition or subtraction, depending on the particular combination of signs.

1. ADDITION OF POSITIVE NUMBERS

To add **positive** numbers to **positive** numbers, add all numbers together and give the sum a plus sign.

EXAMPLE 1-1: Add +4 and +7.

$$\begin{array}{r} +4 \\ +\ \ +7 \\ \hline +11 \ \ (\text{sum}) \end{array}$$

2. ADDITION OF NEGATIVE NUMBERS

To add **negative** numbers to **negative** numbers, add all numbers together and give the sum a minus sign.

EXAMPLE 1-2: Add −8 and −4.

$$\begin{array}{r} -8 \\ +\ \ -4 \\ \hline -12 \end{array}$$

3. ADDITION OF POSITIVE NUMBERS AND NEGATIVE NUMBERS

To add a **positive** number to a **negative** number, and vice versa, subtract the smaller number from the larger, ignoring the signs, and give the sum the sign of the larger number.

EXAMPLE 1-3: Add +8 and −5.

$$\begin{array}{r} +8 \\ +\ \ -5 \end{array}$$

Ignore the signs and subtract the smaller number from the larger.

$$\begin{array}{r} 8 \\ -\ \ 5 \\ \hline 3 \end{array}$$

Give the result the sign of the larger number (+8); hence, the sum is +3.

EXAMPLE 1-4: Add −12 and +3.

$$\begin{array}{r} -12 \\ +\ \ +3 \end{array}$$

Ignore the signs and subtract the smaller number from the larger.

$$\begin{array}{r} 12 \\ -\ \ 3 \\ \hline 9 \end{array}$$

Give the result the sign of the larger number (−12), hence, the sum is −9.

To add several **positive** and **negative** numbers, add all the positive numbers, then add all the negative numbers, and then subtract the smaller sum from the larger and give the final result the sign of the larger sum.

EXAMPLE 1-5: Add +6, −3, −2 and +1.

Add all positive numbers.   Add all negative numbers.

$$\begin{array}{r} +6 \\ +\ +1 \\ \hline +7 \end{array}\qquad\begin{array}{r} -3 \\ +\ -2 \\ \hline -5 \end{array}$$

Subtract the smaller sum from the larger, ignoring the signs.

$$\begin{array}{r} 7 \\ -\ 5 \\ \hline 2 \end{array}$$

Give the final result the sign of the larger sum, in this case +7. The final sum is +2.

Subtraction of Signed Numbers

Remember that subtraction involves the deduction of the value of one number, the **subtrahend,** from the value of another, the **minuend,** to produce a result, the **difference.** In other words, subtract the subtrahend from the minuend to get the difference.

A word of caution—there are two ways to subtract two numbers, depending on which number is the subtrahend and which is the minuend. The subtrahend may not always be the smaller number. Be sure of the direction of all subtraction operations.

When subtracting signed numbers, change the sign of the subtrahend and add according to the rules of addition.

1. SUBTRACTION OF A POSITIVE NUMBER FROM A POSITIVE NUMBER

To subtract a **positive** number from a **positive** number, change the sign of the subtrahend and add.

EXAMPLE 1-6: Subtract +8 from +15.

In this example, +8 is being subtracted from +15. Hence, +15 is the minuend and +8 is the subtrahend.

$$\begin{array}{r} +15 \text{ (minuend)} \\ -\ +8 \text{ (subtrahend)} \\ \hline \end{array}$$

Change the sign of the subtrahend (+8) and add.

$$\begin{array}{r} +15 \text{ (minuend)} \\ +\ -8 \text{ (subtrahend)} \\ \hline +7 \text{ (difference)} \end{array}$$

If this is not clear, study the explanation in Examples 1-3, 1-4, and 1-5.

EXAMPLE 1-7: Subtract +15 from +8.

This example may seem to be the same as Example 1-6. However, here the minuend is +8 and the subtrahend is +15. The difference is not the same.

$$\begin{array}{r} +8 \text{ (minuend)} \\ -\ +15 \text{ (subtrahend)} \\ \hline \end{array}$$

Change the sign of the subtrahend ($+15$) to -15; then add.

$$\begin{array}{r} +8 \\ + -15 \\ \hline \end{array}$$

Following the rules of the addition of positive and negative numbers, ignore the signs of the numbers and subtract the smaller number from the larger.

$$\begin{array}{r} 15 \\ - 8 \\ \hline 7 \end{array}$$

Give the answer the sign of the larger number (-15). Hence, the difference is -7.

2. SUBTRACTION OF A NEGATIVE NUMBER FROM A NEGATIVE NUMBER

To subtract a **negative** number from a **negative** number, change the sign of the subtrahend and add.

EXAMPLE 1-8: Subtract -15 from -28.

In this example, -15 is being subtracted from -28. Hence, -15 is the subtrahend and -28 is the minuend.

$$\begin{array}{r} -28 \\ - -15 \\ \hline \end{array}$$

Change the sign of the subtrahend (-15) and add.

$$\begin{array}{r} -28 \\ + +15 \\ \hline \end{array}$$

To add a positive number to a negative number, ignore the signs of the numbers and subtract the smaller number from the larger.

$$\begin{array}{r} 28 \\ - 15 \\ \hline 13 \end{array}$$

Give the result the sign of the larger number. In this case the larger number is -28; therefore the difference is -13.

If Example 1-8 is reversed and -28 is subtracted from -15, a different answer results.

EXAMPLE 1-9: Subtract -28 from -15.

Here, -28 is being subtracted from -15. The subtrahend is -28, and the minuend is -15.

$$\begin{array}{r} -15 \\ - -28 \\ \hline \end{array}$$

Change the sign of the subtrahend (-28) to $+28$; then add.

$$\begin{array}{r} -15 \\ + +28 \\ \hline \end{array}$$

To add a positive number to a negative number, subtract the smaller number from the larger number, ignoring the signs, and give the sum the sign of the larger number.

$$
\begin{array}{r}
28 \\
-\ 15 \\
\hline
13
\end{array}
$$

In the *addition* portion of this calculation, +28 is the larger number, hence the difference is +13.

3. SUBTRACTION OF A NEGATIVE NUMBER FROM A POSITIVE NUMBER

To subtract a **negative** number from a **positive** number, change the sign of the subtrahend and add.

In this kind of calculation the result is always positive. This is because the subtrahend is negative and its sign is changed to positive according to the rule.

EXAMPLE 1-10: Subtract −14 from +9.

In this example, the subtrahend is −14 and the minuend is +9. If the signs are ignored, the subtrahend is larger than the minuend. However, the same rule as with other subtraction problems still applies. To subtract numbers, change the sign of the subtrahend, add, and give the result the sign of the larger number.

$$
\begin{array}{r}
+9 \ \text{(minuend)} \\
-\ -14 \ \text{(subtrahend)}
\end{array}
$$

Change the sign of the subtrahend (−14) to +14; then add.

$$
\begin{array}{r}
+9 \\
+\ +14 \\
\hline
+23
\end{array}
$$

4. SUBTRACTION OF A POSITIVE NUMBER FROM A NEGATIVE NUMBER

To subtract a **positive** number from a **negative** number, change the sign of the subtrahend and add.

This always results in a negative number as the difference.

EXAMPLE 1-11: Subtract +85 from −100.

$$
\begin{array}{r}
-100 \ \text{(minuend)} \\
-\ +85 \ \text{(subtrahend)}
\end{array}
$$

Change the sign of the subtrahend (+85) to −85; then add.

$$
\begin{array}{r}
-100 \\
+\ -85 \\
\hline
-185
\end{array}
$$

Multiplication and Division of Signed Numbers

The manipulation of signed numbers in multiplication and division is less complicated than with addition and subtraction. Two rules always apply in multiplication and division.

1. The multiplication or division of *like* signs always produces a **positive** result.
2. The multiplication or division of *unlike* signs always produces a **negative** result.

Follow these rules consistently. Study the following examples:

EXAMPLE 1-12: Multiply +4 by +7.

$$+4 \times +7 = +28$$

Multiplication of a positive number by a positive number gives a positive product.

EXAMPLE 1-13: Divide −34 by −2.

$$-34 \div -2 = +17$$

Division of a negative number by a negative number produces a positive quotient.

EXAMPLE 1-14: Multiply +18 by −3.

$$+18 \times -3 = -54$$

Multiplication of a positive number by a negative number results in a negative product.

EXAMPLE 1-15: Divide +25 into −100.

$$-100 \div +25 = -4$$

Division of a negative number by a positive number produces a negative quotient.

The material in this section must be well understood before continuing with the study of laboratory mathematics. It includes many basic concepts that give students problems. Be sure you understand this section before continuing.

SECTION 1.4 FRACTIONS

The word **fraction** refers to a part of a whole. In mathematics, fractions refer to the division of some value into any number of equal parts.

There are two common forms of expression of fractions, common and decimal.

Common Fractions

A **common fraction** is written in two parts, one over the other. The lower number is the **denominator;** the upper number is the **numerator.**

The denominator is the number of parts into which 1 is divided. The numerator is the number of these parts in the fraction.

A **proper fraction** is one in which the numerator is smaller than the denominator. The value of any proper fraction is always less than 1.

$$\frac{1}{2} \qquad \frac{4}{5} \qquad \frac{6}{13} \qquad \frac{227}{2,000}$$

An **improper fraction** is one in which the numerator is equal to or greater than the denominator. The value of any improper fraction is always 1 or greater than 1.

$$\frac{4}{4} \qquad \frac{7}{5} \qquad \frac{18}{16}$$

A **whole number** is any number in which the denominator is 1. This denominator is rarely expressed, but is understood.

$$4 = \frac{4}{1} \qquad 16 = \frac{16}{1} \qquad 2{,}000 = \frac{2{,}000}{1}$$

A **mixed number** is a whole number plus a fraction. This number always has a value of more than 1.

$$2\frac{1}{8} \qquad 10\frac{6}{9} \qquad 15\frac{1}{3}$$

A mixed number can be changed to an improper fraction by multiplying the whole number by the denominator of the fraction, adding the product to the numerator, and using the result as a new numerator over the original denominator.

$$2\frac{2}{5} = \frac{2 \times 5 + 2}{5} = \frac{10 + 2}{5} = \frac{12}{5}$$

An improper fraction can be changed to a whole or mixed number by dividing the numerator by the denominator.

$$\frac{20}{5} = 20 \div 5 = 4 \qquad\qquad \frac{9}{5} = 1\frac{4}{5}$$

A **complex fraction** is one in which the numerator, the denominator, or both are fractions.

$$\frac{2\frac{1}{2}}{3} \qquad \frac{6}{\frac{2}{5}} \qquad \frac{\frac{3}{8}}{\frac{4}{9}}$$

Equivalent fractions are fractions having the same value but different forms.

A fraction can be converted to an equivalent fraction by multiplying or dividing the numerator and denominator by the same number. This does not change the value.

$$\frac{1}{3} \times \frac{2}{2} = \frac{2}{6} \qquad\qquad \frac{12}{18} \div \frac{3}{3} = \frac{4}{6}$$

$$\frac{1}{3} = \frac{2}{6} \qquad\qquad \frac{12}{18} = \frac{4}{6}$$

Addition and Subtraction with Common Fractions

When the denominators of fractions are the same, they are called **common denominators.** The term **like fractions** has been used to describe fractions that have a common denominator. **Unlike fractions** are fractions with denominators that are not alike.

To add or subtract fractions, it is necessary that the denominators of all fractions in the operation be the same.

1. To add or subtract **like** fractions, add or subtract the numerators and place the result over the denominator. Do not change (do not add or subtract) the denominator.

EXAMPLE 1-16: Add ¾ and ¼.

$$\frac{3}{4} + \frac{1}{4} = \frac{4}{4}$$

EXAMPLE 1-17: Add ⁹⁄₁₆ and ⁵⁄₁₆.

$$\frac{9}{16} + \frac{5}{16} = \frac{14}{16}$$

EXAMPLE 1-18: Subtract ¹²⁄₃₃ from ¹⁹⁄₃₃.

$$\frac{19}{33} - \frac{12}{33} = \frac{7}{33}$$

EXAMPLE 1-19: Subtract ⁵⁄₁₃ from ⁸⁄₁₃.

$$\frac{8}{13} - \frac{5}{13} = \frac{3}{13}$$

2. To add or subtract **unlike** fractions, it is necessary to change the unlike fractions to like fractions; then proceed as with like fractions.

This means that a common denominator must be found for all fractions in the calculation. It is better if the common denominator is the least common denominator. The **least common denominator** (LCD) is the smallest denominator into which all the denominators can be evenly divided. The LCD can often be found easily.

EXAMPLE 1-20: Find the sum of ½, ¾, and ⅜.

Since these are unlike fractions, find the LCD. It is obvious that both 2 and 4 can be evenly divided into 8. Thus the LCD for this problem is 8.

The next step is to find the fraction with a denominator of 8 that is equivalent to each of the fractions in the problem. To do this, divide each denominator into the LCD and multiply the result by the numerator. This will give the new numerator.

Place this new numerator over the LCD. This will give the equivalent fraction.

$$\frac{1}{2}; \qquad 8 \div 2 = 4; \qquad 4 \times 1 = 4; \qquad \frac{1}{2} = \frac{4}{8}$$

$$\frac{3}{4}; \qquad 8 \div 4 = 2; \qquad 2 \times 3 = 6; \qquad \frac{3}{4} = \frac{6}{8}$$

Hence,

$$\frac{4}{8} + \frac{6}{8} + \frac{3}{8} = \frac{13}{8} = 1\frac{5}{8}$$

In those problems in which the least common denominator is not obvious, the following procedures may be used.

Place all the denominators in a line. If possible, divide the numbers in this line by a number that will divide at least two of the denominators evenly. Bring down all numbers that cannot be divided. Continue this procedure until all denominators are reduced to a quotient of 1. Multiply all numbers used as divisors together. This number is the LCD.

EXAMPLE 1-21: Find the LCD for ½, ⅔, ⅚, and 4/9.

$$2\ \overline{)2\ 3\ 6\ 9}$$
$$3\ \overline{)1\ 3\ 3\ 9}$$
$$3\ \overline{)\ \ 1\ 1\ 3}$$
$$1$$
$$2 \times 3 \times 3 = 18$$

The LCD for these fractions is 18.

Another method to find a common denominator is to multiply all denominators together. This does not always produce the least common denominator, but it can be used to produce equivalent like fractions.

EXAMPLE 1-22: Add 4/7, ⅝, and ⅗.

First find a common denominator for these fractions. This can easily be done by multiplying all three denominators together.

$$7 \times 8 \times 5 = 280$$

Now find the numerator for each fraction.

$$\frac{4}{7}; \qquad 280 \div 7 = 40; \qquad 40 \times 4 = 160; \qquad \frac{4}{7} = \frac{160}{280}$$

$$\frac{5}{8}; \qquad 280 \div 8 = 35; \qquad 35 \times 5 = 175; \qquad \frac{5}{8} = \frac{175}{280}$$

$$\frac{3}{5}; \qquad 280 \div 5 = 56; \qquad 56 \times 3 = 168; \qquad \frac{3}{5} = \frac{168}{280}$$

Add the fractions.

$$\frac{160}{280} + \frac{175}{280} + \frac{168}{280} = \frac{503}{280} = 1\frac{223}{280}$$

Multiplication with Common Fractions

To multiply one fraction by another, simply multiply the numerators together and multiply the denominators together. This can be done with like or unlike fractions.

EXAMPLE 1-23: Multiply ¼ by ¾.

$$\frac{1}{4} \times \frac{3}{4} = \frac{3}{16}$$

EXAMPLE 1-24: Multiply 4/11 by ⅞.

$$\frac{4}{11} \times \frac{7}{8} = \frac{28}{88}$$

If mixed numbers are involved in a multiplication, convert them to an improper fraction before multiplying the numbers.

EXAMPLE 1-25: Multiply 5⅞ by 3⅖ by 7½.

$$5\frac{7}{8} \times 3\frac{2}{5} \times 7\frac{1}{2}$$

Convert to improper fractions.

$5\frac{7}{8}$; $(8 \times 5) + 7 = 47$; $5\frac{7}{8} = \frac{47}{8}$

$3\frac{2}{5}$; $(5 \times 3) + 2 = 17$; $3\frac{2}{5} = \frac{17}{5}$

$7\frac{1}{2}$; $(2 \times 7) + 1 = 15$; $7\frac{1}{2} = \frac{15}{2}$

Multiply numerators by numerators and denominators by denominators.

$$\frac{47}{8} \times \frac{17}{5} \times \frac{15}{2} = \frac{11{,}985}{80} = 149\frac{65}{80} = 149\frac{13}{16}$$

Division with Common Fractions

As in multiplication, unlike fractions can be divided without being converted to like fractions. To divide one fraction by another, invert the fraction doing the dividing (divisor) by making the numerator the denominator and vice versa. Multiply the resulting fractions.

EXAMPLE 1-26: Divide 3⁄6 by 4⁄5.

$$\frac{3}{6} \div \frac{4}{5} = \frac{3}{6} \times \frac{5}{4} = \frac{15}{24}$$

To divide mixed numbers, convert them to improper fractions and proceed as directed.

EXAMPLE 1-27: Divide 5 7⁄8 by 3 1⁄5.

Convert to improper fractions.

$$5\frac{7}{8} = \frac{47}{8} \qquad 3\frac{1}{5} = \frac{16}{5}$$

$$\frac{47}{8} \div \frac{16}{5}$$

Invert the divisor and multiply.

$$\frac{47}{8} \times \frac{5}{16} = \frac{235}{128} = 1\frac{107}{128}$$

Comparison of Fractional Values

It is often necessary to determine whether one common fraction is greater or less than another. This is the *relative* value of fractions. To find the relative value of two common fractions use the following rules.

1. If the denominators of two fractions are the same, the fraction with the larger numerator is the **larger** fraction (3⁄4 is greater than 1⁄4).

EXAMPLE 1-28: Compare 7⁄20, 4⁄20, 15⁄20, and 12⁄20.

$$\frac{15}{20} > \frac{12}{20} > \frac{7}{20} > \frac{4}{20}$$

2. If the numerators of two fractions are equal, the fraction with the greater denominator has the **lesser** value.

EXAMPLE 1-29: Compare ⅓, ⅙, ¼, and ⅒.

$$\frac{1}{10} < \frac{1}{6} < \frac{1}{4} < \frac{1}{3}$$

3. If the fractions being compared have different denominators and numerators, change them to like fractions and proceed as shown in Steps 1 and 2.

EXAMPLE 1-30: Which is greater, ⁹⁄₁₆ or ⅝?

The least common denominator is 16.

$$\frac{9}{16} = \frac{9}{16} \qquad \frac{5}{8} = \frac{10}{16}$$

$$\frac{10}{16} > \frac{9}{16}$$

$$\frac{5}{8} > \frac{9}{16}$$

NOTE: Small differences in statements using fractions can make a great difference in the meaning conveyed. For example:

1. *What is ¼ of ½?* This is a multiplication problem, the same as "What is 50% of 100 (0.50 × 100)?" or "What is ½ of 2 (½ × 2)?"

$$\frac{1}{4} \times \frac{1}{2} = \frac{1}{8}$$

¼ of ½ is ⅛

In this case the numbers happen to be fractions; however, the principle and solution are the same.

2. *¼ is what part of ½?* In this situation the fractions are treated as a common fraction. ½ represents the total number of parts and is the denominator; ¼ is the part represented and is the numerator.

$$\frac{¼}{½} = \frac{1}{4} \div \frac{1}{2} = \frac{1}{4} \times \frac{2}{1} = \frac{2}{4} = \frac{1}{2}$$

¼ is ½ of ½

Decimal Fractions

A **decimal fraction** is a fraction with a denominator of 10 or some even multiple of 10. This denominator is expressed by using the decimal point instead of writing it under the numerator. The expressed number of a decimal fraction indicates the numerator. This form of writing fractions generally allows for easier calculation. The decimal point is the point of reference used to determine the place value of a digit in a number. Study the following chart.

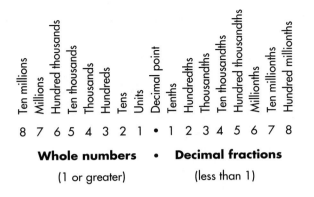

Digits to the left of the decimal point indicate values of 1 or greater, whereas digits to the right of the decimal point indicate values of less than 1.

A decimal number having a value of less than 1 is a proper fraction or pure decimal. A decimal number greater than 1 is a mixed fraction.

Pure decimals:	0.83	0.9	0.5
Mixed fractions:	1.9	7.38	2.251

Some of these examples are read as follows:

0.83	"Eighty-three hundredths" or "zero point eighty-three"
0.9	"Nine tenths" or "zero point nine"
2.251	"Two and two hundred fifty-one thousandths" or "two point two five one"

Decimal fractions can be converted to common fractions and vice versa. The understood denominator of a decimal fraction is 10, 100, 1,000, etc., depending on the number of places in the fractions.

1. CHANGING DECIMAL FRACTIONS TO COMMON FRACTIONS

To convert a decimal fraction to a common fraction, delete the decimal point and place the number over its understood denominator.

$$0.4 = \frac{4}{10} = \frac{2}{5} \qquad 16.25 = 16\frac{25}{100} = 16\frac{1}{4} = \frac{65}{4}$$

2. CHANGING COMMON FRACTIONS TO DECIMAL FRACTIONS

To convert a common fraction to a decimal fraction, divide the numerator by the denominator.

$$\frac{1}{2} = 2\overline{)1.0}^{\,0.5} = 0.5 \qquad \frac{4}{5} = 5\overline{)4.0}^{\,0.8} = 0.8 \qquad 7\frac{3}{4} = \frac{31}{4} = 4\overline{)31.00}^{\,7.75} = 7.75$$

$$\begin{array}{r} 28 \\ \hline 30 \\ 28 \\ \hline 20 \\ 20 \\ \hline \end{array}$$

NOTE: Adding zeros to the right of a decimal fraction does not change the value of the fraction.

$$0.2 = 0.20 = 0.200$$

Often a common fraction cannot be converted into a decimal exactly. In such cases the numbers should be rounded off according to rules discussed on p. 27.

$$\frac{1}{3} = 0.333333333 = 0.33 = 0.3$$

$$\frac{2}{3} = 0.666666666 = 0.67 = 0.7$$

3. ADDITION OR SUBTRACTION OF NUMBERS CONTAINING DECIMALS

Align the decimal point of each number, one directly under the other, and add or subtract as discussed earlier. The decimal point of the answer will remain aligned with the points of the numbers of the problem.

It is important to be neat with this type of calculation.

$$\begin{array}{r} 0.62 \\ 0.103 \\ + \ 0.01 \\ \hline 0.733 \end{array} \qquad \begin{array}{r} 0.762 \\ - \ 0.15 \\ \hline 0.612 \end{array}$$

4. MULTIPLICATION OF NUMBERS CONTAINING DECIMAL FRACTIONS

The number of digits to the right of the decimal point of the answer equals the total number of digits to the right of the decimal points of the numbers involved in the calculation.

$$\begin{array}{r} 7.43 \\ \times \ 3.45 \\ \hline 3715 \\ 2\ 972 \\ 22\ 29 \\ \hline 25.6335 \end{array}$$

5. DIVISION OF ONE DECIMAL NUMBER BY ANOTHER

Arrange the numbers as if whole numbers were being divided.

$$6.78)\overline{74.934}$$

Move the decimal point of the divisor (the number by which division is being made) to the right of the last digit. Now move the decimal point of the dividend (the number being divided) to the right the same number of spaces the decimal point of the divisor was moved.

$$6.78.)\overline{74.93.4}$$

Place the decimal point of the answer directly above the new position of the decimal point of the dividend.

$$678)\overline{7493.4}$$

Complete the calculations.

$$
\begin{array}{r}
11.05 \\
678)\overline{7493.4} \\
\underline{678} \\
713 \\
\underline{678} \\
3540 \\
\underline{3390} \\
150
\end{array}
$$

NOTE: The number of decimal places can be increased by placing a zero after the remainder and continuing the division process.

Percent

A **percent** is a peculiar kind of fraction. It is indicated by the symbol % and means *per 100;* therefore a number given as a percentage is understood to mean that many parts of 100. In other words, a number expressed as a percentage can be thought of as a numerator with an understood denominator of 100. This section discusses the general relationships of calculations with percent values.

3% means 3 parts in 100 total parts

$$3\% = \frac{3}{100} = 0.03$$

Percent values are much used in laboratory work, and many of their uses can be very confusing. Usually there is more unsaid in a percentage number than just the "per 100." For example, a 10% salt solution usually means 10 grams of sodium chloride in 100 milliliters of solution. However, it can mean 10 grams of sodium chloride in 100 grams of water or 10 grams of sodium chloride in 90 grams of water. Or it could mean something else. There can be a lot more to be understood about percentages than just parts per 100. Generally, when a percentage is used in a particular situation, its meaning is well understood. However, one should be careful to know the full meaning of a percent value in that particular situation. Many specific uses of percentages are discussed at length in Chapter 6, pp. 135-138.

There is another need for caution with percent values; when using percent values in calculations, be sure that every percentage used in one mathematical operation is compatible with the others and that the entire calculation is logical. One cannot multiply a 10% salt solution by a 5% red-light transmission and produce a sensible answer. Understand the full meaning of percent values before doing calculations with them.

1. CHANGING PERCENTAGES TO COMMON FRACTIONS

To change a percentage to a common fraction, simply use the percent value as a numerator over a denominator of 100. This is the same as dividing the number by 100. Reduce the resulting fraction to its lowest terms.

EXAMPLE 1-31: Convert 2% to a common fraction.

$$2\% = \frac{2}{100} = \frac{1}{50}$$

EXAMPLE 1-32: Convert $\frac{1}{10}$% to a common fraction.

$$\frac{1}{10}\% = \frac{\frac{1}{10}}{100} = \frac{1}{10} \div \frac{100}{1} = \frac{1}{10} \times \frac{1}{100} = \frac{1}{1,000}$$

2. CHANGING PERCENTAGES TO DECIMAL FRACTIONS

To change a percentage to a decimal fraction, divide the number by 100 and leave off the percent sign.

This can easily be done by moving the decimal point two places to the left. If the number does not have two places to the left, make them by adding zeros.

EXAMPLE 1-33: Change 29% to a decimal fraction.

$$29\% = \frac{29}{100} = 0.29$$

EXAMPLE 1-34: Change 3% to a decimal fraction.

$$3\% = \frac{3}{100} = 0.03$$

EXAMPLE 1-35: Change 0.5% to a decimal fraction.

$$0.5\% = \frac{0.5}{100} = 0.005$$

If the percent value is written as a common fraction, one may change the common fraction to a decimal fraction by dividing the denominator into the numerator.

EXAMPLE 1-36: Convert $\frac{1}{4}$% to a decimal fraction.

$$\frac{1}{4}\% = 4\overline{)1.00}^{.25} = 0.25\%$$

Move the decimal point two places to the left and drop the percent sign.

$$0.25\% = \frac{0.25}{100} = 0.0025$$

3. CHANGING FRACTIONS TO PERCENTAGES

To change a common or decimal fraction to a percentage, multiply by 100 and add the percent sign.

This rule comes from the relationship in a ratio-proportion setup.

0.5 is to 1 as x is to 100

$$\frac{0.5}{1} = \frac{x}{100}$$

$$1x = 0.5 \times 100$$

$$x = 50, \qquad \frac{50}{100} = 50\%$$

The same answer results when you follow the rule: $0.5 \times 100 = 50\%$

EXAMPLE 1-37: Convert ⅟₅₀ to a percentage.

Using ratio and proportion:

1 is to 50 as x is to 100

$$\frac{1}{50} = \frac{x}{100}$$

$$50x = 100$$

$$x = 2, \qquad \frac{2}{100} = 2\%$$

Or using the rule:

$$\frac{1}{50} \times \frac{100}{1} = \frac{100}{50} = 2\%$$

EXAMPLE 1-38: Convert ⅔ to a percentage.

$$\frac{2}{3} \times \frac{100}{1} = \frac{200}{3} = 66.7\%$$

EXAMPLE 1-39: Convert 0.026 to a percentage.

$$0.026 \times 100 = 2.6\%$$

EXAMPLE 1-40: Convert 1.09 to a percentage.

$$1.09 \times 100 = 109\%$$

4. ADDING OR SUBTRACTING PERCENT VALUES

Since percent values represent parts per 100, the understood denominator is always the same; therefore all percent values represent like fractions.

Add or subtract as with simple numbers.

EXAMPLE 1-41: Add 5% and 19%.

$$5\% + 19\% = 24\%$$

EXAMPLE 1-42 Subtract 10% from 20%.

$$20\% - 10\% = 10\%$$

NOTE: This of course applies only if the understood units of both percentages are the same (see Chapter 6, pp. 135-138).

5. MULTIPLYING USING PERCENT

A. Multiplying a nonpercent number by a percentage

Two methods may be used to multiply a number by percentage. The first is to convert the percentage to a decimal and multiply. The second method is to multiply a number by the percentage and divide the product by 100.

The first method is preferred because it generally leads to fewer errors. The percentage is converted to a decimal fraction before it is used in calculations. The result is converted to a percentage after the calculation. The second method gives an intermediate result, which is a nonsense value that has to be converted to a percentage to have a meaningful result. Use care with this method.

EXAMPLE 1-43: What is 32% of 78?

Using the first method, convert the percentage to a decimal fraction and multiply.

$$32\% = \frac{32}{100} = 0.32$$

$$0.32 \times 78 = 24.96$$

Using the second method, multiply the number by the percentage and divide by 100.

$$32\% \times 78 = 2496$$

$$2496 \div 100 = 24.96$$

Both methods are really the same. Only the order of operations has been changed.

B. Multiplying a percentage by a percentage

When multiplying a percentage by a percentage, convert both percentages to decimal fractions and multiply. The product is a decimal fraction. You may then convert the result to a percentage by multiplying the product by 100.

EXAMPLE 1-44: What is 50% of 50%?

$$50\% = \frac{50}{100} = 0.5$$

$$0.5 \times 0.5 = 0.25 = \frac{25}{100} = 25\% \qquad \text{or:}$$

$$0.25 \times 100 = 25\%$$

6. DIVIDING USING PERCENT

A. Dividing a nonpercent number by a percentage

To divide a number by a percentage or to divide a number into a percentage, first convert the percentage to a fraction and follow the applicable procedure.

EXAMPLE 1-45: Divide 248 by 50%.

$$248 \div 50\% = 248 \div 0.5 = \frac{248}{0.5} = 496$$

B. Dividing a percentage by a percentage

When dividing a percentage by a percentage, convert both percentages to decimal fractions and divide. The quotient is a decimal fraction. You may then convert the result to a percentage by multiplying the quotient by 100.

EXAMPLE 1-46: Divide 25% by 50%.

$$25\% = \frac{25}{100} = 0.25$$

$$50\% = \frac{50}{100} = 0.5$$

$$0.25 \div 0.5 = \frac{0.25}{0.5} = 0.50 = \frac{50}{100} = 50\% \qquad \text{or:}$$

$$0.5 \times 100 = 50\%$$

Notice that when a number is *multiplied* by a proper fraction (a percentage of less than 100), the answer is less than the number. When a number is *divided* by a proper fraction, the result is greater than the number. A percentage value is just a form of a fraction.

NOTE: *The presence or absence of the % sign is extremely important. It can change the entire meaning of a value.*

$$0.026 \quad \text{means } {}^{26}\!/_{1,000} \text{ or } \; {}^{2.6}\!/_{100} \text{ or } 0.026$$

$$0.026\% \text{ means } \qquad {}^{0.026}\!/_{100} \text{ or } 0.00026$$

This is a very simple difference, but it is also the source of many errors.

SECTION 1.5 ORDER OF CALCULATIONS

Sometimes in a problem it may be necessary to carry out several types of computations. There is an established *order* in which these operations should be carried out.

1. Order of operations when there are no parentheses: multiply and divide from left to right; then add and subtract.

$$3 \times 4 + 6 - 8 \div 2 + 1 \times 4$$

Multiply and divide first from left to right.

$$(3 \times 4) + 6 - (8 \div 2) + (1 \times 4)$$
$$12 \quad + 6 - \quad 4 \quad + \quad 4$$

$$12 + 6 + 4 - 4$$
$$22 - 4 = 18$$

2. Order of operations within parentheses: do operations within the parentheses first; then treat the result as one number in the operation.

$$(3 + 6 - 2) + (4 \times 2 + 1) - (6 - 4 \div 2)$$
$$(7) \quad + [(4 \times 2) + 1] - [6 - (4 \div 2)]$$
$$(7) \quad + \quad (8 + 1) - (6 - \quad 2)$$
$$(7) \quad + \quad (9) \quad - \quad (4)$$

$$7 + 9 - 4$$
$$16 - 4 = 12$$

3. Order of operations for groupings within a grouping: simplify the innermost grouping first and work outward; then proceed as in Step 1.

$$\{9 - [7 + (6 \div 3) - 1]\}$$
$$[9 - (7 + \quad 2 \quad - 1)]$$

$$9 - \quad 8 \quad = 1$$

4. Order of operations when there are exponents: simplify the exponents first; then proceed with the other operations.

$$7^2 + 3 \times 2^3 + 4$$
$$49 + 3 \times 8 + 4$$
$$49 + (3 \times 8) + 4$$
$$49 + \quad 24 \quad + 4 = 77$$

SECTION 1.6 ALGEBRA

Algebra is a direct outgrowth of arithmetic in which letters or other symbols are used to represent real numbers. This part of mathematics provides a method to describe the order and kind of basic operations necessary to solve a problem.

The fundamental tool of algebra is the **equation.** An equation is a mathematical expression that is divided into two parts separated by an equal sign ($=$). These two parts are equal in value. The part of the equation that is not known is represented as x, y, or some other letter.

The parts of an equation can be moved from one side to the other by following the proper procedures. This allows the equation to be changed to a form that allows one to solve the problem.

The following general rules are used in solving problems set up as equations.

1. Both sides of the equation must produce the same value when solved.

$$x = 2 + 3$$
$$x = 5$$
$$5 = 2 + 3$$
$$5 = 5$$

2. Generally, it is easier to solve a problem if all known material is moved to one side of the equation and all unknown material is moved to the other side.

3. When a part to be added or subtracted in an equation is moved to the other side of the equal sign, the sign of the part being moved is changed.

$$4 + x = 2 + 3 \qquad\qquad x - 7 = 17$$
$$x = 2 + 3 - 4 \qquad\qquad x = 17 + 7$$
$$x = 5 - 4 \qquad\qquad\quad x = 24$$
$$x = 1$$

Proof:

$$4 + 1 = 2 + 3 \qquad\qquad 24 - 7 = 17$$
$$5 = 5 \qquad\qquad\qquad\quad 17 = 17$$

4. When numbers of an equation are to be multiplied or divided, they can be more easily handled if they are expressed as common fractions.

$$x \div 7 = 9 \times 3 \div 4$$
$$\frac{x}{7} = \frac{9 \times 3}{4}$$

5. When such fractional expressions are moved from one side of an equation to the other, they are inverted.

$$\frac{x}{7} = \frac{9 \times 3}{4}$$
$$x = \frac{9 \times 3}{4} \times \frac{7}{1}$$
$$x = \frac{189}{4}$$
$$x = 47.25$$

6. If both sides of an equation are turned over, the equality remains the same.

$$\frac{x}{7} = \frac{27}{4} \qquad\qquad \frac{7}{x} = \frac{4}{27}$$

$$4x = 27 \times 7 \qquad\qquad 4x = 7 \times 27$$

$$x = \frac{27 \times 7}{4} \qquad\qquad x = \frac{7 \times 27}{4}$$

$$x = \frac{189}{4} \qquad\qquad x = \frac{189}{4}$$

$$x = 47.25 \qquad\qquad x = 47.25$$

This is a short introduction to a very broad and complex field of mathematics. Much of the mathematics demonstrated in this book is algebra. A more thorough treatment of algebra is beyond the scope of this book. However, students are encouraged to gain as much skill in this area of mathematics as is practical.

SECTION 1.7 RECIPROCALS

A **reciprocal** is the multiplicative inverse of a number.

To calculate the reciprocal of a number, divide it into +1. The product of a number and its reciprocal is always equal to +1. A number and its reciprocal have the same sign.

The reciprocal of 2 is ½ or 0.5. $(1 \div 2 = \frac{1}{2} = 0.5)$

$$2 \times \frac{1}{2} = \frac{2}{2} = 1$$

$$2 \times 0.5 = 1$$

The reciprocal of 8 is ⅛ or 0.125. $(1 \div 8 = \frac{1}{8} = 0.125)$

$$\frac{8}{1} \times \frac{1}{8} = \frac{8}{8} = 1$$

$$8 \times 0.125 = 1$$

The reciprocal of -7 is $-\frac{1}{7}$. $(1 \div -7 = \frac{1}{-7} = -\frac{1}{7})$

$$-\frac{7}{1} \times -\frac{1}{7} = +\frac{7}{7} = +1$$

The reciprocal of $-\frac{2}{3}$ is $-\frac{3}{2}$. $(1 \div -\frac{2}{3} = \frac{1}{-\frac{2}{3}} = 1 \times -\frac{3}{2} = -\frac{3}{2})$

$$-\frac{2}{3} \times -\frac{3}{2} = +\frac{6}{6} = +1$$

SECTION 1.8 SIGNIFICANT FIGURES

A number is an expression of a quantity. The terms *figure* and *digit* are used to indicate any of the characters from 0 through 9. **Significant figures** are the digits of a whole number or a number written in decimal form, beginning with the leftmost nonzero digit and extending to the right to the precision limit of the measuring devices used to obtain the number. In other words, these are the digits of a number that are known to be reliable.

Since all measurements are limited in accuracy and precision by human error, instrument limitations, reagent reliability, etc., a reported result should have some indication of its reliability and precision by the number of significant figures in the value.

The determination of the significant figures in a number can be made by using the following rules.

1. All nonzero digits in a number are significant. In the number 12.34, all digits are significant because none are zero.

2. All zero digits between two nonzero digits are significant.

According to this rule, all the digits in the numbers 100.1, 120.01, and 110.101 are significant.

3. Zero digits to the right of a nonzero digit but to the left of an understood decimal point may or may not be significant.

This is determined by the ability of the measuring instruments and procedures. One common way to indicate the significant figures in such a number is to place a bar over the rightmost zero considered to be significant. Hence, the number $120\overline{0}0$ contains four significant figures.

4. All zeros both to the right of a decimal point and to the right of a nonzero digit are significant.

Each of the following numbers has four significant figures: 12.00, 0.1200, 1.200, and 120.0. The significant zeros to the right of the decimal point serve to indicate the precision of the number. If they do not do this, they should not be reported in the number.

5. All zeros to the left of a nonzero digit but to the right of a decimal point are not significant if there is not a significant digit to their left.

Each of the following numbers has three significant digits: 0.0123, 0.000123, 0.000000123, and 0.123. This rule is usually the most difficult to understand. A complete explanation of the reasons for this rule is beyond the scope of this book. However, stated simply, such zeros indicate only the decimal place of the other digits in the number and do not confer value to the number. The single zero to the left of the decimal point in this kind of number serves no purpose other than to bring attention to the decimal point and is never significant.

In summary, when zeros appear in a number, they may present a problem when one is trying to determine the number of significant figures. Zeros to the right of the decimal point are always significant if they follow the digits and are not significant if they precede a digit and if the total number is less than 1. Thus 0.072 contains two significant figures; 0.720 contains three significant figures; and 1.072 contains four significant figures. A report of 220 does not indicate whether the measurement was to the nearest tens or to the nearest ones, and the zero is not significant unless it has a bar over it ($22\overline{0}$). If there are digits on both

Table 1-1

Result	Number of significant figures	Implied limit of reliability
11	2	10.5 to 11.5
11.5	3	11.45 to 11.55
11.50	4	11.495 to 11.505

sides of the zero, as 202, it is a significant figure. If the zero is followed by a decimal point and digits or zeros, as 220.1, the zero is a significant figure.

Again, the significant figures reported in a value should reflect the precision of the test that produced the value. For example, if the result of a test was reported as 11.5, this should mean that the result was accurate to the nearest tenth and that the exact value was between 11.45 and 11.55. If this result had been reliable to the nearest hundredth, it would have been reported as 11.50. The number of significant figures is different in each example. The number 11.5 contains three significant figures, but 11.50 contains four significant figures. Table 1-1 gives the implied limits of reliability of a result reported to different significant figures.

Rules for Rounding Off Numbers

Often, as the result of mathematical computations, test results are acquired that produce insignificant digits. It then becomes necessary to *round off* the number to the chosen number of significant figures before reporting results. This is done so one does not imply an accuracy or precision greater than the test is capable of delivering. However, each analyst should follow the same procedures for rounding off to permit consistency in reporting results. The following rules describe the universal system.

1. If the digit to be dropped is less than 5, the preceding figure is not altered.

2. If the digit to be dropped is more than 5, the preceding figure is increased by 1.

3. If the digit to be dropped is 5, the preceding figure is increased by 1 if it is an odd number, and the preceding figure is not altered if it is an even number.

The following numbers have been rounded off to one decimal place:

$$3.24 = 3.2$$
$$3.16 = 3.2$$
$$3.15 = 3.2$$
$$3.25 = 3.2$$

If this system is followed by each analyst, no bias will be introduced into calculations of large amounts of data in small quality-control procedures.

Rules for Figure Retention

1. Retain as many significant figures in data and result as is necessary to give only one uncertain figure.

EXAMPLE 1-47: The number 36.24 ml was recorded using a buret on which the smallest scale divisions were in tenths. Which figures are significant?

All figures are significant, since 36.2 represents actual scale divisions. The 4 represents interpolation between two scale divisions and is the only one that is uncertain. Another analyst may have read the same setting as 36.23 or 36.25.

2. For all of the digits in a number to be significant, every digit except the last must be correct, and the error in the last digit must not be greater than one half of the lowest unit that occupies that space.

EXAMPLE 1-48: The number 36.24 ml has four significant figures, as stated previously. What is the error in this figure?

The 3, 6, and 2 are correct, and the 4 states that the number is closer to 36.24 than it is to 36.235 or 36.245. The lowest unit in the space is 0.01 or $\frac{1}{100}$, and the error is less than or equal to 0.005.

3. In adding or subtracting numbers with differing numbers of digits, retain the significant figures in each number and in the final answer only to the point corresponding to the least number of significant figures occurring after the decimal point.

EXAMPLE 1-49: Add 0.0212, 29.64, and 1.056931.

In these three numbers, 29.64 has the least significant digits (2) to the right of the decimal. Hence, all figures in this calculation should be rounded off to two digits to the right of the decimal and added as follows:

$$
\begin{array}{rcl}
0.0212 & = & 0.02 \\
29.64 & = & 29.64 \\
1.056931 & = & \underline{1.06} \\
& & 30.72
\end{array}
$$

Because 29.64 only goes into the hundredths column and any following figures are unknown, it is useless to extend the digits of the other numbers past the hundredths column.

4. In multiplying and dividing numbers with differing numbers of digits, for practical purposes retain as many significant figures as are found in the factor having the least number of significant figures.

EXAMPLE 1-50: What are the significant figures in $0.0211 \times 25.63 \times 1.05881$?

0.0211	has three significant figures
25.63	has four significant figures
1.05881	has six significant figures

In this calculation, 0.0211 is the governing factor, and the problem looks like this:

$$0.0211 \times 25.6 \times 1.06$$

5. If routine systems for multiplication and division are used, reject all superfluous digits at each stage of the operation.

6. When using logarithm tables for multiplying numbers, retain as many figures in the mantissa of the logarithm of each factor as are found in the factors themselves under Rule 4. (Logarithms are discussed at length in Chapter 7.)

EXAMPLE 1-51: Calculate $0.0211 \times 25.6 \times 1.06$.

$$\log 0.0211 = 8.324 - 10$$
$$\log 25.6 = 1.408$$
$$\log 1.06 = \underline{0.025}$$

Sum of logarithms $= 9.757 - 10 =$ logarithm of product

Antilog $9.757 - 10 = 0.572$

SECTION 1.9 EXPONENTS

Exponents are used to indicate that a number is to be multiplied by itself as many times as is indicated by its exponent. The number to be multiplied by itself is called the **base.** Small superior digits written directly to the right of the base are used to indicate the value of the exponent. This digit is commonly referred to as the **power** of the base. The exponent may have a plus or a minus sign before it. The plus sign is almost always understood and does not appear.

An exponent having a plus sign or no sign is a **positive exponent.** The exponent indicates the number of times *the base* is to be multiplied by itself.

$$10^2 = 10 \times 10 = 100$$
$$10^4 = 10 \times 10 \times 10 \times 10 = 10,000$$
$$6^3 = 6 \times 6 \times 6 = 216$$

An exponent having a minus sign is a **negative exponent.** This indicates the number of times *the reciprocal of the base* is to be multiplied by itself; stated another way, a negative exponent indicates a fraction.

$$10^{-1} = \frac{1}{10} = 0.1$$

$$10^{-3} = \frac{1}{10} \times \frac{1}{10} \times \frac{1}{10} = \frac{1}{1,000} = 0.001$$

$$2^{-3} = \frac{1}{2} \times \frac{1}{2} \times \frac{1}{2} = \frac{1}{8} = 0.125$$

Rules of Exponents

Numbers with exponents can be multiplied or divided by one another by adding or subtracting the exponents using the rules of exponents. In stating these rules, the letters *m* and *n* are usually used to indicate the exponents. Be sure to follow the rules for signed numbers when making these calculations.

1. To multiply two numbers *having the same base*, write the base with the exponents added.

$$a^m \times a^n = a^{m+n}$$
$$6^2 \times 6^3 = 6^{2+3} = 6^5$$
$$10^2 \times 10^{-3} = 10^{2+(-3)} = 10^{-1}$$

2. To raise an exponential number to a higher power, multiply the two exponents.

$$(a^m)^n = a^{m \times n}$$
$$(6^2)^3 = 6^{2 \times 3} = 6^6$$

3. To divide one number by another number *having the same base*, write the base with the exponent of the divisor subtracted from the exponent of the dividend.

$$\frac{a^m}{a^n} = a^{m-n}$$

$$\frac{6^3}{6^2} = 6^{3-2} = 6^1 = 6$$

$$\frac{2^2}{2^{-4}} = 2^{2-(-4)} = 2^{2+4} = 2^6$$

4. To multiply or divide numbers *having different bases,* it is necessary to convert the exponent numbers to the corresponding simple numbers. Then complete the calculations using these numbers.

EXAMPLE 1-52: $2^3 \times 10^2$

$$2^3 = 2 \times 2 \times 2 = 8$$
$$10^2 = 10 \times 10 = 100$$
$$8 \times 100 = 800$$

5. To add or subtract numbers having exponents, it is necessary to convert these numbers to simple numbers before doing the calculations.

EXAMPLE 1-53: $3^3 + 2^2$

$$3^3 = 3 \times 3 \times 3 = 27$$
$$2^2 = 2 \times 2 = 4$$
$$27 + 4 = 31$$

SECTION 1.10 SCIENTIFIC NOTATION

Often it is necessary to work with numbers that have a string of zeros behind them or that are just too large to handle efficiently. **Scientific notation** has been devised as a kind of shorthand way of writing such numbers. In this system the powers of 10 are used. For example, one hundred is 10×10 (100) or 10^2, one thousand is $10 \times 10 \times 10$ (1,000) or 10^3, and one million is $10 \times 10 \times 10 \times 10 \times 10 \times 10$ (1,000,000) or 10^6.

A number written in scientific notation consists of two parts multiplied together. The first part has all the significant figures expressed as a number with one place to the left of the decimal point. The second part is a power of 10 that restores the original value to the number.

$$100 = 1 \times 10^2$$
$$278 = 2.78 \times 10^2$$
$$376,000 = 3.76 \times 10^5$$

To convert a number greater than 1 to scientific notation, count the number of places required to move the decimal point to obtain a number having one place to the left of the decimal point. That number will be the correct positive power of 10.

$$100 = 1 \times 10^2$$
$$2$$
$$1,000 = 1 \times 10^3$$
$$3$$
$$13,600 = 1.36 \times 10^4$$
$$4$$
$$2,618,000,000 = 2.618 \times 10^9$$
$$9$$

A number less than 1 is indicated by a negative power of 10. To convert such a number to scientific notation, place the decimal to the right of the first nonzero digit of the number. Count the places the decimal point was moved. Use this value with a minus sign as the exponent of 10 in the converted number. Said another way, count the number of places the decimal must be moved to the right to obtain a number between 1 and 10. This will be the correct negative power of 10.

$$0.001 = 1 \times 10^{-3}$$
$$3$$
$$0.0000431 = 4.31 \times 10^{-5}$$
$$5$$
$$0.00000000918 = 9.18 \times 10^{-9}$$
$$9$$

Multiplication in Scientific Notation

1. POSITIVE POWER OF 10

To multiply numbers expressed as **positive** powers of 10, first multiply the numbers (between 1 and 10) that appear to the left of the 10 to a power; then *add* the exponents.

EXAMPLE 1-54: Multiply 15,100 by 200,000.

Convert the numbers to scientific notation.

$$15,100 = 1.51 \times 10^4$$
4

$$200,000 = 2.0 \times 10^5$$
5

Multiply the numbers between 1 and 10.

$$
\begin{array}{r}
1.51 \\
\times \quad 2.0 \\
\hline
3.020
\end{array}
$$

Add the exponents of 10.

$$10^4 \times 10^5 = 10^{4+5} = 10^9$$

Multiply the two parts.

$$3.02 \times 10^9 = 3,020,000,000$$

2. NEGATIVE POWER OF 10

To multiply numbers expressed as **negative** powers of 10, first multiply the numbers (between 1 and 10) that appear to the left of the 10 to a negative power; then add the negative exponents.

EXAMPLE 1-55: Multiply 0.000192 by 0.000000008.

$$0.000192 = 1.92 \times 10^{-4}$$
4

$$0.000000008 = 8.0 \times 10^{-9}$$
9

$$(1.92 \times 10^{-4}) \times (8.0 \times 10^{-9}) = (1.92 \times 8.0) \times (10^{-4} \times 10^{-9}) =$$
$$(1.92 \times 8.0) \times (10^{(-4)+(-9)}) = (1.92 \times 8.0) \times 10^{-13} = 15.36 \times 10^{-13} = 1.536 \times 10^{-12}$$

Division in Scientific Notation

The same general rules are followed when dividing in scientific notation; however, when dividing exponents *with the same base, subtract* the exponent of the divisor from the exponent of the dividend. First divide the numbers (between 1 and 10) that appear to the left of the powers of 10; then subtract the power of 10 in the denominator from that in the numerator.

Be careful. The answer should be logical.

EXAMPLE 1-56: Divide 540,000 by 2,100.

$$540,000 = 5.4 \times 10^5$$
5

$$2,100 = 2.1 \times 10^3$$
3

$$(5.4 \times 10^5) \div (2.1 \times 10^3) = (5.4 \div 2.1) \times (10^{5-3}) = (5.4 \div 2.1) \times 10^2 = 2.57 \times 10^2$$

EXAMPLE 1-57: Divide 0.00913 by 0.0000014.

$$0.00913 = 9.13 \times 10^{-3}$$
$$\underset{3}{\underset{\uparrow}{\rule{0pt}{0pt}}}$$
$$0.0000014 = 1.4 \times 10^{-6}$$
$$\underset{6}{\underset{\uparrow}{\rule{0pt}{0pt}}}$$

$$\frac{9.13 \times 10^{-3}}{1.4 \times 10^{-6}} = \frac{9.13}{1.4} \times (10^{(-3)-(-6)}) = \frac{9.13}{1.4} \times 10^3 = 6.52 \times 10^3$$

Addition and Subtraction with Scientific Notation

Generally, it is not wise to add and subtract numbers in scientific notation. These are tricky operations, and errors are likely. It is almost always advisable to convert the numbers to their conventional forms before adding or subtracting.

SECTION 1.11 RATIO AND PROPORTION

A **ratio** is an amount of one thing *relative* to an amount of something else. Ratios are frequently used to describe amounts and magnitude of the things and systems dealt with in laboratories. A ratio *always* describes a *relative* amount. At least two values are always involved in a ratio statement. Both of these amounts may be stated in the expression of a ratio, or one may be implied. On the other hand, **absolute values** describe an amount of something without any direct or implied reference to any other values.

Proportion in this sense refers to two or more ratios that have the same relative meaning but different numbers. In effect, proportion is a statement that two ratios are equal. The ratio and proportion procedure is one of the most used mathematical procedures in laboratory work. It is a way to calculate an amount of something relative to an amount of something else based on a known relationship between the two things. A thorough knowledge of this procedure is necessary for the competent laboratory worker.

Ratios

As stated above, a ratio is an expression of one amount *relative* to another. It considers the relative sizes of two numbers. A ratio is found by dividing one number by the number with which it is being compared. A ratio may be indicated in several ways, as seen by the following methods of expressing a comparison of 5 to 4.

1. An indicated quotient using the division sign ($\div$) is $5 \div 4$.
2. An indicated quotient using the ratio sign (:) is $5:4$. This is the most common and the preferred means of expressing a ratio.
3. The common fractional form is 5/4. When a ratio is written in fractional form, it may then be treated like any other fraction. However, if it is not being used in a mathematical computation, the ratio sign (:) should be used, and the slash mark (/) should be reserved for use with dilutions (Chapter 5, pp. 92-93).
4. The decimal fractional form is 1.25 ($5 \div 4 = 1.25$). This is the same as $1.25:1$. The 1 to the right of the ratio sign is simply understood.

A ratio is expressed exactly as the words describing it are written. *This is very important.* A ratio of 4 to 10 is written 4:10 (the 4 comes first in the statement; therefore it also comes first in the written ratio). A ratio of 6 to 2 is written 6:2.

> EXAMPLE 1-58: A given test tube contains 6 ml of saline and 3 ml of serum. What is the saline to serum ratio?
>
> The ratio of saline to serum is 6:3. The word *saline* comes first in the question; therefore the amount corresponding to saline must come first in the written ratio.

In reality, a ratio is a quantity of something compared with a quantity of something else. Be careful to ascertain exactly what is being compared and then express it in the proper manner. Consider 9 milliliters of saline and 1 milliliter of serum in a test tube (9 + 1 = 10 ml total volume). The following expressions are correct.

1. The serum to saline ratio is 1:9.
2. The saline to serum ratio is 9:1.
3. The saline to total volume ratio is 9:10.
4. The total volume to saline ratio is 10:9.
5. The serum to total volume ratio is 1:10.
6. The total volume to serum ratio is 10:1.

Consider a gathering of 10 men and 5 women. The following expressions are correct.

1. The men to women ratio is 10:5.
2. The women to men ratio is 5:10.
3. The men to total attendance ratio is 10:15.
4. The total attendance to men ratio is 15:10.
5. The women to total attendance ratio is 5:15.
6. The total attendance to women ratio is 15:5.

Why each of the written ratios above are expressed as they are and what each one means should be understood before continuing.

Ratio and Proportion Procedure

The same relationship can be expressed with more than one ratio. Consider the ratio 1:2. If a ratio is expressed as a fraction, it can be compared with another equal ratio.

$$1/2 = 5/10$$

The two fractions, 1/2 and 5/10, are the same thing; they are two ratios that have the same relationship, only they are expressed in different ways. In reality the relationship between the two numbers of each ratio is the same (2 is twice as great as 1, and 10 is twice as great as 5).

Ratio and proportion calculations are used with many laboratory procedures. In this calculation an existing ratio is used to calculate a new ratio with the same relationship as the first. In discussions of ratio and proportion, the **known ratio** is an existing ratio and the **unknown ratio** is a ratio to be calculated.

If one desires to make more or less of the same thing *without changing concentration* (or any other kind of relative relationship), it can usually be done using ratio and proportion.

The more common method to express a ratio and proportion is to set up an equality between the ratios written as fractions. To do the ratio-proportion procedure this way, use the following format.

$$A \text{ is to } B \text{ as } C \text{ is to } D$$

$$A/B \quad = \quad C/D$$

This format is in the form of an equation. If three of the four values are known, the fourth can be found by calculation.

In setting up the ratio and proportion, the known and unknown ratios must be written in the same order and must be in the same units.

EXAMPLE 1-59: Using ratio and proportion, calculate how many grams would be in 20 ml if there are 20 g in 100 ml.

Putting the information about one solution in one ratio and the information about the other solution in another ratio produces the following statement: if there are 20 g in 100 ml there are x g in 20 ml. The known ratio here is 20 g in 100 ml. The unknown ratio is x in 20 ml.

$$\frac{20 \text{ g}}{100 \text{ ml}} = \frac{x \text{ g}}{20 \text{ ml}}$$

Solve the equation:

$$100x = 20 \times 20$$

$$100x = 400$$

$$x = \frac{400}{100}$$

$$x = 4 \text{ g } (4 \text{ g in 20 ml})$$

When ratio and proportion problems are written or verbally stated, the order of the values may or may not be in the order for calculation. In setting up the format of the problem, always place the values in each ratio in the same relationship. This is necessary if correct results are expected.

EXAMPLE 1-60: Six grams of substance make 10 ml of a given solution; how many milliliters can be made from 15 g?

Note that the two ratios are stated differently in this problem. *Grams* is stated first in the first ratio and *milliliters* is stated first in the second ratio; however, the problem should be set up as follows:

Known ratio		Unknown ratio
$\dfrac{6 \text{ g}}{10 \text{ ml}}$	=	$\dfrac{15 \text{ g}}{x \text{ ml}}$

Place the value in one ratio directly across the equal sign from the equivalent value in the other ratio (that is, grams across from grams and milliliters across from milliliters), and complete the calculation.

$$\frac{6}{10} = \frac{15}{x}$$

$$6x = 10 \times 15$$

$$6x = 150$$

$$x = \frac{150}{6}$$

$$x = 25$$

The 15 g of substance will make 25 ml of solution.

EXAMPLE 1-61: How many grams would it take to make 100 ml of solution if 5 g made 20 ml?

$$\frac{x \text{ g}}{100 \text{ ml}} = \frac{5 \text{ g}}{20 \text{ ml}}$$

$$20x = 5 \times 100$$

$$x = \frac{500}{20}$$

$$x = 25$$

It would take 25 g to make 100 ml of solution.

When ratios are used in general descriptions of relationships, they are usually expressed as some number to one, or as a single number with the one understood. To do this, you simply set up your ratio and proportion problem to give the information desired.

EXAMPLE 1-62: A blood sample was found to have 2,850 white blood cells and 5,000,000 red blood cells. How does this compare with normal blood having a 1,000:1 ratio of red cells to white cells?

In this problem, the observed ratio of red cells to white cells is 5,000,000 to 2,850. Determine the number of red cells for every one white cell. Remember to keep the order of the numbers the same as the order of the words.

Set up the ratio and proportion:

In this problem the known ratio is 5,000,000 red cells to 2,850 white cells, and the unknown ratio is x red cells to 1 white cell. Solve for x.

$$\frac{5,000,000 \text{ red cells}}{2,850 \text{ white cells}} = \frac{x \text{ red cells}}{1 \text{ white cell}}$$

$$2,850x = 5,000,000 \times 1$$

$$x = \frac{5,000,000}{2,850}$$

$$x = 1,754$$

This shows that the ratio of red cells to white cells in this sample is 1,754:1. It may also be stated that the red cells to white cells ratio is 1,754 (with the 1 understood).

An older method of expressing a ratio and proportion problem is through the use of colons. Consider the proportion 1 is to 2 as 5 is to 10.

$$\text{1 is to 2 as 5 is to 10}$$

$$1:2 \quad :: \quad 5:10$$

$$1:2 :: 5:10$$

Here, two ratios, 1:2 and 5:10, are shown connected by a double colon (::). The double colon is sometimes called the proportion symbol. To solve this type of set-up, you multiply the first and fourth values together, then multiply the second and third values together, and connect the two with an equal sign.

$$1:2 \; :: \; 5:10$$

$$1 \times 10 = 2 \times 5$$

This is actually the same as the current method that uses fractions; it is simply spread out on a single line.

Current method	Older method
$\dfrac{1}{2} = \dfrac{5}{10}$	$1:2 \; :: \; 5:10$
$1 \times 10 = 2 \times 5$	$1 \times 10 = 2 \times 5$
$10 = 10$	$10 = 10$

The following example is calculated by using the current and older methods of notation.

EXAMPLE 1-63: If 6 g of a substance make 10 ml of a particular solution, 30 ml could be made from how many grams?

Determine the known and unknown ratios, and make a proportion statement. The known ratio is 6 g of substance in 10 ml of solution. The unknown ratio is x g of substance in 30 ml of solution. The proportion statement:

6 g are to 10 ml as x g are to 30 ml.

Solve using the two methods of notation.

Current method	Older method
$\dfrac{6 \text{ g}}{10 \text{ ml}} = \dfrac{x \text{ g}}{30 \text{ ml}}$	$6 \text{ g} : 10 \text{ ml} \; :: \; x \text{ g} : 30 \text{ ml}$
$10x = 6 \times 30$	$10x = 6 \times 30$
$10x = 180$	$10x = 180$
$x = 18$	$x = 18$

18 g make 30 ml.

Use the method that makes the most sense to you.

SUMMARY

Skill in basic mathematics is one of the classic needs for success in any endeavor involving the logical use of information. The laboratory worker has a great need for competence in this area. Effort spent in the improvement of math skill is well spent. This chapter gives only a brief review of basic mathematics. The worker is encouraged to use every available opportunity to extend his skill in this area.

APPENDIXES OF GENERAL INTEREST

    A. Greek Alphabet Table
    B. Math Symbols
    C. Cardinal Numbers: Arabic and Roman
    D. Ordinal Numbers
    E. Denominations above One Million
    Q. Formulas Presented in This Book
    Y. Periodic Chart of the Elements

PRACTICE PROBLEMS

Calculate the answer for each problem. Understand each portion of the calculation, and determine whether the answer is logical. *Just because an answer can be calculated does not mean that it is reasonable.*

Roman Numerals

Convert to Roman numerals:

1. 3	5. 173	8. 1,020
2. 43	6. 568	9. 1,652
3. 51	7. 704	10. 52,371
4. 96		

Convert to Arabic numerals:

11. MCXVII	15. DCCLXXVII	18. XLIII
12. XLV	16. LXV	19. XVI
13. CDXLII	17. XCII	20. MCD
14. VI		

Manipulation of signed numbers

Add:

21. $+6$ and $+10$	25. -6 and -2	29. -21 and $+8$
22. $+7$ and -2	26. $+18$ and -3	30. -13 and -46
23. -3 and $+8$	27. -12 and -18	31. $+7$ and -32
24. -10 and $+4$	28. $+21$ and -30	32. $+49$ and -20

Subtract:

33. $+3$ from $+21$	39. -6 from -2	44. $-5 - (-10)$
34. $+18$ from $+10$	40. -11 from -19	45. $-30 - (-4)$
35. $+4$ from -20	41. $+42 - +26$	46. $+6 - (+20)$
36. $+16$ from -3	42. $-17 - +32$	47. $+18 - (+6)$
37. -18 from $+14$	43. $+10 - (-6)$	48. $-21 - (-7)$
38. -5 from $+7$		

Multiply:

49. $+18 \times +5$	52. -7×-40	55. -2×-40
50. $+9 \times -4$	53. -9×-2	56. -10×-5
51. $-3 \times +22$	54. $+7 \times -6$	

Divide:

57. $+10 \div +2$
58. $+6 \div +8$
59. $+25 \div -5$

60. $+7 \div -35$
61. $-22 \div +2$
62. $-6 \div +10$

63. $-28 \div -7$
64. $-4 \div -40$

Common fractions

Match the following (some answers may be used more than once):

65. Common fraction _____
66. Proper fraction _____
67. Improper fraction _____
68. Whole number _____
69. Mixed number _____
70. Complex fraction _____
71. Equivalent fractions _____
72. Decimal fraction _____
73. List choices *a* thru *n* (to the right) in ascending order of magnitude.

a. $\frac{4}{4}$
b. $1\frac{3}{8}$
c. 0.75
d. $\dfrac{3}{\frac{1}{4}}$
e. $\frac{2}{5}$
f. 22
g. $\frac{3}{4}$
h. 6
i. $1\frac{3}{8}$
j. 0.09
k. $\frac{9}{12}$
l. $\dfrac{\frac{3}{8}}{2}$
m. $10\frac{1}{4}$
n. $\dfrac{\frac{1}{4} + \frac{1}{2}}{\frac{4}{7}}$

Find the lowest common denominator (LCD):

74. $\frac{1}{2}, \frac{1}{4}, \frac{5}{8}$
75. $\frac{1}{32}, \frac{3}{4}, \frac{7}{16}$
76. $\frac{1}{3}, \frac{5}{6}, \frac{1}{2}, \frac{4}{9}$

77. $\frac{1}{16}, \frac{3}{5}, \frac{2}{10}, \frac{3}{4}, \frac{8}{17}$
78. $\frac{3}{50}, \frac{2}{3}, \frac{5}{7}, \frac{11}{18}$

Add:

79. $\frac{3}{5} + \frac{4}{5}$
80. $1\frac{2}{8} + \frac{3}{8}$
81. $\frac{3}{6} + \frac{4}{8} + \frac{1}{3}$
82. $\frac{5}{2} + \frac{5}{16} + \frac{5}{10}$
83. $1\frac{2}{9} + 1\frac{2}{3}$

84. $\frac{7}{12} + \frac{3}{9}$
85. $3\frac{1}{4} + 2\frac{3}{4}$
86. $5\frac{6}{8} + 7\frac{17}{24}$
87. $2\frac{4}{9} + (-\frac{5}{8})$
88. $\frac{3}{16} + 1\frac{3}{4}$

Subtract:

89. $\frac{3}{7} - \frac{2}{7}$
90. $\frac{4}{15} - \frac{7}{15}$
91. $\frac{5}{12} - (-\frac{1}{2})$
92. $\frac{6}{8} - \frac{9}{4}$
93. $3\frac{5}{7} - \frac{1}{2}$

94. $1\frac{3}{6} - \frac{4}{24}$
95. $1\frac{3}{8} - 3\frac{1}{8}$
96. $4\frac{1}{2} - 2\frac{4}{5}$
97. $\frac{3}{11} - (-2\frac{1}{8})$
98. $1\frac{3}{6} - 1\frac{3}{6}$

Multiply:

99. $\frac{2}{7} \times \frac{5}{7}$
100. $\frac{6}{8} \times \frac{4}{13}$
101. $1\frac{2}{5} \times -5\frac{3}{5}$
102. $8\frac{2}{6} \times 5\frac{1}{3}$
103. $\frac{9}{8} \times (-\frac{9}{2})$

104. $\frac{3}{8} \times \frac{9}{6}$
105. $-\frac{8}{3} \times 1\frac{6}{8}$
106. $4\frac{3}{8} \times 2\frac{1}{3}$
107. $3\frac{2}{9} \times \frac{6}{8}$
108. $-\frac{4}{5} \times -\frac{3}{7}$

Divide:

109. $\frac{5}{9} \div \frac{3}{9}$
110. $\frac{9}{12} \div -\frac{3}{6}$
111. $1\frac{2}{3} \div 3\frac{1}{3}$
112. $4\frac{7}{8} \div 2\frac{3}{6}$
113. $-\frac{9}{10} \div 4$

114. $-\frac{4}{7} \div \frac{9}{3}$
115. $1\frac{1}{8} \div \frac{3}{4}$
116. $\frac{2}{3} \div -3\frac{1}{6}$
117. $5\frac{1}{8} \div 3\frac{3}{8}$
118. $-7 \div (-\frac{6}{7})$

Circle the equivalent fractions:
119. $\frac{1}{3}$, $\frac{2}{4}$, $\frac{2}{6}$, $\frac{5}{10}$, $\frac{4}{15}$, $\frac{6}{18}$
120. $1\frac{1}{3}$, $2\frac{2}{3}$, 4, $\frac{4}{3}$, $\frac{3}{4}$, $\frac{12}{9}$, $2\frac{2}{6}$

Arrange in ascending order of magnitude:
121. $\frac{2}{18}$, $\frac{15}{18}$, $\frac{6}{18}$, $\frac{10}{18}$, $\frac{7}{18}$, $\frac{4}{18}$, $\frac{20}{18}$, $\frac{25}{18}$, $\frac{9}{18}$, $\frac{13}{18}$
122. $\frac{9}{16}$, $\frac{9}{2}$, $\frac{9}{4}$, $\frac{9}{21}$, $\frac{9}{14}$, $\frac{9}{16}$, $\frac{9}{10}$, $\frac{9}{20}$, $\frac{9}{7}$, $\frac{9}{13}$
123. Answers to questions 79 to 88
124. Answers to questions 89 to 98
125. Answers to questions 99 to 108
126. Answers to questions 109 to 118

Convert to common fractions, mixed numbers, or both if applicable:
127. 0.42   130. 11.45   133. 100.03
128. 3.9   131. 0.9072   134. 2.018
129. 0.006   132. 0.01902

Convert to decimal fractions:
135. $\frac{1}{6}$ 137. $1\frac{1}{4}$ 139. $\frac{9}{7}$
136. $\frac{7}{8}$ 138. $13\frac{2}{7}$ 140. $\frac{15}{23}$

Indicate the equivalent decimals:
141. 2.0   142. 1.5
     0.2   1.555
     0.02   1.50
     0.20   1.505
     0.2000   1.5000
     0.002   1.005

Decimal fractions

Add:
143. 0.08 + 0.90
144. 0.08 + (−0.90)
145. −1.93 + 3.768
146. 0.00945 + 0.0173 + 0.246
147. 9.736 + (−0.03434)
148. −2.14 + (−4.18)
149. 9.0004 + 4.0543
150. 0.00038 + 0.00820
151. 0.992 + (−0.0400) + 0.046 + 0.00200
152. 0.0270 + (−3.897) + 1.543 + (−0.0487)

Subtract:
153. 1.078 − 0.0640   158. −0.0669 − 0.0390
154. −1.83 − 0.984   159. 0.0389 − (−0.0669)
155. 1.008 − (−0.0834)   160. 5.14 − 4.57
156. −0.073 − (−0.084)   161. 0.00840 − 0.000363
157. 8.850 − 9.037   162. −3.61 − 3.17

Multiply:

163. 5.31×0.238
164. 0.427×-0.0835
165. -0.014×-0.36
166. -321×-0.0385
167. -0.864×8.880

168. 0.0445×-0.240
169. 4.97×0.000443
170. 0.002×0.007
171. -0.0130×22.800
172. -0.351×0.0940

Divide:

173. $0.948 \div 0.809$
174. $6.13 \div 1.06$
175. $-0.458 \div 0.535$
176. $-3.11 \div -1.64$
177. $\dfrac{7.087}{0.116}$
178. $\dfrac{0.671}{0.0437}$

179. $\dfrac{0.00520}{0.161}$
180. $\dfrac{-0.00717}{0.00493}$
181. $\dfrac{0.35}{-0.58}$
182. $\dfrac{-0.430}{-9.0300}$

Percent

State as percentages:

183. 2 parts in 100 total parts
184. 0.03 parts in 100 total parts
185. 100 total parts containing 6.3 parts
186. 18 parts + 82 parts

187. 5 parts in 50 total parts
188. 0.06 parts in 40 total parts
189. 1.1 parts + 26 parts
190. 0.002 parts in 25 total parts

Change to common fractions:

191. 2%
192. 1.006%
193. 0.08%
194. 32.9%

195. 0.25%
196. $\frac{1}{10}$%
197. $3\frac{1}{8}$%
198. $\frac{25}{30}$%

Change to decimal fractions:

199. 38%
200. 0.07%
201. 2.9%
202. 1.00065%

203. 0.092%
204. $\frac{1}{8}$%
205. $2\frac{1}{5}$%
206. $\frac{8}{10}$%

Change to percentages:

207. $\frac{1}{2}$
208. $9\frac{2}{3}$
209. $\frac{3}{10}$
210. $\frac{4}{5}$
211. $7\frac{1}{8}$
212. $\dfrac{\frac{1}{2}}{\frac{1}{4}}$

Change to percentages:

213. 0.29
214. 5
215. 16.2

216. 0.0138
217. 1.0006
218. 592.98

Add:

219. 3% + 10%
220. 4.9% + 2%
221. 0.26% + 0.04%
222. $\frac{1}{8}$% + 12%
223. 35% + $\frac{5}{6}$%
224. $\frac{2}{3}$% + $\frac{1}{4}$%

Subtract:

225. 25% − 5%
226. 2.9% − 0.8%
227. $\frac{3}{8}$% − $\frac{1}{16}$%
228. 0.29% − $\frac{1}{4}$%
229. 3% − 0.6%
230. 12$\frac{1}{2}$% − $\frac{4}{9}$%

Multiply:

231. 65 × 10%
232. 4 × 0.6%
233. $\frac{3}{7}$% × 1$\frac{1}{8}$%
234. 200% × 9.9%

Divide:

235. 30 ÷ 15%
236. 5.5 ÷ 40%
237. 1.3 ÷ $\frac{1}{4}$%
238. $\frac{9}{16}$ ÷ 3%
239. 0.75% ÷ 1$\frac{1}{8}$%
240. 20% ÷ $\frac{5}{9}$%

Order of calculations

Solve the following:

241. $3 \times 5 + 6 - 7 \div 3 + 1 \times 5$
242. $7 \div 1 \times 3 - 8 + 6 \times 4$
243. $9 + 3 \times 7 \div 3 - 6 + 1 - 8 \times 3$
244. $10 + 2 - 8 \times 7 + 6 \div 3 - 2 \times 4$
245. $(2 + 7 - 1) + (3 \times 6 + 4) - (6 - 5 \div 3)$
246. $(6 \times 7 \div 4 + 1) - (3 + 7 - 6) + (4 \times 1 - 3 \div 2)$
247. $(1 + 2) \times (8 \div 2 - 7 + 6 \times 4) - (8 \times 7 - 6) \div (9 \times 4 - 3 \div 7 + 1)$
248. $7 \times 8 - 2 \div 6 + (4 - 1 + 8 \div 7 \times 4) \times (2 \div 6 \times 5 \div 4 + 1 - 3)$
249. $8 + [7 \times (6 - 1 \div 4)] \div (8 - 2) + 4 - (6 \times 3 \div 2)$
250. $[3 \div 7 \times (4 - 1 \div 2 \times 3)] + [(9 - 3) \times 4 \div (8 - 2 + 4)] - 8 \times 6 \div 3$
251. $\{[(3 - 1) + 4] \div 5\} \times (8 \div 4) - 1$
252. $4 \times \{6 + [8 - (6 \div 2 + 2)] - 8\} + \{(3 - 1) \div 7 \times 4 + 2\} - 8 \div 2$

Equations

Indicate which of the following are true:

253. $5 + 6 = 12 - 1$
254. $5 \times \frac{3}{8} = 3 \times \frac{5}{8}$
255. $\frac{1}{2} \times \frac{1}{2} = 0.2500$

Solve for x:

256. $4x = 500$
257. $10 \times 0.6 = 7 \times x$
258. $x \div 4 = 9 \times 2 \div 3$
259. $\dfrac{0.4}{x} = 9.7$
260. $\frac{1}{3} \times \frac{4}{5}x = 120 \times 32$
261. $\dfrac{140}{x} = \dfrac{50}{2{,}000}$
262. $\dfrac{150}{20} \times \dfrac{1}{x} = 3{,}200$
263. $4.5 \times \dfrac{x}{20} = \dfrac{210}{15}$

Reciprocals

Give the reciprocal of the following as common and decimal fractions:

264. 2
265. −8
266. ⅖
267. ¹⁰⁄₇
268. −⁸⁄₁₅

269. 2⅓
270. −4.5
271. −0.012
272. 1.19
273. 0.7

Significant figures

Give the number of significant figures in each of the following:

274. 126
275. 3
276. 0.04
277. 1.920
278. 10.3
279. 10

280. 100.0420
281. 73.03
282. 0.0006
283. 1$\overline{0}$0
284. 3.7281

Rules for rounding off numbers

Report to the nearest tenth:

285. 7.64
286. 7.56

287. 7.55
288. 7.65

Report to the nearest hundredth:

289. 13.182
290. 44.096

291. 7.115
292. 123.185

Rules for figure retention

Calculate the following:

293. $0.0613 + 32.73 + 1.09257$
294. $19.42736 - 4.9$

295. $0.0711 \times 14.17 \times 3.01644$
296. $32.973 \div 4.3$

Exponents

Give the corresponding whole number or fraction:

297. 8^8
298. 10^4
299. 10^{-6}
300. 5^6

301. 3^{-2}
302. 10^{-3}
303. 10^{-4}
304. 9^{-7}

Express as whole, decimal, or fractional numbers:

305. 10^4
306. 10^{-6}
307. $10^2 + 10^3$
308. $10^{-6} + 10^{-2}$
309. $6^6 \times 6^3$

310. $5^4 \times 5^{-2}$
311. $10^7 \div 10^3$
312. $10^{-4} \div 10^2$
313. $7^6 \times 3^4$

Perform the following:

314. $6^3 + 6^5$
315. $a^2 \times a^7$
316. $b^3 \times c^6$
317. $2^7 - 8^4$
318. $d^9 \div d^6$
319. $(7^2)^3$
320. a^8/a^4
321. $(a^b)^c$

322. $10^4 + 10^5$
323. $8^{-6} + 8^{-8}$
324. $4^6 \times 4^3$
325. $8^7 \times 8^{-2}$
326. $5^7 \div 5^3$
327. $13^{-8} \div 13^4$
328. $9^8 \times 3^4$
329. $(9^6)^{-2}$

Scientific notation

Express in scientific notation:

330. 1,000
331. 100,000
332. 326
333. 15.9
334. 3,561
335. 2,826,000,000
336. 33,000

337. 1,010,100
338. 0.001
339. 0.00001
340. 0.0421
341. 0.397000
342. 0.000000000000723
343. 0.101

Perform the following using scientific notation:

344. $942,000 + 62,700$
345. $1,000,000,000 - 33,700$
346. $642,000 \times 3,739,000$
347. $15,000 \times 150,000$
348. 0.000942×0.00784

349. $493,000 \div 25,000$
350. $\dfrac{0.00000008}{0.00313}$
351. $420 \div 1,732,000$

Ratio and proportion

352. Express the ratio 3 to 9 four different ways.
353. A solution is made using 4 ml of serum and 10 ml of saline. Give the following:
    a. Saline to serum ratio
    b. Serum to saline ratio
    c. Total volume to serum ratio
    d. Serum to total volume ratio
    e. Total volume to saline ratio
    f. Saline to total volume ratio
354. Solve the following proportions for x:
    a. $3/9 = x/27$
    b. $x/12 = 2/6$
    c. $10/x = 5/4$
    d. $4/20 = 10/x$
355. Solve the following proportions for x.
    a. $3:9 :: 1:x$
    b. $x:12 :: 17:1$
    c. $13:2 :: 52:x$
    d. $10:x :: 5:4$
    e. $4:20 :: 10:x$
    f. $1.7:0.8 :: x:1$
356. If there are 5 g in 20 ml of solution, how many grams are present in 100 ml of solution?
357. If 3 g make 24 ml of solution, how many grams are required to make 72 ml of solution?
358. If there are 4 g in 80 ml of solution, how many grams are in 4 ml of solution?
359. How many grams are required to make 40 ml of solution if 10 g make 60 ml?

360. If 2,500 ml of urine contain 150 mg/100 ml of a substance, how many milligrams does the entire sample contain?

361. Fill in all blanks with equivalent answers:

Common fraction	Decimal fraction	Percentage (%)	Ratio			
			:	÷	Fraction	Decimal
¾						
	0.06					
	1.15					
		1.8%				
⁶⁄₇						
		21%				
	0.13					
1⅕						
		132%				
³⁰⁄₂₀						

2

Systems of Measure

To have successfully learned the material in this chapter, the student should be able to do the following properly:

- ◆ Describe the concept of measurement and the need of measurement in the clinical laboratory.
- ◆ Describe the metric system, its organization of prefixes, and the manner of assigning abbreviations and symbols to metric units.
- ◆ Convert metric values from prefix level to prefix level.
- ◆ Explain the organization and philosophy of the *Système International d'Unités* (SI).
- ◆ Demonstrate an understanding of basic and derived properties and their SI units by explanation and appropriate calculation.
- ◆ Describe the organization of the major nonmetric systems of measure, and relate these systems to the SI system and other metric systems used in clinical laboratories.
- ◆ Convert values given in one system of measure to equivalent values in other systems.
- ◆ Describe units of measure commonly used in the clinical laboratory in terms of their relationship to the applicable system of measure and the relationship of the unit to the system.

SECTION 2.1 INTRODUCTION

Measurement can be defined as the description of something in terms of number values. It is the determination of the magnitude of some property. **Properties** are the traits and attributes of something. Those properties that can be measured are **quantitative properties;** those that cannot be measured are **qualitative properties.**

A **unit of measure** is a precisely defined amount of some quantitative property. The meter, foot, yard, and mile are all units of length. A group of units of measure used together is a **system of measure.** Many systems of measure have been developed. However, most of these have fallen into disuse. Only three major systems of measure are still used to any appreciable extent. The most commonly used system of measure in the world is the international system, commonly called the *metric system.* The other two systems in use today are the United States Customary System and the British Imperial System. These two systems are being replaced with the metric system in almost all laboratory work. However, they are still widely used in many areas, and one should be familiar with them.

Units of measure are assigned symbols consisting of letters or other symbols. Appendix I is a listing of many common symbols of units of measure used in laboratories. In using these symbols, be sure of the recommended form. For example, the proper symbol for gram is *g,* written as lower case and without a period. The symbol *gr,* which is sometimes used for gram, is really the symbol for grain in the avoirdupois system. All metric units and most other kinds of units have only one recommended symbol. The use of the proper symbol for each unit of measure will improve laboratory communication and reduce confusion.

SECTION 2.2 METRIC SYSTEM

The **metric system** is a system of measure specifically designed to be used with decimal notation. This system consists of one primary unit for each quantitative property and a set of prefixes. Metric prefixes are used in combination with the primary units to create other units. Each prefix indicates a factor by which the primary unit is to be multiplied to produce larger or smaller units of a property. In this way the number of totally different units can be kept to a minimum. Table 2-1 is an outline of the metric prefixes with their values. Notice that the factor of each prefix is a multiple of 10. When a prefix is added to a primary unit, a new unit is made that has a value of the prefix factor times the factor of the primary unit (which is always 1). For example, 1 kilometer is equal to 1,000 meters, 1 milliliter is equal to 1/1,000 liter, and 1 microgram is equal to 1/1,000,000 gram. The primary units are equivalent to the multiple 10^0, or 1, and do not carry a prefix.

Table 2-1

Prefix	Symbol	Exponent factor (power of 10)	Decimal factor
Exa	E	10^{18}	1,000,000,000,000,000,000.0
Peta	P	10^{15}	1,000,000,000,000,000.0
Tera	T	10^{12}	1,000,000,000,000.0
Giga	G	10^9	1,000,000,000.0
Mega	M	10^6	1,000,000.0
Kilo	k	10^3	1,000.0
Hecto[*]	h	10^2	100.0
Deca[*]	da	10^1	10.0
Primary unit (no prefix)		10^0	1.0
Deci[*]	d	10^{-1}	0.1
Centi[*]	c	10^{-2}	0.01
Milli	m	10^{-3}	0.001
Micro	μ	10^{-6}	0.000001
Nano	n	10^{-9}	0.000000001
Pico	p	10^{-12}	0.000000000001
Femto	f	10^{-15}	0.000000000000001
Atto	a	10^{-18}	0.000000000000000001

[*]These four prefixes are not recommended for use as much as those above and below them. Use has shown that factors that are powers of 10 with exponents that are simple multiples of 3 provide enough units for convenient work.

Table 2-2 contains examples of some of the more common units of measure used in the biological laboratory. Notice that the table does not include all possible combinations of the primary units and prefixes. This is simply because all combinations are unnecessary for the convenient use of the metric system.

The units of measure in Table 2-2 and the prefixes in Table 2-1 conform to the latest recommendations of the International Union of Pure and Applied Chemistry (IUPAC) and the International Federation of Clinical Chemistry (IFCC).

There are several other units of measure that are based on the metric system but do not strictly conform to the rules of the system. Some of these units are designed to meet a specialized need. The most common example of this is the Angström unit. This is a unit of length nearly equal to 0.1 nanometer. This unit of measure was developed for use in the study of wavelengths of light. It is also a convenient unit of measure for use with molecules and cell organelles.

There are other units commonly used in biological laboratories that do not meet all the current rules of the metric system. These units developed through tradition and specific application of some of the basic concepts during the original development of the metric system. The units micron, lambda, and gamma are examples of such development. These are the traditional names of micrometer, microliter, and microgram, and have the symbols μ, λ, and γ, respectively. The proper name for such units of 1/1,000,000 primary unit includes the prefix *micro* and the unit name. The symbols for these three units are composed of μ and the symbol of the primary unit (Table 2-2). The use of the traditional units is technically incorrect but functionally useful. The laboratory worker should recognize both forms of these units and know their values.

Another traditional use of the metric system that is not considered correct is the use of combinations of prefixes. Units such as millimicrometer refer to the product of the combinations of prefixes. *Milli* refers to 1/1,000 and *micro* to 1/1,000,000; hence, *millimicro* refers to 1/1,000 $\times$ 1/1,000,000 or 1/1,000,000,000, so millimicrometer is a unit denoting 1/1,000,000,000 meter. This of course is equal to 1 nanometer. The use of such combinations of prefixes should be recognized, understood, and discouraged. The established prefixes in

Table 2-2

Multiple	Mass	Length	Volume
1,000	Kilogram (kg)	Kilometer (km)	Kiloliter (kl)
1 (primary unit)	Gram (g)	Meter (m)	Liter (L)
1/10	Decigram (dg)	Decimeter (dm)	Deciliter (dl)
1/100	Centigram (cg)	Centimeter (cm)	Centiliter (cl)
1/1,000	Milligram (mg)	Millimeter (mm)	Milliliter (ml)
1/1,000,000	Microgram (μg)	Micrometer (μm)	Microliter (μl)
1/1,000,000,000	Nanogram (ng)	Nanometer (nm)	Nanoliter (nl)
1/10,000,000,000		Angstrom (Å)	
1/1,000,000,000,000	Picogram (pg)	Picometer (pm)	Picoliter (pl)

Table 2-1 provide ample latitude in the development of acceptable units for almost any situation.

SECTION 2.3 SI SYSTEM

In 1960, the Conférence Générale des Poids et Mesures (CGPM) agreed to adopt the Système International d'Unités (International System of Units), which is abbreviated *SI* in all languages. The International Organization for Standardization (ISO), which is the international authority for standardization of names and symbols of physical properties, has also endorsed the system. Most other international scientific organizations have also endorsed this system of measure. The SI system was developed for use in physics; however, it has been recommended for the clinical laboratory with some modification. Such modifications are necessary to make the system convenient to laboratory work. Efforts have been made to adhere as closely as possible to the strict system and still make its use in the clinical laboratory practical.

The SI system is organized around a few basic properties. A **basic property** is one that is defined without using any other quantitative properties. Each basic property is assigned one unit. These are the **basic units.** No other units are used for the basic properties. Table 2-3 is a list of the basic properties and units of the SI system.

All other properties are called **derived properties.** These properties are described by using combinations of the basic properties. Units used to describe derived properties are called **derived units.** Derived units are either coherent or noncoherent with the SI system. **Coherent derived units** are those defined by using only the basic units and without using any factor other than 1. **Noncoherent derived units** are defined as units derived from units other than the basic SI units or involving a factor other than 1.

Consider the property of volume. Volume is the amount of space something takes up. It is not a basic property. Some combination of the basic units needs to be used to define volume. This can be done using the basic property of length in three dimensions. Volume is defined as length × length × length, or length cubed. Since the only basic SI unit of length is the meter, then the only *coherent* SI unit of volume is the cubic meter (meter × meter × meter). However, 1 cubic meter is the volume of a load for a small pickup truck. This is somewhat ridiculous for a unit of volume in a laboratory. The common unit of volume in

Table 2-3 Basic SI Properties

Basic property	Property symbol	Basic unit	Basic unit symbol
Length	*l*	meter	m
Mass	*m*	kilogram	kg
Time	*t*	second	s
Electrical current	*I*	ampere	A
Thermodynamic temperature	*T*	degree Kelvin	K
Luminous intensity	*I*	candela	cd
Amount of substance	*n*	mole	mol

laboratories is the liter. A liter is defined as 1 cubic decimeter or 0.001 cubic meters; hence, the liter is *not coherent* with the SI system. If it is defined as 1 cubic decimeter, then a unit other than the basic SI unit is used. If it is defined as 0.001 cubic meters, then a factor other than 1 is used. Either way, a liter cannot be a coherent SI unit.

Concentration of solutions is another derived property. It is the amount of solute per amount of solvent or per amount of total solution. If a concentration is defined as the amount of solute per mass of solvent, then the only coherent derived SI unit would be a number of moles of solute per kilogram of solvent. This is the definition of molality. Molality is the unit for the concentration of solutions that is coherent with the SI system. Again, this is inconvenient for common use in laboratories. The much more common unit for concentration of solutions is molarity. Molarity is defined as the number of moles of solute per liter of solution. Because liter is not a coherent SI unit, any unit defined with liter is not a coherent unit. Hence, molarity is a noncoherent derived unit.

Most units used in the clinical laboratory are being changed to units coherent with the SI system. However, as stated, strict adherence to this system for all laboratory work is not practical, and many recommended units are still not coherent with the SI system.

Table 2-4 lists most of the units in the modified SI system that are recommended for use in the clinical laboratory.

Definitions of Terms Used in Table 2-4 and Appendix DD

amount of substance   Number of formula units (atoms or molecules) in a given mass of matter.

arbitrary kind of quantity   Kind of quantity used when the result of a measurement is not a part of a recognized kind of quantity. For example, *titer* is a much-used arbitrary unit in serology. It is used to express the end point of a titration. Since the end point of a titration is not a recognized kind of quantity, titer is an arbitrary kind of unit.

area   Amount of surface. The surface may be on a plane or on a solid figure.

bar   Derived unit for pressure not coherent with the SI system, equal to 100,000 newtons per square meter (1 bar = 10^5 Pa = 10^5 N/m²). The use of "bar" is no longer recommended. It should be replaced by the coherent SI unit *pascal* (Pa), which is newtons per square meter (N/m²).

catalytic activity (catalytic amount)   The catalyzed rate of reaction for a specific chemical reaction, produced in a specific assay system.

catalytic activity concentration   Catalytic activity of the component (enzyme) in a mixture divided by the volume of the mixture. The numerical value depends on the temperature and pressure of the system.

catalytic activity content   Catalytic activity of the component (enzyme) divided by the mass of the system.

clearance   See **mean volume rate.**

density (mass density)   Mass of a system or object divided by its volume. The numerical value depends on the temperature and pressure of the system. *Mass density* should not be confused with *weight density,* which is the weight of a system divided by its volume.

density (relative density)   Ratio of the density of a system to the density of a reference or standard system under specified conditions for both systems. The numerical value depends on the temperature and pressure of each of the two systems.

enzyme unit   Amount of enzyme that will catalyze the transformation of 1 micromole (μmol) of substrate per minute under standard conditions. It has been recommended that the term *enzyme unit* (U) be discouraged so that it may eventually be abandoned. For a given method 1 U $\triangleq$ 1 μmol/min = 10^{-6} mol/min = $1/(10^6 \times 60)$ mol/s = 16.67 nmol/s $\triangleq$ 16.67 nkat.

international unit   Arbitrary units having a definition recognized by international agreement.

katal   Unit of catalytic activity of any catalyst (including any enzyme) that catalyzes a reaction rate of 1 mol/s.

Kelvin scale   Thermodynamic scale of temperature in which 0 K is the temperature of absolute zero and 273.16 K is the temperature of the triple point of pure water. The unit Kelvin (K) is defined as the fraction 1/273.16 of the thermodynamic temperature of the triple point of pure water.

kilogram   Basic SI unit for mass. It is equal to the mass of the international kilogram prototype kept at Sévres, France.

kind of quantity   The abstract concept of a property, common to a number of real phenomena (quantities). Examples: length, substance concentration, and pressure.

length   Basic kind of quantity, being the distance between two points.

liter   Unit of volume equal to 1 cubic decimeter or 1/1,000 of 1 cubic meter. The symbol for liter and the numeral 1 should be given distinctly different symbols. It is recommended in the United States that the capital L be the accepted symbol for liter, because most typescript gives insufficient distinction in the lower case.

mass   Basic kind of quantity, being the amount of matter in something. *Mass* should not be confused with *weight,* which is a derived kind of quantity.

mass concentration   Mass of a component in a mixture divided by the volume of the mixture. The numerical value depends on the temperature and pressure of the system.

mass fraction   Mass of the component divided by the mass of the system. The numerical value is independent of the temperature and pressure of the system.

mean catalytic activity rate   Catalytic activity of the component changed in or moved to or from a system divided by the time interval during which the component was changed or moved.

mean mass rate   Mass of a component changed in or moved to or from a system divided by the time interval during which the component was changed or moved.

mean substance rate   Amount of substance of the component changed in or moved to or from a system divided by the time interval during which the component was changed or moved.

mean volume rate   Volume of a component changed in or moved to or from a system divided by the time interval during which the component was changed or moved. The temperature, and for gases, the pressure of the isolated component should be stated.

   The kind of quantity *clearance* is usually defined as the product of the substance concentration of the component in the specified output and the volume rate of that output, divided by the substance concentration of the component in the specified output. Rephrased, it is the volume of plasma totally cleansed of a specified component divided by the time required. Thus this methodological definition equals *mean volume rate* and this latter name is preferred.

Text continued on p. 62.

Table 2-4 Recommended Units for the Clinical Laboratory

Kind of quantity	Basic or derived quantity	Property symbol	Name of unit	Basic or derived unit
Amount of substance	Basic	n	Mole	Basic
Arbitrary kind of unit	Non-SI basic or derived		International unit	Non-SI basic or derived
			Arbitrary unit	Non-SI basic or derived
Area	Derived	A	Square meter	Derived
Catalytic activity	Derived	z	Katal	Special derived
			Moles per second	Derived
Catalytic activity concentration (catalytic concentration)	Derived	b	Katal per liter	Special derived
			Moles per second liter	Derived
Catalytic activity content	Derived	z_c/m_s	Katals per kilogram	Derived
Density (mass density)	Derived	ρ	Kilograms per liter	Derived
Density (relative density)	Derived	d	Unity	Derived

*The symbol for liter (l) and the numeral one (1) should be given distinctly different symbols. It is recommended in the United States that the capital L be the accepted symbol for liter because most typescript gives insufficient distinction in the lower case.

Coherent or noncoherent unit	Unit symbol*	Symbols for multiples or fractions*		
		Recommended		Not recommended
	mol	mol mmol μmol nmol		M, *M*, eq, val, g-mol mM, meq, mval μM, uM, μeq, μval nM, neq, nval
	Int. unit			iu, u, IU, I.U.
	Arb. unit			
Coherent	m^2	m^2 mm^2 μm^2		cm^2 μ^2
Coherent	kat	kkat kat mkat	kmol/s mol/s mmol/s	kU
Coherent	mol/s	μkat nkat	μmol/s nmol/s	U mU
Noncoherent	kat/L	kkat/L kat/L mkat/L	kmol $\cdot$ s^{-1} $\cdot$ L^{-1} mol $\cdot$ s^{-1} $\cdot$ L^{-1} mmol $\cdot$ s^{-1} $\cdot$ L^{-1}	kmol/s/L mol/s/L mmol/s/L
Noncoherent	mol $\cdot$ s^{-1} $\cdot$ L^{-1}	μkat/L nkat/L	μmol $\cdot$ s^{-1} $\cdot$ L^{-1} nmol $\cdot$ s^{-1} $\cdot$ L^{-1}	U/ml U/L	μmol/s/L nmol/s/L
Coherent	kat/kg			
Noncoherent	kg/L	kg/L g/L mg/L		g/ml mg/ml μg/ml
Coherent	1	$\times$1 $\times 10^{-3}$		

Continued.

Table 2-4 Recommended Units for the Clinical Laboratory—cont'd

Kind of quantity	Basic or derived quantity	Property symbol	Name of unit	Basic or derived unit
Length	Basic	l	Meter	Basic
Mass	Basic	m	Kilogram	Basic
Mass concentration	Derived	ρ	Kilograms per liter	Derived
Mass fraction	Derived	w	Unity	Derived
Mean mass rate	Derived	$\Delta m/\Delta t$	Kilograms per second	Derived
			Kilograms per day	Derived

Coherent or noncoherent unit	Unit symbol[*]	Symbols for multiples or fractions[*]	
		Recommended	**Not recommended**
	m	m mm µm nm	cm µ, u mµ, mu
	kg	kg g mg µg ng pg	Kg, K gr., gm., gms., GR, GRM mgm, mgms γ, ug mµg, mug µµg, uug
Noncoherent	kg/L	kg/L g/L mg/L µg/L ng/L	g/ml %, g%, %$^{(w/v)}$, g/100 ml, g/dl ‰, g‰, ‰$^{(w/v)}$ mg%, mg%$^{(w/v)}$, mg/100 ml, mg/dl ppm, p.p.m.$^{(w/v)}$, mg‰ µg%, µg%$^{(w/v)}$, µg/100 ml, µg/dl mµg/ml µµg/ml, uug/ml
Coherent	1	×1 ×10^{-3} ×10^{-6} ×10^{-9} ×10^{-12}	kg/kg g/g %, %$^{(w/w)}$ g/kg ‰, ‰$^{(w/w)}$ mg/kg p.p.m., p.p.m.$^{(w/w)}$, ppm µg/kg p.p.b., p.p.b.$^{(w/w)}$, ppb ng/kg

Coherent	kg/s	kg/s
		     kg/min
		     kg/h
		     kg/d
		     kg/a
		g/s
		     g/min
		     g/h
		     g/d
			kg/sec.
			     kg/min.
			     kg/hr.
			     kg/da.
			     kg/yr.
			gm/sec.
			     gm/min.
			     g/hr.
			     g/da.

Noncoherent	kg/d	mg/s
		     mg/min
		     mg/h
		µg/s
		     µg/min.
		ng/s
		     ng/min
			
			     mg/min
			     mg/hr.
			
			     µg/min.
			
			     ng/min.

Continued.

Table 2-4 Recommended Units for the Clinical Laboratory—cont'd

Kind of quantity	Basic or derived quantity	Property symbol	Name of unit	Basic or derived unit
Mean catalytic activity rate	Derived	$\Delta z/\Delta t$	Katals per second	Derived
Mean substance rate	Derived	$\Delta n/\Delta t$	Moles per second	Derived
			Moles per day	Derived
Mean volume rate	Derived	$\Delta V/\Delta t$	Liters per second	Derived
			Liters per day	Derived
Molality	Derived	m	Moles per kilogram	Derived
Mole fraction (Substance fraction)	Derived	x	Unity	Derived

Coherent or noncoherent unit	Unit symbol[*]	Symbols for multiples or fractions[*]	
		Recommended	Not recommended
Coherent	kat/s		

Coherent	mol/s	mol/s
		    mol/min
		    mol/d
		mmol/s
		    mmol/min
		    mmol/h
		    mmol/d
			mol/sec., eq/sec.
			    mol/min., eq/min.
			    mol/da.
			mmol/sec., meq/sec.
			    mmol/min., meq/min.
			    mmol/hr., meq/hr.
			    mmol/da., meq/da.

Noncoherent	mol/d	μmol/s
		    μmol/min
		    μmol/h
		nmol/s
		    nmol/min
			μmol/min.
			    μmol/hr.
			    nmol/min.

Noncoherent	L/s	L/s
		    L/min
		    L/h
		    L/d
		ml/s
			L/sec.
			    L/min.
			    L/hr.
			    L/da.
			ml/sec.

Noncoherent	L/d	ml/min
		    ml/h
		μl/s
		    μl/min
		nl/s
		    nl/min
			ml/min.
			    ml/hr.
			    μl/min.
			    nl/min.

Coherent	mol/kg	mol/kg mmol/kg μmol/kg	m, m, mmol/g, μmol/mg mm, mm μm, μm
Coherent	1	$\times 1$ $\times 10^{-3}$ $\times 10^{-6}$	mol/mol %, mol% mmol/mol ‰, mol‰ μmol/mol

Continued.

Table 2-4   Recommended Units for the Clinical Laboratory—cont'd

Kind of quantity	Basic or derived quantity	Property symbol	Name of unit	Basic or derived unit
Number (of entities)	Derived	N	Unity	Derived
Number concentration	Derived	C	One per liter	Derived
Number fraction	Derived	δ	Unity	Derived
Partial pressure	Derived	p	Pascal	Derived
			Newtons per square meter	Derived
Pressure	Derived	p	Pascal	Derived
			Newtons per square meter	Derived
Relative kind of quantity	Derived		Unity	Derived

Coherent or noncoherent unit	Unit symbol*	Symbols for multiples or fractions*	
		Recommended	**Not recommended**
Coherent	1	$\times 10^9$ $\times 10^6$ $\times 10^3$ $\times 1$ $\times 10^{-3}$	
Noncoherent	L^{-1} or $1/L$	$\times 10^9 L^{-1}$ $\times 10^9 /L$ $\times 10^6 L^{-1}$ $\times 10^6 /L$ $\times 10^3 L^{-1}$ $\times 10^3 /L$ L^{-1} $\times 1/L$ $\times 10^{-3} L^{-1}$ $\times 10^{-3}/L$	$\times 1/\mu 1, \times 1/ul, \mu 1^{-1}$ $\times 1/ml, ml^{-1}$
Coherent	1	$\times 1$ $\times 10^{-3}$ $\times 10^{-6}$	% ‰
Coherent	Pa	MPa MN/m^2 kPa kN/m^2	atm bar, b
Coherent	N/m^2	 Pa N/m^2	mm Hg, Torr mbar, mb mm H_2O pascal μbar, μb
Coherent	Pa	MPa MN/m^2 kPa kN/m^2	atm bar, b
Coherent	N/m^2	 Pa N/m^2	mm Hg, Torr mbar, mb mm H_2O pascal μbar, μb
Coherent	1	$\times 1$ $\times 10^{-3}$ $\times 10^{-6}$ $\times 10^{-9}$	% ‰ p.p.m., ppm p.p.b., ppb

Continued.

Table 2-4 Recommended Units for the Clinical Laboratory—cont'd

Kind of quantity	Basic or derived quantity	Property symbol	Name of unit	Basic or derived unit
Substance concentration	Derived	c	Moles per liter	Derived
Substance content	Derived	n_c/m_s	Moles per kilogram	Derived
Temperature, Celsius	Derived	θ	Degree Celsius	Derived
Temperature difference	Derived	ΔT	Kelvin	Derived
Temperature, thermodynamic	Basic	T	Kelvin	Basic
Time	Basic	t	Second	Basic
			Minute	Derived
			Hour	Derived
			Day (24 hours)	Derived
			Year	Derived
Volume	Derived	V	Cubic meter	Derived
			Liter	Derived
Volume content	Derived	V_c/m_s	Liters per kilogram	Derived
Volume fraction	Derived	φ	Unity	Derived

Coherent or noncoherent unit	Unit symbol*	Symbols for multiples or fractions*	
		Recommended	Not recommended
Noncoherent	mol/L	mol/L mmol/L μmol/L nmol/L	M, *M*, eq/L, val/L, N, *N*, n mM, m*M*, meq/L, mval/L, mN, etc. μM, uM, μeq/L, etc. nM, neq/L, etc.
Coherent	mol/kg		
Special coherent	°C	°C, K m°C, mK	C, °, C°, centigrade
Coherent	K	K mK	°C °K, C, °, C°, centigrade m°C mdeg
	K	K mK	°K, °, K°, °C
	s	Ms a	yr.
Noncoherent	min	d	da.
Noncoherent	h	h ks	hr.
Noncoherent	d	min s ms	min., m. sec., s.
Noncoherent	a	μs	us

Coherent	m³	m³
		   L
		   ml
			dm³ l.
			           dl
			cm³, cc, ccm

Noncoherent	L	mm³ μl
		     nl
		     pl
		μm³ fl
			λ, ul
			$\mu\mu$l, uul
			μ^3, u³

Noncoherent	L/kg		
Coherent	1	×1 ×10⁻³ ×10⁻⁶	L/L, ml/ml %, %$^{(v/v)}$, vol% ml/L ‰, ‰$^{(v/v)}$, vol‰ μl/L p.p.m., p.p.m.$^{(v/v)}$, ppm

meter   Basic SI unit for length, being the length of 1,650,763.73 wavelengths of the radiation of krypton 86.

molality   Amount of substance of a solute in a solution divided by the mass of the solvent. The numerical value is independent of the temperature and pressure of the solution.

mole   Basic unit of an *amount of substance* equal to the mass of any substance containing the same number of formula units (atoms or molecules) as there are in 0.012 kilogram (12 grams) of pure carbon 12. This is equivalent to the number of grams of any substance equal to the numerical value of the atomic or molecular weight.

mole fraction   Amount of substance of the component divided by the amount of substance of all components of the system. The numerical value is independent of the temperature and pressure of the system.

newton   Force that when applied to a body having a mass of 1 kilogram, gives it an acceleration *in vacuo* of 1 m/s^2.

number (of entities)   Any kind of defined entity or mixture of entities. This kind of quantity was called *number of particles* in QU-R66-4.5.

number concentration   Number of stated particles of the component divided by the volume of the system. The numerical value depends on the temperature and pressure of the system.

number fraction   Number of defined particles of a component in a system divided by the total number of defined particles in the system. This kind of quantity had the name *particle fraction* in QU-R66-4.15.

partial pressure   Pressure of a component in a gaseous mixture measured as the product of the mole fraction of the component and the total pressure of the mixture. The temperature of the system should be stated.

pascal   Newtons per square meter (N/m^2).

pressure   Force exerted at right angles to a surface divided by the area of the surface. The numerical value depends on the temperature of the system.

relative kind of quantity   Ratio between a kind of quantity referring to a specified kind of system and an identical kind of quantity referring to another standard system.

second   Basic SI unit for time, being the amount of time required for 9,192,631,770 cycles of transition between the energy levels of cesium 133.

substance concentration   Amount of substance in a mixture divided by the volume of the mixture. The numerical value is dependent on the temperature and pressure of the system. In QU-R66 the term *molar concentration* was used.

substance content   Amount of substance of the component divided by the mass of the system. This kind of quantity should not be confused with molality.

temperature, Celsius   Temperature normally encountered in most clinical and biological systems. Degree Celsius is the temperature scale at which the triple point of pure water has the temperature of 0.01° and the steam point has the temperature of 100°. The name *customary temperature* was used in QU-R66.

temperature, thermodynamic   Basic kind of quantity, being the tendency of a body to lose heat relative to absolute zero.

temperature difference   Arithmetic difference between two temperatures using the same scale.

time   Basic kind of quantity that is the duration of some event.

unity   Dimensionless unit being the ratio of some value to 1 and usually having the 1 understood.

volume   Amount of space occupied by something.

volume content   Volume of the isolated component at specified conditions divided by the mass of the system.

volume fraction   Volume of an isolated component of a mixture divided by the volume of the mixture, both at specified conditions. The numerical value depends on the temperature and pressure of the component and the system.

SECTION 2.4 NONMETRIC SYSTEMS OF MEASURE

Nonmetric systems of measure are much more complex in their organization than the decimal-based metric system. There is little consistency in the relative magnitude of the units of measure of any one property. Appendix J gives the units of the apothecary, avoirdupois, and troy systems of measure. Appendix K gives the relative values of many systems and units of measure used in these systems. Tradition, established procedures, and other factors may require that laboratory personnel use nonmetric units of measure. However, the metric system should be used whenever possible because it has much greater compatibility with decimal-based mathematics and is used more in other countries.

The system of measure used in this country is a conglomeration of older systems. This system is usually called the **English system** because most of the system was used in England at the time of the development of the United States. However, today the system of measure used in the United States has several significant differences from the British Imperial System that was official in England until the 1970s. The **United States Customary System** is the proper name for this system of measure.

As a matter of practical consideration, there are a few units that are much used in this country. The following units of measure are the ones most commonly seen in the laboratory. The memorization of these units will save the laboratory worker time and energy in calculations involving measurement. Again the values of many other units of measure are found in Appendix K.

Weight	Volume	Length
1 gram = 15.4 grains	1 fluid dram = 3.7 milliliters	1 inch = 2.54 centimeters
1 avoirdupois ounce = 28.35 grams	1 fluid ounce = 29.6 milliliters	1 foot = 0.305 meters
1 avoirdupois pound = 16 avoirdupois ounces	1 gallon = 128.0 fluid ounces	
1 kilogram = 2.2 pounds		

SECTION 2.5 CONVERSIONS FROM ONE UNIT OF MEASURE TO ANOTHER

Laboratory calculations often involve the conversion of one unit of measure to another. For example, one may need to convert 250 milliliters to liters or 0.028 inches to millimeters. In general, units of measure can be converted only to units of the same property. Kilograms cannot be converted to liters, or yards cannot be converted to meters per second. All units of length are compatible; that is, they are all units of length and any unit of length can be converted to any other unit of length. However, units of length cannot be converted to units of another property.

One common exception to this involves the conversion of units of weight to units of mass. Pounds are converted to kilograms, and ounces are converted to grams. Pounds and ounces are units of *weight* in the avoirdupois system. Kilograms and grams are units of *mass* in the metric system. **Weight** is defined as the force of gravity on something, whereas **mass** is defined as the amount of matter in something. However, in common usage pounds and ounces are also used as units of mass. The units of weight in the United States Customary system are also used as units of mass. Hence, pounds can be converted to kilograms.

There are two common methods used to convert one unit to another. The ratio and proportion procedure is probably the most flexible method to accomplish this. The use of conversion factors is the other commonly used method. This is an abbreviated form of the ratio and proportion procedure. Either method can be used as long as it is done correctly.

Conversion of Metric Units to Metric Units

The ratio and proportion procedure is probably the most useful way to convert one unit of measure to another. Remember that this procedure is a way to make a known ratio proportional, or equivalent to, an unknown ratio.

To convert one metric unit to another using ratio and proportion, obtain the known ratio between one of the units to the other from some reference. Now make the unknown ratio by setting the known number of the units given against x units desired. Solve for x. Study the following examples.

EXAMPLE 2-1: How many milligrams equal 0.025 g?

From Appendix K it is found that 1 g is equal to 1,000 mg. Hence, the known ratio is 1 g to 1,000 mg.

The unknown ratio is 0.025 g to x mg.

Make a ratio and proportion statement.

0.025 g is to x mg as 1 g is to 1,000 mg.

$$\frac{0.025 \text{ g}}{x \text{ mg}} = \frac{1 \text{ g}}{1,000 \text{ mg}}$$

$$x = 0.025 \times 1,000$$

$$x = 25 \text{ mg}$$

Hence, 25 mg = 0.025 g.

EXAMPLE 2-2: Convert 250,000 m to kilometers.

From Appendix K find that 1,000 m equal 1 km.

Make a ratio and proportion statement.

250,000 m is to x km as 1,000 m is to 1 km.

Set up the ratio and proportion and solve for x.

$$\frac{250,000 \text{ m}}{x \text{ km}} = \frac{1,000 \text{ m}}{1 \text{ km}}$$

$$1,000x = 250,000 \times 1$$

$$x = \frac{250,000}{1,000}$$

$$x = 250 \text{ km}$$

250,000 m are equal to 250 km.

Another way to convert one kind of unit to another is to use a conversion factor. These are numbers by which a number of one kind of unit is multiplied to convert it to another similar value. Factors are discussed at length in Chapter 4 of this book. Many factors can be found in references such as Appendixes K and T, or they may be calculated as shown in the next examples.

One major advantage of the metric system results from the relationship of the prefixes to the power of 10. This allows the conversion from one compatible unit to another by moving decimal points or by the manipulation of exponents of 10. Note the exponent of 10 for each prefix of the metric units in Table 2-1. You would do well to memorize these values.

> To determine the factor between two metric units of a property, divide the prefix value of the given unit by the prefix value of the desired unit. To obtain the number of desired units, multiply the number of the existing units by this factor.

Since the prefix values are whole number powers of 10, one can do this by subtracting the exponent of the desired unit from the exponent of the existing unit by using the rules for subtraction of signed numbers discussed in Chapter 1, pp. 7–9. *Ten to the power of this result is equal to the conversion factor.* This number is then converted to a decimal number and used to convert one metric unit to another.

Study the following examples.

EXAMPLE 2-3: How many nanograms are equal to 0.0078 mg?

The existing unit prefix is milli- (10^{-3}), and the desired unit prefix is nano- (10^{-9}).

$$10^{-3} \div 10^{-9} = 10^{-3-(-9)} = 10^6$$

$$[-3 - (-9) = -3 + 9 = 6]$$

The factor for converting milligrams to nanograms is $10^6 = 1,000,000$; hence, 0.0078 mg $\times$ 1,000,000 = 7,800 ng.

EXAMPLE 2-4: How many milligrams are equal to 0.0078 ng?

The existing unit prefix is nano- (10^{-9}), and the desired unit prefix is milli- (10^{-3}).

$$10^{-9} \div 10^{-3} = 10^{-9-(-3)} = 10^{-6}$$

$$[-9 - (-3) = -9 + 3 = -6]$$

The factor for converting nanograms to milligrams is 10^{-6} or 0.000001; hence, 0.0078 ng $\times$ 0.000001 = 0.0000000078 mg.

EXAMPLE 2-5: How many liters equal 38,967 ml?

The existing unit is 10^{-3}, and the desired unit is 10^0.

$$10^{-3} \div 10^0 = 10^{-3-(0)} = 10^{-3}$$

$$[-3 - 0 = -3]$$

The factor for converting milliliters to liters is 10^{-3} or 0.001; hence, 38,967 ml $\times$ 0.001 = 38.967 L.

EXAMPLE 2-6: How many kilometers would it take to make 46,520 dm?

The existing unit is 10^{-1}, and the desired unit is 10^3.

$$10^{-1} \div 10^3 = 10^{-1-(+3)} = 10^{-4}$$

$$[-1 - (+3) = -4]$$

The factor for converting decimeters to kilometers is 10^{-4} or 0.0001; hence, 46,520 $\times$ 0.0001 = 4.652 km.

This procedure to convert a number of one metric unit to an equivalent number of another metric unit may be summarized by the following formulas.

$$\frac{\text{Exponent of 10}}{\text{of existing unit}} - \frac{\text{Exponent of 10}}{\text{of desired unit}} = \frac{\text{Exponent of 10}}{\text{of the factor}}$$

Factor $\times$ number of existing units = number of desired units

Consider Example 2-3: How many nanograms are equal to 0.0078 mg?

$$-3 - (-9) = -3 + 9 = 6$$

The factor is 10^6.

$$10^6 \times 0.0078 = 7{,}800 \text{ ng}$$

This same procedure may be modified and used to change one metric unit of area or volume to another unit of the same property. Since these properties are linear measure taken in two and three dimensions, respectively, the exponents of the factors must be multiplied by either 2 for area or 3 for volume.

EXAMPLE 2-7: Convert 0.78 m^2 to *square* centimeters.

Determine the exponent of 10 for the factor between meters and centimeters.

$$10^0 \div 10^{-2}$$

$$0 - (-2) = +2$$

Multiply this exponent as a number times 2.

$$2 \times 2 = 4$$

The factor between square meters and square centimeters is 10^4, or 10,000.

Multiply this factor times the existing number.

$$10{,}000 \times 0.78 \text{ m}^2 = 7{,}800 \text{ cm}^2.$$

0.78 m^2 is equal to 7,800 cm^2.

EXAMPLE 2-8: Convert 15,000 mm^3 to *cubic* decimeters.

Determine a factor between millimeters and decimeters.

$$10^{-3} \div 10^{-1}$$
$$-3 - (-1) = -3 + 1 = -2$$

Multiply this by 3.

$$-2 \times 3 = -6$$

The factor to convert cubic millimeters to cubic decimeters is 10^{-6}.

Multiply the existing number by this factor.

$$10^{-6} \times 15,000 = 0.015$$

There are 0.015 dm^3 in 15,000 ml^3.

Conversion with Nonmetric Units

Unlike the metric systems, the nonmetric systems of measure do not have consistent relationships among their units. The relationship between any two particular units has to be obtained from references. Use this relationship as the known ratio of a ratio and proportion to convert from one unit to another.

EXAMPLE 2-9: How many fluid drams are in 3.8 fluid ounces?

From Appendix J, find that 1 fluid ounce is equal to 8 fluid drams.

Make the ratio and proportion statement.

x fluid drams are to 3.8 fluid ounces as 8 fluid drams are to 1 fluid ounce.

Set up the ratio and proportion and solve for x.

$$\frac{x \text{ fl dr}}{3.8 \text{ fl oz}} = \frac{8 \text{ fl dr}}{1 \text{ fl oz}}$$
$$x = 3.8 \times 8$$
$$x = 30.4 \text{ fl dr}$$

There are 30.4 fluidrams in 3.8 fluidounces.

Sometimes a reference does not give a relationship between two units directly. However, a relationship can often be found by using some thought.

EXAMPLE 2-10: Convert 2,500 grains to avoirdupois ounces.

Appendix J does not show how many grains equal 1 oz. However, it does show that 1 dram equals 27.344 grains and 1 oz equals 16 drams. One way to make this conversion is to convert 2,500 grains to the equivalent number of drams and then convert this number of drams to a number of ounces.

First convert grains to drams.

$$\frac{x \text{ dr}}{2,500 \text{ gr}} = \frac{1 \text{ dr}}{27.344 \text{ gr}}$$
$$27.344x = 2500 \times 1$$
$$x = \frac{2500}{27.344}$$
$$x = 91.428 \text{ dr}$$

Now convert drams to ounces.

$$\frac{x \text{ oz}}{91.428 \text{ dr}} = \frac{1 \text{ oz}}{16 \text{ dr}}$$

$$16x = 91.428$$

$$x = \frac{91.428}{16}$$

$$x = 5.714 \text{ oz}$$

A more direct way to solve this problem is to consider that since 1 dram equals 27.344 grains and 1 oz equals 16 drams, then 1 oz equals 16 times 27.344 grains. Hence, the relationship between grains and ounces is 1 oz equals 437.504 grains. Use this for the known ratio.

Set up a ratio and proportion and solve for x.

$$\frac{x \text{ oz}}{2,500 \text{ gr}} = \frac{1 \text{ oz}}{437.504 \text{ gr}}$$

$$437.504x = 2,500$$

$$x = \frac{2,500}{437.504}$$

$$x = 5.714 \text{ oz}$$

It is often necessary to convert nonmetric units to metric units. The procedure for this is the same as that for the conversion of nonmetric units to other nonmetric units. From a reference, find a relationship between the nonmetric and metric unit and complete a ratio and proportion procedure.

EXAMPLE 2-11: How many liters are in 2.4 pints (pt)?

From Appendix K find that 1 pt is equal to 0.473 L.

Set up a ratio and proportion and solve for x.

$$\frac{1 \text{ pt}}{0.473 \text{ L}} = \frac{2.4 \text{ pt}}{x \text{ L}}$$

$$x = 0.473 \times 2.4$$

$$x = 1.135 \text{ L}$$

EXAMPLE 2-12: How many grams are there in 6 lb?

This problem may be done at least two different ways. From the common units given in Section 2.4, one relationship between pounds and kilograms and one relationship between kilogram and grams are shown. Therefore pounds can be converted to kilograms, and then kilograms can be converted to grams using a factor. Additionally, relationships are shown between pounds and ounces and between ounces and grams; therefore pounds can be converted to ounces, and ounces can be converted to grams. Using ratio and proportion, set up the problem.

Method 1

Step 1. 1 kg is to 2.2 lb as x kg are to 6 lb.

$$\frac{1 \text{ kg}}{2.2 \text{ lb}} = \frac{x \text{ kg}}{6 \text{ lb}}$$

$$2.2x = 6$$

$$x = 2.727 \text{ kg}$$

$$6 \text{ lb} = 2.727 \text{ kg}$$

Step 2. Convert kilograms to grams. The multiple of kilo- is 10^3, and the multiple of gram is 10^0.

$$\frac{10^3}{10^0} = 10^{3-0} = 10^3, \qquad \text{factor} = 10^3$$

$$2.727 \text{ kg} \times 1,000 = 2,727 \text{ g}$$

$$6 \text{ lb} = 2,727 \text{ g}$$

Method 2

Step 1. 1 lb = 16 oz; therefore 1 lb is to 16 oz as 6 lb are to x oz.

$$\frac{1 \text{ lb}}{16 \text{ oz}} = \frac{6 \text{ lb}}{x \text{ oz}}$$

$$x = 6 \times 16$$

$$x = 96 \text{ oz}$$

$$6 \text{ lb} = 96 \text{ oz}$$

Step 2. 1 oz = 28.35 g; therefore 1 oz is to 28.35 g as 96 oz are to x g.

$$\frac{1 \text{ oz}}{28.35 \text{ g}} = \frac{96 \text{ oz}}{x \text{ g}}$$

$$1x = 2,721.6 \text{ g}$$

$$6 \text{ lb} = 2,721.6 \text{ g}$$

This problem may also be solved in one step if the relationship between grams and pounds is known.

APPENDIXES RELATED TO THIS CHAPTER

I   Symbols of Units of Measure
J   Apothecary, Avoirdupois, and Troy Systems of Measure
K   Conversion Factors for Units of Measure
T   Conversions Among Metric Prefixes
U   Conversions Among Square Metric Units
V   Conversions Among Cubic Metric Units
W   Conversions Between Liter Units and Cubic Metric Units
DD Clinical Tests with Units, Normal Values, and Conversion Factors

PRACTICE PROBLEMS

Calculate the answer for each problem. Understand each portion of the calculation and determine whether the answer is logical. *Just because an answer can be calculated does not mean that it is reasonable.*

Metric system

1. Give the metric prefix and power of 10 that corresponds to the following symbols:

m	da	n	h
a	c	k	f
T	p	d	P
M	G	μ	E

2. Give the correct metric prefix for the following:

μ	millimicro
λ	micromicro
γ	

Express the following (use Appendix K or T):

3. 300 dg as micrograms
4. 3 mg as centigrams
5. 15 dag as milliliters
6. 16,000 nm as millimeters
7. 0.8 pg as femtograms
8. 0.0004 hl as deciliters
9. 167 ng as micrograms
10. 16 kg as decagrams
11. 3265 pl as deciliters
12. 0.1829 mm as attometers

13. 10,000 lambda as liters
14. 560 lambda as milliliters
15. 400 mg as decimeters
16. 3,200 μg as centigrams
17. 0.07 dl as nanoliters
18. 9,000 cm as kilometers
19. 0.048 kg as milliliters
20. 52 dl as milliliters
21. 8 dal as centiliters
22. 30.0097 dm as millimeters

23. How many milligrams are in 5.7 g?
24. How many grams does 66 mg represent?
25. 10^{-9} equals:
   a. 0.0000000009
   b. 0.000000001
   c. 0.000000009
   d. 0.0000000001
26. 6×10^{-3} g is equivalent to:
   a. 60 mg
   b. 0.0006 g
   c. 0.06 g
   d. 6.0 mg
27. 5×10^4 mg is equivalent to:
   a. 5000 mg
   b. 50 g
   c. 500 mg
   d. 5 g
28. Which of the following is the smallest unit?
   a. kilometer
   b. decimeter
   c. micrometer
   d. meter
   e. decameter
   f. centimeter
29. One micron equals:
   a. 0.000001 mm
   b. 1,000 m
   c. 0.001 mm
   d. 0.001 m

Nonmetric conversions (use Appendix K)

Convert the following:
30. 35 kg to pounds (avdp)*
31. 10 kg to ounces (avdp)

*avdp, avoirdupois system; apoth, apothecary system; US, United States Customary System.

32. 32 g to ounces (avdp)
33. 432 g to pounds (apoth)
34. 16 m to feet
35. 320 grains to grams
36. 231 lb (avdp) to kilograms
37. 1 lb (avdp) to pounds (apoth)
38. 300 ml to fluid ounces (US)
39. 3 qt to deciliters
40. 13 L to gallons (US)

41. One inch equals:
    a. 0.254 cm   c. 25.4 mm
    b. 0.254 mm   d. 2.54 m
42. Which pair below is *not* matched correctly?
    a. 1 L = 0.946 qt   c. 1 m = 39.4 in
    b. 1,000 mm = 100 cm   d. 1 lb (avdp) = 454 g
43. Which pair below is *not* equivalent?
    a. 1 ft = 0.305 m   c. 200 cm = 78.8 in
    b. 1 L = 1,000 cm^3 d. 0.1 kg = 0.022 lb (avdp)
44. Which pair below is *not* equivalent?
    a. 1 mm = 0.0394 in   c. 1 fl oz = 29.6 ml
    b. 1.0 ml = 1.0 cc   d. 1.0 cc = 1.0 mm^3
45. 1 L of water (at 4°C) weighs:
    a. 1,000,000 mg   c. 1 lb
    b. 0.1 lb   d. 100 g
46. 12 g = _____ oz (avdp)
47. 20 lb (apoth) = _____ g
48. 4 kg = _____ oz (apoth)
49. 100 oz = _____ gal
50. 2.6 gal = _____ drams
51. You use 200 ml/wk of a solution that requires 192 g of solute per Liter to make up. You ordered 5 lb of solute. It costs 5¢ per gram. How long will it last and how much will it cost?

3

Temperature Conversions

EDUCATIONAL OBJECTIVES

To have successfully learned the material in this chapter, the student should be able to do the following properly:

♦ Differentiate between temperature and heat.
♦ Differentiate among the Fahrenheit, Celsius, and Kelvin temperature scales.
♦ Relate the size and reference point of the degrees among the three scales.
♦ Convert temperatures given in one scale to equivalent values in the other two scales.

SECTION 3.1 INTRODUCTION

Heat is energy. Heat may be a kind of electromagnetic energy with a lower frequency than light, or it may be the energy in matter that results in the constant motion of the particles of the matter. This latter form of heat is sometimes called **thermal energy. Temperature** is a measure of the tendency of a body to gain or lose thermal energy. If one body of matter has a higher temperature than another, heat will move from the warmer to the cooler body. The total amount of energy is not the only determinant for the temperature of a body. Different substances hold different amounts of heat at a given temperature. However, substances with higher temperatures always lose heat to substances with lower temperatures.

There are three scales used to measure temperature in the United States. These are the **Fahrenheit, Celsius,** and **Kelvin** scales. The *centigrade scale* is an old name for the Celsius scale. The Fahrenheit scale is considered to be part of the English system of measure and is commonly used in the United States and a few other countries. The Celsius scale is the common temperature scale of those countries that use the metric system. The Kelvin scale is preferred for physics and is the scale that must be used in direct and indirect proportion calculations involving temperature change.

All three temperature scales are divided into units called **degrees.** The size of each degree of the Celsius and Kelvin scales are the same, but they are different from Fahrenheit degrees. The zero point is different for all three scales. Zero degrees Celsius is the temperature of freezing water. Zero degrees Fahrenheit is the lowest temperature that can be attained by mixing table salt and ice. The zero point of the Kelvin scale is absolute zero. This is the lowest theoretical temperature. It is considered to be the temperature of a body that has no more heat to lose. Fig. 3-1 gives the temperature of five natural phenomena on each of the three scales.

Notice that 0 K is −273°C and that 273 K is 0°C. The size of each degree of the Celsius and Kelvin scales are the same. In other words, a change of 1°C is equal to a change of 1 K. The scales just start at a different place. Fahrenheit degrees are different. Notice that 0°C is 32°F, but 0°F is −17.78°C. The Fahrenheit scale has both different sized degrees and a different starting point from the other two scales. A change of 1°F is not equal to a change of 1°C or 1 K.

In the United States, laboratory procedures are written using any one of these three temperature scales. Often it becomes necessary to convert temperature values from one scale to another. The simplest way to do this is to use a temperature conversion table found in a reference book. Two such tables are found in Appendixes N and O in this book. If a reference is not available, temperatures can be converted from one scale to another by calculation.

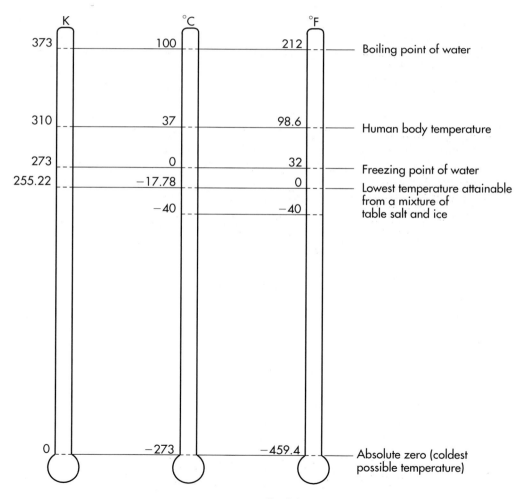

Fig. 3-1.

Table 3-1

	Kelvin	Celsius	Fahrenheit
Boiling point of water	373	100°	212°
Freezing point of water	273	0°	32°
Number of degrees from boiling point to freezing point	100	100°	180°

Conversion between the Celsius and Kelvin scales is relatively simple. This simplicity is possible because the degrees of the two scales are equal. A 100° temperature change is the same with either scale. Water at standard pressure boils at 100°C or 373 K. The difference between the boiling point and freezing point of water is 100° using either the Kelvin or Celsius scale (Table 3-1).

Conversions between the Celsius and Fahrenheit scales are somewhat more complicated. The Fahrenheit scale has the zero point set at the lowest temperature attainable from a mixture of table salt and ice. One hundred degrees Fahrenheit was set at the body temperature of a small animal. This scale was later standardized against the Celsius scale. The freezing point of water is 32°F, whereas the boiling point of water at standard pressure is 212°F. This results in degree increments of a magnitude different from the other two scales. Hence, the conversion between the Fahrenheit scale and the other scales is somewhat complicated. Table 3-1 shows the boiling and freezing points of water in these three scales.

There are 100° (or units) on the Celsius scale from the boiling point to the freezing point of water. In the equivalent range on the Fahrenheit scale, there are 180 units. To compare the two, one may use a ratio-proportion method; that is, 100°C is to 180°F as 1 is to x.

$$\frac{100°C}{180°F} = \frac{1°C}{x°F}$$

$$100x = 180$$

$$x = \frac{180}{100}$$

$$x = 1.8 = 1\frac{4}{5} = \frac{9}{5}$$

Therefore 1°C is equal to 1.8°F. Using common fractions, it can be seen that 1°C is equal to $\frac{9}{5}$°F.

Similarly, 180°F is to 100°C as 1 is to x.

$$\frac{180°F}{100°C} = \frac{1°F}{x°C}$$

$$180x = 100$$

$$x = \frac{100}{180}$$

$$x = 0.556 = \frac{5}{9}$$

Therefore 1°F is equal to 0.556°C, or 1°F is equal to $\frac{5}{9}$°C.

Notice that this comparison begins at the freezing point of water on both scales and not at the zero point. This means that 0°F and 0°C are different temperatures. *This difference must be adjusted in the conversion from one scale to the other.*

SECTION 3.2 CONVERSION BETWEEN DEGREES CELSIUS AND DEGREES KELVIN

To convert degrees Kelvin to degrees Celsius, subtract 273 from the value in degrees Kelvin. To convert degrees Celsius to degrees Kelvin, add 273 to the value in degrees Celsius.

$$°C = K - 273$$

$$K = °C + 273$$

SECTION 3.3 CONVERSION BETWEEN DEGREES CELSIUS AND DEGREES FAHRENHEIT

To Convert Degrees Celsius to Degrees Fahrenheit

Since one Celsius degree is equal to $\frac{9}{5}$ (or 1.8) Fahrenheit degrees, one must multiply the degrees Celsius readings by $\frac{9}{5}$ (or 1.8) to convert it to units of the magnitude of the Fahrenheit degree. This figure is then adjusted to the zero point of the Fahrenheit scale by the addition of 32 (Fig. 3-2).

$$°F = \left(°C \times \frac{9}{5}\right) + 32$$

$$°F = (°C \times 1.8) + 32$$

EXAMPLE 3-1: Convert 37°C to °F.

$$°F = (°C \times 1.8) + 32$$

$$°F = (37 \times 1.8) + 32$$

$$°F = 66.6 + 32$$

$$°F = 98.6$$

To Convert Degrees Fahrenheit to Degrees Celsius

First adjust the zero point of the Fahrenheit scale to the zero point on the Celsius scale by subtracting 32 from the Fahrenheit value. Since 1°F is equal to $\frac{5}{9}$°C or 0.556°C, multiply the adjusted Fahrenheit value by $\frac{5}{9}$, or (0.556) to get degrees Celsius.

$$°C = (°F - 32) \times \frac{5}{9}$$

$$°C = (°F - 32) \times 0.556$$

EXAMPLE 3-2: Convert 98.6°F to °C.

$$°C = (°F - 32) \times \frac{5}{9}$$

$$°C = (98.6 - 32) \times \frac{5}{9}$$

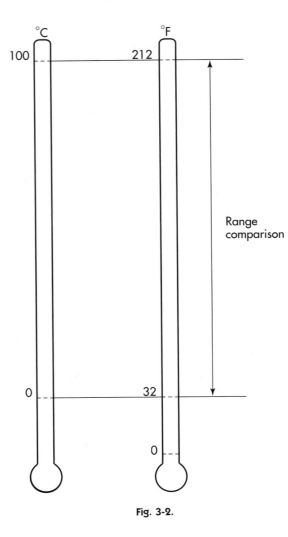

Fig. 3-2.

$$°C = 66.6 \times \frac{5}{9}$$

$$°C = \frac{333}{9}$$

$$°C = 37$$

The simplified formula, $9C = 5F - 160$, can be extracted from the following formula. This simple formula can be easily remembered and is useful for conversion in either direction between the Celsius and Fahrenheit scales.

$$°C = (°F - 32) \times \frac{5}{9}$$

$$9C = (°F - 32) \times 5$$
$$9C = 5(F - 32)$$
$$9C = 5F - 160$$

EXAMPLE 3-3A: Convert 37°C to °F.

$$9C = 5F - 160$$
$$9(37) = 5F - 160$$
$$333 = 5F - 160$$
$$5F - 160 = 333$$
$$5F = 333 + 160$$
$$F = \frac{493}{5}$$
$$F = 98.6$$
$$37°C = 98.6°F$$

EXAMPLE 3-3B: Convert 98.6°F to °C.

$$9C = 5F - 160$$
$$9C = 5(98.6) - 160$$
$$C = \frac{493 - 160}{9}$$
$$C = \frac{333}{9}$$
$$C = 37$$
$$98.6°F = 37°C$$

Another simple means of converting between Fahrenheit and Celsius scales was offered by Martinek (1972). The temperature of −40° is the same on the Celsius and the Fahrenheit scales (Fig. 3-1). This conversion method and these equations for conversions between degrees Celsius and degrees Fahrenheit are based on the 9⁄5 and 5⁄9 relationships and the number 40.

To convert degrees Fahrenheit to degrees Celsius, add 40 to the original temperature, multiply by 5⁄9 and subtract 40 from this product. To convert degrees Celsius to degrees Fahrenheit, add 40 to the beginning temperature, multiply by 9⁄5 and subtract 40 from the result.

$$°C = \left[(°F + 40) \times \frac{5}{9}\right] - 40$$
$$°F = \left[(°C + 40) \times \frac{9}{5}\right] - 40$$

EXAMPLE 3-4A: Convert 100°F to °C

$$°C = \left[(°F + 40) \times \frac{5}{9}\right] - 40$$
$$°C = \left[(100 + 40) \times \frac{5}{9}\right] - 40$$
$$°C = \left[140 \times \frac{5}{9}\right] - 40$$
$$°C = 77.8 - 40$$
$$°C = 37.8$$

EXAMPLE 3-4B: Convert 37°C to °F

$$°F = \left[(°C + 40) \times \frac{9}{5}\right] - 40$$
$$°F = \left[(37 + 40) \times \frac{9}{5}\right] - 40$$
$$°F = \left[77 \times \frac{9}{5}\right] - 40$$
$$°F = 138.6 - 40$$
$$°F = 98.6$$

NOTE: If you are not sure which fraction to use, choose a familiar conversion point, such as 100°C = 212°F; it is obvious that to get from 100°C to 212°F one had to multiply by the larger fraction, 9⁄5. Therefore to convert degrees Celsius to degrees Fahrenheit, use 9⁄5.

SECTION 3.4 CONVERSION BETWEEN DEGREES FAHRENHEIT AND DEGREES KELVIN

To Convert Degrees Fahrenheit to Degrees Kelvin

The simplest method to convert degrees Fahrenheit to degrees Kelvin is to first convert degrees Fahrenheit to degrees Celsius and then add 273 to the result.

EXAMPLE 3-5: Convert 100°F to K.

$$9C = 5F - 160$$
$$9C = 5(100) - 160$$
$$9C = 500 - 160$$
$$9C = 340$$
$$C = \frac{340}{9}$$
$$°C = 37.78$$
$$K = °C + 273$$
$$K = 37.78 + 273$$
$$K = 310.78$$
$$100°F = 310.78 \ K$$

To Convert Degrees Kelvin to Degrees Fahrenheit

Reverse the process given above.

First convert degrees Kelvin to degrees Celsius by subtracting 273, then convert degrees Celsius to degrees Fahrenheit.

EXAMPLE 3-6: Change 310 K to °F.

$$310 \ K - 273 = 37°C$$

Now convert 37°C to °F.

$$9C = 5F - 160$$
$$9 \times 37 = 5F - 160$$
$$5F - 160 = 9 \times 37$$
$$5F = (9 \times 37) + 160$$
$$5F = 333 + 160$$
$$5F = 493$$
$$F = \frac{493}{5}$$
$$F = 98.6$$
$$310 \ K = 98.6° \ F$$

SECTION 3.5 REVIEW

The following formulas have been presented. Use any of them; however, try to *understand* the underlying principle.

1. $°C = (°F - 32) \times \dfrac{5}{9}$

2. $°C = \left[(°F + 40) \times \dfrac{5}{9}\right] - 40$

3. $°F = \left(°C \times \dfrac{9}{5}\right) + 32$

4. $°F = \left[(°C + 40) \times \dfrac{9}{5}\right] - 40$

5. $9C = 5F - 160$

6. $°C = K - 273$

7. $K = °C + 273$

APPENDIXES RELATED TO THIS CHAPTER

N Temperature Conversion Table
O Fahrenheit-Celsius Conversions: 96.0°F to 108.0°F (in tenths)

PRACTICE PROBLEMS

Calculate the answer for each problem. Understand each portion of the calculation and determine whether the answer is logical. *Just because an answer can be calculated does not mean that it is reasonable.*

Convert the following:

1. 30 K to °C
2. −11 K to °C
3. 0 K to °C
4. 340 K to °C
5. −80 K to °C
6. 20°C to K
7. −50°C to K
8. 0°C to K
9. 120°C to K
10. −4°C to K

11. 40°C to °F
12. −21°C to °F
13. 1°C to °F
14. 200°C to °F
15. −150°C to °F
16. 142°F to °C
17. −51°F to °C
18. 0°F to °C
19. 400°F to °C
20. −16°F to °C

21. 60°F to K
22. −10°F to K
23. 0°F to K
24. 250°F to K
25. −100°F to K
26. 172 K to °F
27. −90 K to °F
28. 0 K to °F
20. 40 K to °F
30. −3 K to °F

4

Factors

EDUCATIONAL OBJECTIVES

To have successfully learned the material in this chapter, the student should be able to do the following properly:

- Define *factor* as the term is used in applied mathematics and give some examples of the use of factors in the clinical laboratory.
- Calculate the factor that can be used to express a quantity of one substance as an equivalent quantity of a related substance.
- Calculate the factor that will accommodate differences in the color equivalents of two substances.
- Develop a factor that will combine a string of calculations into a single calculation.
- Develop a factor to correct for a variation in a procedure or reagent.

SECTION 4.1 INTRODUCTION

As the term is used in the clinical laboratory, a **factor** is a number used to produce a result in a single calculation that otherwise involves several steps. As long as factors are used appropriately and the details of the calculation remain the same, they are a useful tool for repetitious procedures. However, caution is needed to avoid the inappropriate use of a particular factor. Should any part of a procedure be different, the factor may give an erroneous result. For this reason, the worker should understand the derivation of the factors used. Four common uses of factors in the clinical laboratory are:

1. Expressing a quantity of one substance as an equivalent quantity of another substance
2. Allowing for differences in color equivalents or molecular differences
3. Combining many calculations into a single process
4. Correcting for variation in procedure quantities

It is useful for the student to understand how a factor is developed and how it relates to a procedure. One can accept a factor on simple faith or laziness and have it work as long as everything is used correctly and there is nothing unusual in the particular test. However, the possibility for error is significant under these conditions. This possibility is greatly decreased if the worker fully understands the procedures used to develop the factor.

Factors are useful in procedures that are done often. Many calculations that use a factor can be done by using ratio and proportion. If a particular calculation is to be done once or a very few times, it is not practical to produce a factor. However, if a calculation is to be done often, then factors that simplify the process are a convenience. The purpose of this chapter is to help you understand the derivation and use of factors.

SECTION 4.2 FACTORS USED TO EXPRESS A QUANTITY OF ONE SUBSTANCE AS AN EQUIVALENT QUANTITY OF ANOTHER SUBSTANCE

The following are some general considerations in this use of factors:

1. To calculate a factor of this type, there must be some known basis of comparison between the two substances, for example, their molecular weights.
2. In using a conversion factor in this manner, multiply the known quantity by the conversion factor. The product is the equivalent value.
3. When this type of factor is used, quantities of the two substances must be expressed in the same units, that is, *milligrams* of urea nitrogen to *milligrams* of urea or *grams* of urea nitrogen to *grams* of urea.

The kind of factor described in this section can be obtained at least three ways: (1) by looking it up in some reference source, (2) by using ratio and proportion and setting the known relationship against x to 1, and (3) by setting up the known relationship as a common fraction and converting it to a decimal number.

The first method, the use of a reference source, is excusable if the reference can be easily obtained and if the worker has no professional curiosity.

The second method, the use of ratio and proportion, may be explained using a very common factor of this type, 2.14, for converting an amount of urea nitrogen to an equivalent amount of urea. The structure of urea is as follows:

$$
\begin{array}{ccc}
\text{H} & \text{O} & \text{H} \\
\diagdown & \| & \diagup \\
\text{N} - & \text{C} - & \text{N} \\
\diagup & & \diagdown \\
\text{H} & & \text{H}
\end{array}
$$

The molecular weight of urea is calculated by the following procedure (which is explained in Chapter 6, p. 138):

Element	Number of atoms	$\times$	Atomic weight	$=$	Weight of molecule
Carbon	1		12		12
Oxygen	1		16		16
Nitrogen	2		14		28
Hydrogen	4		1		4
			Molecular weight of urea $=$		60

The molecular weight of the nitrogen in the urea molecule is 28 (2×14). Therefore there are 28 parts of urea nitrogen in 60 parts of urea. The ratio-proportion formula for the determination of the amount of urea equivalent to one part of urea nitrogen is as follows: 60 parts of urea are to 28 parts of urea nitrogen as x parts of urea are to 1 part of urea nitrogen.

$$\frac{60 \text{ parts urea}}{28 \text{ parts urea nitrogen}} = \frac{x \text{ parts urea}}{1 \text{ part urea nitrogen}}$$

$$60 \times 1 = 28x$$

$$28x = 60$$

$$x = 2.14$$

One part of urea nitrogen is contained in 2.14 parts of urea. Therefore if the amount of urea nitrogen is multiplied by 2.14, the result equals the amount of urea to which the known quantity of urea nitrogen is equivalent. For example:

$$\text{Milligrams of urea nitrogen} \times 2.14 = \text{milligrams of urea}$$

$$\text{Grams of urea nitrogen} \times 2.14 = \text{grams of urea}$$

This is a use of ratio and proportion in which the known part of a relationship is set against 1 and the desired part of the relationship is set against x. The result of such calculations is the amount of the desired substance that is equal to one unit of the known substance.

$$\frac{60}{28} = \frac{x}{1}$$

Hence, in the preceding example the answer is the conversion factor used to convert a value for urea nitrogen to an equivalent value for urea.

The important thing is to make what is to be changed equivalent to 1 and to make the desired value equivalent to x. Note that if the *entire* ratio-proportion setup is turned over, the answer remains the same.

$$\frac{60}{28} = \frac{x}{1} \qquad \frac{28}{60} = \frac{1}{x}$$

$$x = 2.14 \qquad x = 2.14$$

The third method to obtain a factor of this type is to write the known relationship as a common fraction and convert this to a decimal number. To arrive at a conversion factor in this manner, divide the number that represents the comparative amount of the existing material into the number that represents the comparative amount of the desired material. This answer is the conversion factor. Care should be taken to use the known relationship properly. This method can be used to produce two conversion factors from one relationship between two substances. Be sure that the conversion factor calculated is the one that converts the value for the existing material to the value for the desired material and not vice versa. Use common sense.

EXAMPLE 4-1: Find the amount of NaCl that is equivalent to 100 mg of Cl.

Divide the number that represents the comparative amount of the existing material (Cl) into the number that represents the comparative amount of the desired material (NaCl).

Molecular and atomic weights or mass represent comparative amounts of chemical substances. Appendix Z gives atomic weights. Molecular weight is the sum of the atomic weights of the atoms making up a molecule. The atomic weights of sodium and chlorine are about 23 and 35.5 respectively. Hence, the molecular weight of sodium chloride is about 58.5.

$$\frac{58.5 \ (\text{the comparative amount of the desired material})}{35.5 \ (\text{the comparative amount of the existing material})} = 1.65$$

The factor to convert an amount of chlorine to an equivalent amount of sodium chloride is 1.65.

Multiply this factor by the amount of existing material to find the equivalent amount of the desired material.

$$1.65 \times 100 \ \text{mg Cl} = 165 \ \text{mg NaCl}$$

This method is actually a shortened ratio and proportion procedure. The known ratio, 58.5/35.5, is shown, and the unknown ratio, $x/1$, is understood. Note that when a number is used as a numerator over 1, the resulting fraction is equal to the numerator. Again, an important consideration of this method of calculating factors is that because only part of a ratio and proportion procedure is used, this relationship *cannot* be turned over without changing the factor.

$$\frac{58.5}{35.5} = 1.65$$

Turned over:

$$\frac{35.5}{58.5} = 0.61$$

If you cannot remember this rule, use common sense and good logic. Example 4-2 works through the logic of this problem.

EXAMPLE 4-2: Find the amount of NaCl that is equivalent to 100 mg Cl.

The amount of Cl is the existing value, whereas the amount of NaCl is the desired value.
1. The atomic weight of Cl is about 35.5, and the molecular weight of NaCl is about 58.5.
2. The number representing NaCl is greater than the number representing Cl.

$$58.5 > 35.5$$

3. Therefore if one wants to change 100 mg Cl into an equivalent amount of NaCl, the answer must be greater than the amount of Cl present.

$$100 \text{ mg Cl} = x \text{ mg NaCl}$$

$$x \text{ must be} > 100 \text{ mg}$$

4. To get a larger number, one must multiply the amount of Cl present by a factor greater than 1.

$$100 \text{ mg Cl} \times \text{factor} = x \text{ mg NaCl}$$

$$\text{factor must be} > 1$$

5. To get a factor greater than 1, divide the larger number of the comparison by the smaller; that is, $58.5 \div 35.5$.

$$\frac{58.5}{35.5} = 1.65$$

$$1.65 > 1$$

6. The factor used to change an amount of Cl to an equivalent amount of NaCl is 1.65.
7. To use the factor, multiply the existing value by the factor to get the equivalent value.

$$100 \text{ mg Cl} \times 1.65 = 165 \text{ mg NaCl}$$

$$165 \text{ mg} > 100 \text{ mg}$$

EXAMPLE 4-3: Change 200 mg NaCl to mg Cl.

1. The molecular weight of NaCl is 58.5, and the atomic weight of Cl is 35.5.

$$NaCl = 58.5$$

$$Cl = 35.5$$

2. The number representing Cl is smaller than the number representing NaCl.

$$35.5 < 58.5$$

3. Therefore the final amount of Cl must be less than the 200 mg NaCl.
4. To get a smaller amount, multiply the amount of NaCl by a factor of less than 1.

$$200 \text{ mg NaCl} \times \text{factor} = \text{mg Cl}$$

$$\text{factor must be} < 1$$

5. To get a factor of less than 1, divide the smaller comparative number by the larger; that is, $35.5 \div 58.5$.

$$\frac{35.5}{58.5} = 0.61$$

$$0.61 < 1$$

$$200 \text{ mg NaCl} \times 0.61 = 122 \text{ mg Cl}$$

$$122 \text{ mg} < 200 \text{ mg}$$

IN REVIEW:

1. This type of factor may be figured by using ratio and proportion.

> If the ratio-proportion procedure is to be used, put down the known relationship; fill in the opposite side of the problem, making the substance to be changed equivalent to 1; and solve for x; the answer is the factor. If this relationship is turned upside down, the same answer will still be received, providing the ratio-proportion procedure is correct.

2. This type of factor may also be figured by using only the known relationship as a fraction and converting this to a decimal number.

> In using the comparative relationships only, always put the number that corresponds to the *basis* for comparison or change (that is, the standard or the substance being changed) on the bottom and the other number on the top; then reduce the fraction. The resulting answer is the factor. This type of problem *may not* be turned upside down without changing the result.

These two methods are presented in parallel in Examples 4-4, 4-5, and 4-6.

EXAMPLE 4-4: What is the conversion factor for converting milligrams of urea to milligrams of urea nitrogen?

Ratio and proportion	**Known relationship only**

$$\frac{28 \text{ mg urea nitrogen}}{60 \text{ mg urea}} = \frac{x \text{ mg urea nitrogen}}{1 \text{ mg urea}} \qquad\qquad \frac{28}{60}\; \frac{\text{mg urea nitrogen}}{\text{mg urea (to be changed)}}$$

$$60x = 28$$

$$x = \frac{28}{60} \qquad\qquad\qquad\qquad\qquad\qquad \frac{28}{60} = 0.467$$

$$x = 0.467$$

$$\text{mg urea} \times 0.467 = \text{mg urea nitrogen} \qquad\qquad \text{mg urea} \times 0.467 = \text{mg urea nitrogen}$$

EXAMPLE 4-5: What is the conversion factor for converting milligrams of Cl to milligrams of NaCl?

Ratio and proportion

$$\frac{58.5 \text{ mg NaCl}}{35.5 \text{ mg Cl}} = \frac{x \text{ mg NaCl}}{1 \text{ mg Cl}}$$

$$35.5x = 58.5$$

$$x = \frac{58.5}{35.5}$$

$$x = 1.65$$

$$\text{mg Cl} \times 1.65 = \text{mg NaCl}$$

Known relationship only

$$\frac{58.5}{35.5} \quad \frac{\text{mg NaCl}}{\text{mg Cl (to be changed)}}$$

$$\frac{58.5}{35.5} = 1.65$$

$$\text{mg Cl} \times 1.65 = \text{mg NaCl}$$

EXAMPLE 4-6: What is the conversion factor for converting grams of NaCl to grams of Cl?

Ratio and proportion

$$\frac{35.5 \text{ g Cl}}{58.5 \text{ g NaCl}} = \frac{x \text{ g Cl}}{1 \text{ g NaCl}}$$

$$58.5x = 35.5$$

$$x = \frac{35.5}{58.5}$$

$$x = 0.61$$

$$\text{g NaCl} \times 0.61 = \text{g Cl}$$

Known relationship only

$$\frac{35.5}{58.5} \quad \frac{\text{g Cl}}{\text{g NaCl (to be changed)}}$$

$$\frac{35.5}{58.5} = 0.61$$

$$\text{g NaCl} \times 0.61 = \text{g Cl}$$

SECTION 4.3 FACTORS USED TO ALLOW FOR DIFFERENCES IN COLOR EQUIVALENTS OR MOLECULAR DIFFERENCES

Often one reaction may be used to test for a variety of compounds, and if colorimetry is used to evaluate the test results, allowances need to be made in the color equivalent values obtained. The test for sulfonamides is a good example. All the drugs in this group contain the sulfonamide group ($-SO_2NH_2$), which participates in a diazo reaction with the subsequent formation of a colored compound. The sulfa compounds have similar chemical properties but differ from each other in molecular structure and weight. Colorimetry values are often considered to vary directly with the molecular weights (mol wt) of the test materials. In theory, the particular drug being measured should also be used for the standard, because some authors state that the intensity of color produced by a given amount of the different drugs is not always in the calculated proportions to their molecular weights. However, such deviations are usually small, and their consideration is generally not worthwhile. In cases in which a substance different from that being measured is used for the standard, the formula for the factor is as follows:

$$\text{Conversion factor} = \frac{\text{mol wt of drug being measured}}{\text{mol wt of drug used as standard}}$$

To express a quantity of one substance as an equivalent quantity of another substance, a known relationship is needed between the two substances in question. Again, the molecular weights may be used. Using this known relationship, it is possible to work these problems in the same two ways discussed previously in this chapter: (1) by using the ratio-proportion procedure, in which case the ratio-proportion is set up with a comparison of one part standard; and (2) by using the two comparative figures and dividing the molecular weight of the standard into the molecular weight of the drug in question.

EXAMPLE 4-7: If one were measuring sulfanilamide and had used sulfathiazole as the standard, what would be the conversion factor?

$$\text{Mol wt of sulfanilamide} = 172$$

$$\text{Mol wt of sulfathiazole} = 255$$

$$\frac{172}{255} = \frac{x}{1}$$

$$255\,x = 172$$

$$x = 0.674 = \text{conversion factor}$$

One would then multiply the answer derived in the test by the conversion factor.

REMEMBER: When using only the molecular weights, always put the basis for comparison (or change) on the bottom, which in this case is the standard; the reason for this is the same as described on pp. 82–83.

SECTION 4.4 FACTORS USED TO COMBINE MANY CALCULATIONS INTO A SINGLE PROCESS

The factors under this heading need little explanation. The factor is simply the reduction of two or more calculations into a single number.

In any situation in which there are several steps in a calculation that are *always* the same, one may reduce them to a single factor to be used each time, thereby reducing time and work.

One example of this kind of factor is the number 50, used to determine the manual white blood cell count. This procedure is used to ascertain the concentration of white blood cells in a sample of blood. The results are reported as the number of white blood cells per cubic millimeter. To count all the white blood cells in 1 cubic millimeter of blood would be unreasonably difficult for routine work, so a much smaller volume of blood is used. Several factors are used to make the results of the count equivalent to the number of white blood cells per cubic millimeter. The volume of blood is reduced or changed in three ways: (1) the blood is diluted, (2) a greater area than 1 square millimeter is counted, and (3) a depth of blood much less than 1 millimeter is used. Since each of these results in a volume other than 1 cubic millimeter, there are three different factors: (1) dilution, (2) area, and (3) depth.[*] With the usual dilution (1:20) and the area counted (4 mm^2) on a standard counting chamber (depth 0.1 mm) with Neubauer ruling, the total number of cells can be calculated by the following procedure:

$$\text{Cells counted} \times \text{dilution factor} \times \text{area factor} \times \text{depth factor} = \text{cells/mm}^3$$

$$\text{Cells counted} \times 20 \times \tfrac{1}{4} \times 10 = \text{cells/mm}^3$$

[*]These are explained in detail in Chapter 11.

To do this each time would be time consuming and pointless. Since the three factors are always the same under routine conditions, the three individual factors may be combined into a single number.

$$\text{Cells counted} \times (20 \times \tfrac{1}{4} \times 10) = \text{cells/mm}^3$$

$$\text{Final factor} = 20 \times \tfrac{1}{4} \times 10 = 50$$

$$\text{Cells counted} \times 50 = \text{cells/mm}^3$$

If correction factors are constantly changing, it is of no benefit to figure a final factor; however, such a factor may save a great deal of time and effort if the intermediate factors are constant.

EXAMPLE 4-8: To convert milligrams per deciliter of Cl to milliequivalents per liter,[*] the following formula may be used. What factor could be used instead?

$$\text{mEq/L} = \frac{\text{mg/dl} \times 10}{35.5}$$

The 10 and the 35.5 are constant; therefore they may be converted to the following factor:

$$\text{mEq/L} = \text{mg/dl} \times \frac{10}{35.5}$$

$$\text{mEq/L} = \text{mg/dl} \times 0.282 \text{ (factor)}$$

SECTION 4.5 CORRECTION FOR VARIATION IN PROCEDURE QUANTITIES

There are several situations in laboratory work in which a different quantity from the one described in a procedure is used. In such cases, this difference must be considered in the calculations relating to the reporting of the results. Collecting insufficient sample or accidental destruction of some part of a sample are examples of this situation.

The calculations relating to this sort of correction can be summarized by the following general rule.

Divide by what was used and multiply by what should have been used.

This can be done by using one of the following methods.
1. Make a factor from the amounts of what was used and what should have been used. Multiply this factor by the test result to determine the corrected result.
2. Simply divide the test result by the amount used and multiply this quotient by the amount that should have been used. A factor is not made in this method.
3. Use the complete ratio and proportion procedure.

EXAMPLE 4-9: A procedure for sodium determination calls for 5 ml of urine. However, the amount of specimen sent to the laboratory consisted of only 3.5 ml.

To complete this test, 3 ml of urine were diluted with 2 ml of distilled water to make a total of 5 ml. The sodium concentration in this 5 ml was found to be 40 mEq/L. This result must be corrected for the insufficient sample volume.

---

[*]This is explained in detail in Chapter 6.

Correct this result using method 1.

Make a factor from the amounts of what was used and what should have been used.

Make a ratio of the two amounts such that you divide by what was used and make this into a decimal fraction by dividing the bottom into the top.

$$\frac{5}{3} = 1.67$$

Now multiply this factor by the result of the test, 40 mEq/L.

$$1.67 \times 40 = 66.8 \quad \boxed{\text{Report 67 mEq/L}}$$

Correct this result using method 2.

Divide the test result by what was used.

Since 3 ml were used, divide 40 mEq/L by 3.

$$\frac{40}{3} = 13.33$$

Now multiply by what should have been used, 5 ml of urine.

$$13.33 \times 5 = 66.67 \quad \boxed{\text{Report 67 mEq/L}}$$

Correct this result using method 3.

Use the complete ratio and proportion procedure.

Set up a ratio and proportion.

If 3 ml of urine has a concentration of 40 mEq/L, how many mEq/L are in 5 ml of urine?

$$\frac{3}{40 \text{ mEq/L}} = \frac{5 \text{ ml}}{x \text{ mEq/L}}$$

$$3x = 200$$

$$x = 66.65 \quad \boxed{\text{Report 67 mEq/L}}$$

Each of the three methods produces the same result. Understand how each method is really a different form of the same calculation.

APPENDIXES RELATED TO THIS CHAPTER

Z Atomic Weights

PRACTICE PROBLEMS

Calculate the answer for each problem. Understand each portion of the calculation and determine whether the answer is logical. *Just because an answer can be calculated does not mean that it is reasonable.*

Converting to equivalent quantities

Give the factor for converting the following:
1. NaCl to Na
2. NaCl to Cl

3. Cl to NaCl
4. Na to NaCl
5. Ca to CaCl$_2$
6. CaCl$_2$ to Ca
7. K to KCl
8. KCl to K
9. Na to NaOH
10. NaOH to Na
11. Ba to BaCl$_2$
12. BaCl$_2$ to Ba
13. AgNO$_3$ to Ag
14. Ag to AgNO$_3$

15. What is the factor for converting Br to NaBr?
16. What is the factor for converting NaBr to Na?
17. What is the factor for converting HCl to Cl?

Convert to equivalent quantities using a factor:
18. 300 mg of SO$_2$ to milligrams of S
19. 21 g Cu to grams of CuSO$_4$
20. 1300 mg Br to grams of NaBr

21. Using a factor, convert 424 mg Ca to milligrams of CaCO$_3$.
22. Using a factor, convert 300 mg NaHCO$_3$ to milligrams of Na.
23. Convert 300 mg Cl to HCl using the ratio-proportion method and a factor.
24. Convert 100 mg NaBr to Br using the ratio-proportion method and a factor.
25. Using a factor, convert 350 mg K to milligrams of KOH.
26. Using a factor, convert 340 mg Br to milligrams of LiBr.
27. Express 20 mg PO$_4$ as P, using a factor.
28. Using a factor, express 700 mg MgSO$_4$ as milligrams of Mg.

Converting color equivalents

29. You are measuring sulfadiazine (mol wt 250). The answer obtained from a curve using sulfamerazine (mol wt 264) as the standard was 40 mg/dl. Using a factor, derive the correct answer.
30. You are measuring sulfanilamide (mol wt 172). The answer obtained from a curve set up using sulfathiazole (mol wt 255) as standard was 100 mg/dl. Using a factor, give the answer to be reported.
31. Sulfanilamide (mol wt 172) is used as a standard. We measured sulfadiazine (mol wt 250) and read from the curve an answer of 150 mg/dl. What is the correct answer?

Combining many calculations

32. In a certain procedure there are three constant correction factors: 10, ¼, and 50. Derive a single factor.
33. In a certain procedure there are four constant correction factors: 15, ¹⁄₁₀, ⅓, and 50. Derive a single factor.
34. In a certain procedure there are three constant correction factors: 3, 30, and 0.2. What single factor could be used instead?

35. A certain formula is as follows:

$$x = \frac{y \times 5 \times 10}{54}$$

By what factor could y be multiplied instead?

36. Make a factor to use in the following:

   a. $x = \dfrac{\frac{1}{4} \times 50}{10} \times y$

   b. $x = \dfrac{10 \times y \times 50}{2}$

Correcting for variation in procedure quantities

37. You are running a test that calls for 1 ml of spinal fluid. You only use 0.4 ml. The answer you obtain is 12 mg/dl. What would the correct answer be?

38. A sodium determination calls for 10 ml of urine. However, the specimen consisted of only 4.5 ml. The test is performed using 4 ml of urine plus 6 ml of distilled water. The sodium concentration in the diluted sample is 35 mEq/L. What should be reported?

39. A test procedure calls for 1 ml of specimen. The procedure is run with 0.6 ml. The answer obtained is 50 mg/L. What should be reported?

5

Dilutions

EDUCATIONAL OBJECTIVES

To have successfully learned the material in this chapter, the student should be able to do the following properly:

- Describe a particular dilution in terms of its ratio of component substances.
- Recognize various expressions of a dilution as different descriptions of the same mixture.
- Calculate the absolute amount of the substances in a given volume of a dilution.
- Calculate the amount of a substance needed to make a given volume of a particular dilution.
- Determine the final dilution of a mixture after adding substances to a known mixture.
- Make a dilution series, and determine the concentration at each step in the series.
- Calculate the total volume expected from a dilution.
- Describe the procedure for making a dilution series, and calculate the concentration and total volume of each dilution in the series.
- Describe the procedure for making a series of tube dilutions, and determine the concentration and total volume of each dilution in the series.
- Differentiate between tube dilutions and solution dilutions.
- Determine the substance concentration of a dilution.
- Produce dilutions with prescribed concentrations and volumes.
- Describe the procedure for making a two-fold serial dilution.
- Determine the titer of an antibody by dilution.

SECTION 5.1 INTRODUCTION

Many laboratory procedures involve the addition of one substance to another to reduce the concentration of one of the substances. Both these procedures and the resulting mixtures are called **dilutions.** Dilution procedures are used quite often in laboratories, and laboratory personnel should be competent in their use. This requires both skill in manipulating the calculations and a thorough understanding of the procedures and the notation used in describing the mixtures.

The word *dilution* is defined as a weakened solution. It is a statement of the *relative* concentrations of the components of a mixture. *The preferred method used to describe dilutions is to refer to the number of parts of the material being diluted in the total number of parts of the final product.*

A major hindrance in understanding dilutions is the confusion between ratios and dilutions. Ratio is the more general term and refers to an amount of one thing relative to an amount of something else with no other implication. Dilution, as the term is used in laboratories, is more specific. It refers to a number of parts of a substance in the total number of parts of mixture containing the substance, usually along with some implication as to how the mixture was made or how it is to be made. All dilutions are a kind of ratio, but all ratios are not dilutions.

Ratios are discussed completely in Chapter 1, pp. 33-37; however in general, it may be said that a single solution may represent six different ratios. The colon (:) is used as the ratio symbol. Consider a solution consisting of 1 milliliter of serum plus 9 milliliters of saline for a total volume of 10 milliliters. The following ratios correctly describe this solution.

1. The serum to saline ratio is 1:9.
2. The saline to serum ratio is 9:1.
3. The serum to total volume ratio is 1:10.
4. The total volume to serum ratio is 10:1.
5. The saline to total volume ratio is 9:10.
6. The total volume to saline ratio is 10:9.

Dilutions, on the other hand, should represent one thing—the number of *parts* of the substance being diluted in a total number of *parts* of solution. Notice in the above examples (#3) that this is the same as a ratio of the material being diluted to the total amount of the final product. The slash (/) mark is generally considered to be the dilution symbol.

Another source of confusion about dilutions is the terminology of the methods used to give instructions for making dilutions. Consider the following statements:

1. Make a 1 to 10 dilution of serum in saline.
2. Make a 1 in 10 dilution of serum in saline.
3. Make a 1 to 10 dilution of serum with saline.
4. Make a 1/10 dilution of serum with saline.
5. Make a 1:10 dilution of serum using saline.
6. Make a dilution of 1 part serum and 9 parts saline.
7. Make a dilution of 1 part serum to 9 parts saline.
8. Make a 1/10 dilution by diluting 1 part serum up to 10 parts with saline.

These are all instructions for making serum dilutions that have been read in test procedures. When all these procedures were analyzed, it was discovered that they all meant the same thing: Mix 1 milliliter of serum with 9 milliliters of saline to give 10 milliliters total volume.

There should be a consistent use of the words *to* and *in*. Use *to* to mean ":" (part to part) and *in* to mean "/" (part to total volume). However, it appears that this is not the case.

The authors recommend the following to help clarify this problem.

1. *Ratio* should refer to part to part. One simply needs to know what is referred to by each part.
2. *Dilution* should refer to parts in total volume.

3. The consistent use of (:) and *to* to represent ratios.
4. The consistent use of (/) and *in* to represent dilutions.
These recommendations are used in this chapter.

The terms *dilute up to* and *bring up to* also refer to dilutions. Do not confuse these with *to* used to refer to ratios. The following relationship should be thoroughly understood before continuing.

$$\begin{array}{r} 1 \text{ part serum} \\ + \quad \underline{9 \text{ parts saline}} \\ 10 \text{ parts final solution (total volume)} \end{array}$$

$$1{:}9 \text{ ratio of serum to saline} = \frac{1{:}10 \text{ ratio of serum to total}}{\text{volume of solution}} = \frac{1/10 \text{ dilution of serum}}{\text{in saline}}$$

Recall that a dilution is a statement of *relative* concentration. Any combination of units that gives the above relationship will be a 1/10 dilution. Some possibilities are: 2 ounces of serum added to 18 ounces of saline for a total volume of 20 ounces, 10 drams of serum and enough saline to make 100 drams of the final product, 0.1 quarts of iodine solution in a total volume of 1 quart. In all cases there is 1 *part* original substance in 10 *parts* of final solution. Also all parts of each dilution are in the same units; that is, all milliliters, or all ounces, or all quarts, etc. These conditions need to be met to have a 1/10 dilution. You cannot have 5 quarts of iodine solution in a total volume of 50 milliliters and still have a 1/10 dilution. Study the use of the units in the following examples. The calculations are covered later in this chapter.

(1)	(2)
$1/10 = 1 \text{ ml}/x \text{ ml}$	$1/10 = 2 \text{ oz}/x \text{ oz}$
$x = 10 \text{ ml}$	$x = 20 \text{ oz}$
1 ml diluted up to 10 ml = a 1/10 dilution	2 oz diluted up to 20 oz = a 1/10 dilution

(3)	(4)
$1/10 = 10 \text{ drams}/x \text{ drams}$	$1/10 = 0.1 \text{ qt}/x \text{ qt}$
$x = 100 \text{ drams}$	$x = 1 \text{ qt}$
10 drams diluted up to 100 drams = a 1/10 dilution	0.1 qt diluted up to 1 qt = a 1/10 dilution

Notice that the final volume is not the same in each of these examples, although each is a 1/10 dilution. *A dilution is an expression of concentration, not an expression of volume.* This is very important. Any volume of a dilution can be made as long as the *relative* amounts of the components remain the same. Stated another way, a dilution indicates the relative amount of the substances in a solution. The volume may or may not be the same as indicated in the dilution statement.

SECTION 5.2 CALCULATIONS INVOLVING ONE DILUTION

The simplest of the dilution procedures involves the making of a single dilution from a single substance diluted with one other substance.

EXAMPLE 5-1: Dilute 1 ml of serum with 9 ml of saline.

To complete these directions, simply mix the volumes of the two substances in one vessel. This results in a solution having a ratio of one part serum to nine parts saline and a ratio of one part serum to 10 parts of the final solution.

$$
\begin{array}{r}
1 \text{ ml serum} \\
+ \ \underline{9 \text{ ml saline}} \\
10 \text{ ml total volume}
\end{array}
$$

Hence, this is a 1/10 dilution of serum with saline.

EXAMPLE 5-2: Consider the following statement: Dilute 3 ml of serum with 25 ml of saline.

To complete these directions, one would add 3 ml of serum to 25 ml of saline. The total volume of the final solution would be 28 ml.

$$
\begin{array}{r}
3 \text{ ml serum} \\
+ \ \underline{25 \text{ ml saline}} \\
28 \text{ ml total volume of final solution}
\end{array}
$$

$$3:25 \text{ ratio of serum to saline} = 3/28 \text{ dilution}$$

The dilution of serum in this solution is 3/28. However, dilutions are usually easier to understand and compare when they are stated as a 1-in-something (1/x) dilution. To convert a 3/28 dilution to a 1-in-something dilution, set up a ratio-proportion calculation.

3 is to 28 as 1 is to x

$$\frac{3}{28} = \frac{1}{x}$$

$$3x = 28$$

$$x = \frac{28}{3}$$

$$x = 9.33$$

$$3/28 \text{ dilution} = 1/9.33 \text{ dilution}$$

The 3/28 dilution of serum is equivalent to a 1/9.33 dilution.

The serum to saline *ratio* in this example is 3:25 or 1:8.33, found by inspection of the dilution or as follows:

$$\frac{3}{25} = \frac{1}{x}$$

$$3x = 25$$

$$x = \frac{25}{3}$$

$$x = 8.33$$

Hence, a 3:25 serum to saline ratio is equal to a 1:8.33 serum to saline ratio.

EXAMPLE 5-3: Five milliliters of serum is diluted up to 25 ml with saline. What is the serum dilution? What is the serum to saline ratio?

Since there are 5 ml of serum in 25 ml of total solution, this is a 5/25 dilution of serum with saline.

Reduce this to a 1-in-something ($1/x$) dilution.

$$\frac{5}{25} = \frac{1}{x}$$

$$5x = 25$$

$$x = \frac{25}{5}$$

$$x = 5$$

Hence, a 5/25 dilution equals a 1/5 dilution. The serum to saline ratio is $5:20$ or $1:4$.

NOTE: Be sure these relationships are completely understood before continuing.

Volume of Dilutions

The preceding examples are presented in the manner they are for purposes of explanation. This should not be taken to mean that a dilution is always made by adding a given amount of one substance to a given amount of another substance. Quite the contrary: a dilution is usually made by taking the specified amount of the solution or substance to be diluted and adding enough of the diluent to make the desired volume of the final solution. The main reason for this is that 1 part of one substance plus 1 part of another substance does not always equal 2 parts of total volume. For example, 1 liter of water plus 1 liter of alcohol does not yield 2 liters of solution. It yields less than 2 liters because of the positioning of the molecules. For this reason, the suggested technique of diluting up to a final volume, rather than adding a designated amount, should be followed when applicable.

Almost all problems involving the determination of volumes in single dilutions can be solved by the proper use of the ratio-proportion procedures discussed in Chapter 1, pp. 33-37.

EXAMPLE 5-4: Make 250 ml of a 1/10 dilution of serum in saline.

The final mixture in this problem has a relative concentration of 1 part serum in 10 parts of final solution. The final volume of this solution is to be 250 ml. Since an amount of serum is to be diluted up to a final volume with saline, the amount of saline need not be known. The simplest method to use in calculating the amount of serum needed to make 250 ml of solution is the ratio-proportion procedure.

If 1 ml serum is needed for 10 ml total volume, then x ml serum are needed for 250 ml total volume.

$$\frac{1 \text{ part serum}}{10 \text{ parts total volume}} = \frac{x \text{ ml serum}}{250 \text{ ml total volume}}$$

$$10x = 250$$

$$x = 25 \text{ ml}$$

Hence, to produce 250 ml of a 1 in 10 dilution of serum in saline, place 25 ml of serum in a measuring vessel and add enough saline to bring the total volume up to 250 ml.

EXAMPLE 5-5: Determine the amount of serum in 40 ml of a 1/5 dilution of serum in saline.

Since there is 1 part serum in every 5 parts total volume of a 1/5 dilution, there would be x ml of serum in 40 ml of total volume.

$$\frac{1 \text{ part serum}}{5 \text{ parts total volume}} = \frac{x \text{ ml serum}}{40 \text{ ml total volume}}$$

$$5x = 40$$

$$x = \frac{40}{5}$$

$$x = 8$$

There are 8 ml of serum in 40 ml of a 1/5 dilution of serum with saline.

EXAMPLE 5-6: How much of a 1/16 dilution of urine in distilled water could be made with 3 ml of urine?

In a 1/16 dilution there would be 1 ml of urine in 16 ml of total volume; therefore 3 ml of urine make x ml total volume.

Set up a ratio and proportion.

$$\frac{1 \text{ part urine}}{16 \text{ parts total volume}} = \frac{3 \text{ ml urine}}{x \text{ ml total volume}}$$

$$1x = 16 \times 3$$

$$x = 48 \text{ ml}$$

Three milliliters of urine make 48 ml of a 1/16 dilution of urine in distilled water.

Concentration of Dilutions

Use the following rule to calculate the resulting concentration where a dilution has been made.

> The original concentration of a solution times the dilution made equals the concentration of the resulting solution.

The solution being diluted may be any solution that has a known concentration, for example, 0.9% NaCl, 3M KOH, or 1N HCl. Such substances as serum, urine, or absolute ethanol are said to be undiluted. Serum and urine are complex biological solutions, whereas absolute alcohol is a liquid compound and not a solution. However, for purposes of discussions about dilutions, they can be considered solutions with a concentration of 1/1.

The concentration of a dilution has the same units as the concentration of the original solution. If the original concentration was expressed as a percentage, then the concentration of the resulting dilution must be a percentage; if the original concentration was in mg/dl, then the final concentration must be in mg/dl, and so on.

EXAMPLE 5-7: What is the concentration of a 1/10 dilution of a 12% NaCl solution?

$$\text{Original concentration} \times \text{dilution} = \text{final concentration}$$

$$12\% \quad \times \quad 1/10 \quad = \quad x\%$$

$$12 \times \frac{1}{10} = x$$

$$x = \frac{12}{10}$$

$$x = 1.2$$

The concentration of a 1/10 dilution of 12% NaCl is 1.2% NaCl.

Since the original concentration is in terms of a percentage, the concentration of the resulting solution is expressed as a percentage.

EXAMPLE 5-8: A 4N solution of HCl is diluted 3/5. What is the concentration of the resulting solution?

$$4\text{N} \times 3/5 = x\text{N}$$

$$x = 4 \times \frac{3}{5}$$

$$x = \frac{12}{5}$$

$$x = 2.4$$

The resulting concentration of the 3/5 dilution of 4N HCl is 2.4N.

EXAMPLE 5-9: A solution containing 80 mg of glucose in 100 ml of solution is diluted 1/50. What is the resulting concentration?

The concentration of this solution is not expressed simply. However, the problem states that 100 ml of the solution contains 80 mg of glucose. This is an amount of one thing relative to another. This is the definition of concentration. Hence the concentration of the solution could be expressed as 80 mg/100 ml. Multiply this by the dilution to determine the concentration of the resulting solution.

$$\frac{80 \text{ mg}}{100 \text{ ml}} \times \frac{1}{50} = \frac{80 \text{ mg}}{5,000 \text{ ml}} = \frac{1.6 \text{ mg}}{100 \text{ ml}}$$

The resulting solution has a concentration of 1.6 mg/100 ml.

You should understand the following things about dilutions before continuing your study:
1. The meaning of the term *dilution* as it is used in laboratory work (Section 5.1)
2. The difference between a dilution and a ratio (Section 5.1)
3. How to determine amounts needed for a dilution (Section 5.2, Volume of Dilutions)
4. How to determine the concentration of a dilution (Section 5.2, Concentration of Dilutions)

SECTION 5.3 DILUTION SERIES

Many laboratory procedures involve the use of a dilution series. A **dilution series** is a group of solutions having different concentrations of the same substances. The concentration of the solution being diluted decreases with increased dilution. It should be obvious that the concentration of the other component of the dilution then increases.

This is a confusing topic. Most students benefit from reading through this entire section before trying to understand each portion of the discussion. This approach may make the understanding of dilution series less traumatic.

There are two general ways to prepare a dilution series. In the first, each solution in a dilution series can be made by using the original substances and making each dilution independently of the others.

EXAMPLE 5-10: Make the following dilutions of serum in saline: 1/5, 1/10, and 1/100.

In this example, each of the three dilutions of serum is a separate and independent solution. Since no volumes are specified, a convenient volume of each dilution may be selected. A simple way to follow these instructions would be to make 5 ml of a 1/5 dilution of serum in saline in one test tube, then in another tube make 10 ml of a 1/10 dilution of serum in saline, and finally in a third tube make 100 ml of a 1/100 dilution of serum in saline.

Tube #1	Tube #2	Tube #3
1 ml serum	1 ml serum	1 ml serum
+ 4 ml saline	+ 9 ml saline	+ 99 ml saline
5 ml total volume	10 ml total volume	100 ml total volume

This method is not used very often for the actual preparation of dilution series. It is included here and in examples below to demonstrate some calculations. The more common method of making a dilution series is to make the first dilution and then use some of this dilution to make the second dilution, some of the second to make the third, and so on.

EXAMPLE 5-11: A serum sample is diluted with saline 1/5, rediluted 1/10, and again 1/100.

In this example each succeeding dilution is dependent on the previous solution in the series. Again no volumes are specified. To make the first dilution, place 1 part of serum in a container and dilute up to a total volume of 5 parts. This is a 1/5 dilution of serum in diluent. To make the 1/10 dilution take 1 part of the 1/5 solution and dilute it up to a total volume of 10 parts with diluent. To make the last dilution, 1/100, take 1 part of the 1/10 solution and dilute it up to a total volume of 100 parts with diluent. If the volume of each dilution is chosen as the number of milliliters equal to the number of parts of total volume, the following will result.

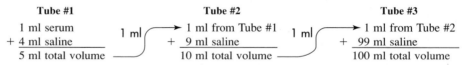

In the first method each dilution is *independent* of the others in the series. In the second, all dilutions except the first are *dependent* on the others in the series. Either method can be used to produce the dilutions in a series. The manner in which the instructions are given sometimes determines the most convenient method to use. However, extreme care must be taken with instructions pertaining to a dilution series. The two examples above appear to be the same. However, as is explained later, the resulting concentrations are quite different. The meaning must be explained or clearly implied in the instructions concerning that particular dilution series.

The following properties for each dilution in a series should be understood. The terms are somewhat arbitrary, but the concepts are important. They relate to dilutions made from some original solution. This original solution may be a simple chemical solution or some complex fluid such as serum or urine.

1. **The total volume** is the final volume of each dilution. Depending on a specific description, this may be the volume immediately after making each dilution or after using some of a dilution to make subsequent dilutions.
2. **The tube dilution** is the dilution in a particular tube as determined by the immediate manner it was made *in that tube*. It may or may not be the same as the solution dilution or the substance concentration.
3. **The solution dilution** is the actual *dilution* of the original solution in a particular tube. If the dilution was made by diluting previous dilutions, then the solution dilution is

the product of all previous tube dilutions. In other words, it is the result of the accumulated dilutions in a particular tube within a series.

4. **The substance concentration** is the *concentration* of the original solution or substance in each tube.

5. **The amount of original solution** is the actual *volume* of the original solution in a particular tube.

These properties relate to each dilution in a series as it was prepared. The value of the properties of a dilution in a dependent series may or may not be equal to the properties of a particular dilution prepared independently.

The value of these properties may be needed to complete some calculation. Since there are many ways to describe and make dilution series, precise directions for every possible situation are not feasible. However, the guidelines presented here should allow for the development of methods to determine the needed values, provided the worker understands the properties and has the ability and will to think carefully through a particular problem.

The worker should be able to calculate the value of the following properties of each step in a dilution series:

1. The total volume of each dilution before and after transfer
2. The concentration of each dilution in terms of tube dilution, solution dilution, and substance concentration
3. The amount of the original solution in each dilution before and after transfer

Each of these kinds of calculations is explained below.

Calculation of Total Volume of Each Dilution in a Series

The volume of a given dilution within a series is dependent on the method used in preparing the series. The volume of each dilution prepared is influenced by the available glassware, laboratory space, the amount of some component of the series, the amount of dilution needed, and several other factors. Usually the volumes of dilutions used in a laboratory procedure are less than 500 milliliters and often less than 1 milliliter. The volumes are often some irregular value. Because of these factors, the competent laboratory worker must think through dilution procedures carefully to produce proper results. Consider the following examples.

EXAMPLE 5-12: Make the following dilutions of serum in saline: 1/5, 1/10, and 1/100.

In this example each of the three dilutions of serum could be a separate and independent solution.

	Tube #1	Tube #2	Tube #3
	1 ml serum	1 ml serum	1 ml serum
	+ 4 ml saline	+ 9 ml saline	+ 99 ml saline
Total volume of dilution in each tube:	5 ml	10 ml	100 ml

Since each dilution was a separate operation and nothing was removed to make the next dilution, the total volume of solution in each tube is not changed by making the other dilutions in the series.

EXAMPLE 5-13: A serum sample is diluted with saline 1/5, rediluted 1/10, and again 1/100.

In this example each succeeding dilution is dependent on the previous dilution in the series.

	Tube #1 1st dilution	Tube #2 2nd dilution	Tube #3 3rd dilution
	1 ml serum + 4 ml saline	1 ml dilution #1 + 9 ml saline	1 ml dilution #2 + 99 ml saline
Total volume of dilution before transfer:	5 ml	10 ml	100 ml
Total volume after some is removed to make next dilution:	4 ml (1 ml removed to make dilution #2)	9 ml (1 ml removed to make dilution #3)	100 ml (None removed)

Some of the previous dilution is used to make each dilution. This means that the volume of all dilutions except the last have less volume than the amount prepared.

Suppose that 100 milliliters of the third dilution is not needed or that there was some other reason not to make this much of the dilution. One would need to calculate the amount of the second dilution to use to make a prescribed amount of the third dilution.

EXAMPLE 5-14: A serum sample is diluted with saline 1/5, rediluted 1/10, and again 1/100. Make 10 ml of the 1/100 dilution.

Calculate the amount of the 1/10 dilution (tube #2) needed to make 10 ml of the 1/100 dilution (tube #3). One would have the following calculation for the last tube.

$$\frac{1}{100} = \frac{x}{10}$$

$$100x = 10$$

$$x = 0.1 \text{ ml } (0.1/10 \text{ dilution} = 1/100 \text{ dilution})$$

0.1 ml of the second dilution will be needed to make 10 ml of the third dilution.

	Tube #1 1st dilution	Tube #2 2nd dilution	Tube #3 3rd dilution
	1 ml serum + 4 ml saline	1 ml dilution #1 + 9 ml saline	0.1 ml dilution #2 + 9.9 ml saline
Total volume of dilution before transfer:	5 ml	10 ml	10 ml
Total volume after some is removed to make next dilution:	4 ml (1 ml removed to make dilution #2)	9.9 ml (0.1 ml removed to make dilution #3)	10 ml (None removed)

In determining the volume of any solution in a series, the worker needs to determine what went into each solution and what came out. Common sense and simple arithmetic are then used to calculate the volume.

Tube Dilution

The tube dilution is the dilution in a particular tube in a series as it was made *in that tube*. It has nothing to do with the tube before it or after it. Do not confuse it with the solution dilution or the substance concentration. They may or may not be the same, as will be seen later. Consider the three following examples.

EXAMPLE 5-15: Make the following dilutions of serum in saline: 1/5, 1/10, and 1/100.

In this example, each of the three dilutions of serum was made as a separate and independent solution.

	Tube #1	Tube #2	Tube #3
Total volume of dilution in each tube:	1 ml serum + 4 ml saline 5 ml	1 ml serum + 9 ml saline 10 ml	1 ml serum + 99 ml saline 100 ml
Tube dilution:	1/5	1/10	1/00

The tube dilution is simply the amount of substance being diluted in the total volume *of that tube*. It has nothing to do with the preceding dilution or whether the dilutions are independent or not.

Study the next two examples, 5-16 and 5-17. Notice that the tube dilutions in these examples are the same *numbers* as the tube dilutions in Example 5-15.

EXAMPLE 5-16: A serum sample is diluted with saline 1/5, rediluted 1/10, and again 1/100.

In this example each succeeding dilution is dependent on the previous solution in the series.

	Tube #1 1st dilution	Tube #2 2nd dilution	Tube #3 3rd dilution
Volume before transfer: Volume after transfer:	1 ml serum + 4 ml saline 5 ml 4 ml	1 ml dilution #1 + 9 ml saline 10 ml 9 ml	1 ml dilution #2 + 99 ml saline 100 ml 100 ml
Tube dilution:	1/5	1/10	1/100

EXAMPLE 5-17: A serum sample is diluted with saline 1/5, rediluted 1/10, and again 1/100. Make 10 ml of the 1/100 dilution.

	Tube #1 1st dilution	Tube #2 2nd dilution	Tube #3 3rd dilution
	①ml serum + 4 ml saline	①ml dilution #1 + 9 ml saline	⓪.①ml dilution #2 + 9.9 ml saline
Volume before transfer: Volume after transfer:	⑤ml 4 ml	⑩ml 9.9 ml	⑩ml 10 ml
Tube dilution:	1/5	1/10	1/100 (0.1/10 = 1/100)

In all of these examples one can see that:

1. The tube dilution has nothing to do with whether the dilutions are dependent or independent of each other.
2. The tube dilution has nothing to do with the preceding tube.
3. The tube dilution is based on the amount of substance diluted in the total volume of the tube before transfer.
4. The tube dilution has nothing to do with the total volume after transfer.

The tube dilution is simply the way a dilution was made in a particular tube.

Solution Dilution

The solution dilution is the actual *dilution* of the original solution in a particular tube. In a series in which each dilution is made directly from the original solution, that is, an independent series, the *solution dilution* is the same as the *tube dilution.*

EXAMPLE 5-18: Make the following dilutions of serum in saline: 1/5, 1/10, and 1/100.

In this example each of the three dilutions of serum was made as a separate and independent solution.

	Tube #1	Tube #2	Tube #3
	1 ml serum + 4 ml saline	1 ml serum + 9 ml saline	1 ml serum + 99 ml saline
Total volume of solution in each tube:	5 ml	10 ml	100 ml
Tube dilution: Solution dilution:	1/5 1/5	1/10 1/10	1/100 1/100

However, in those series in which the dilutions are made from previous dilutions, that is, the dependent series, there is a difference between the solution dilution and the tube dilution. In these series the solution dilution is calculated by multiplying the tube dilutions of all previous solutions in the series together. In other words, to find the solution dilution of the third tube in a series multiply the first tube dilution by the second tube dilution and this result by the third tube dilution and so on.

1st tube dilution × 2nd tube dilution × 3rd tube dilution . . . = solution dilution.

EXAMPLE 5-19: A serum sample is diluted with saline 1/5, rediluted 1/10, and again 1/100. 10 ml of the 1/100 dilution is made. What is the solution dilution of each of these solutions?

	Tube #1 1st dilution	Tube #2 2nd dilution	Tube #3 3rd dilution
	1 ml serum + 4 ml saline	1 ml dilution #1 + 9 ml saline	0.1 ml dilution #2 + 9.9 ml saline
Volume before transfer:	5 ml	10 ml	10 ml
Volume after transfer:	4 ml	9.9 ml	10 ml
Tube dilution:	1/5	1/10	1/100
Solution dilution:	1/5	1/50 (1/5 × 1/10)	1/5,000 (1/5 × 1/10 × 1/100)

In this example, pure serum was used for the first dilution. The first tube dilution was 1/5. As this is the only dilution made to this point in the series, the solution dilution of tube #1 is the same as the tube dilution, 1/5.

To calculate the solution dilution in tube #2, multiply the tube dilutions of all previous solutions in the series with the tube dilution of this tube.

$$1/5 \times 1/10 = 1/50$$

This shows that the solution dilution of the second dilution is 1/50 serum in saline.

To calculate the solution dilution in tube #3, multiply the tube dilutions of all previous solutions in the series with the tube dilution of this solution.

$$1/5 \times 1/10 \times 1/100 = 1/5,000$$

The solution dilution in Tube #3 is 1/5,000 serum in saline

The same kind of calculations can be used to determine the solution dilutions of other types of dilutions.

EXAMPLE 5-20: What is the solution dilution in all tubes of a series resulting from the dilution of a 10% NaCl solution with water 1/2, rediluted 1/5, rediluted 1/10, and again 1/50? Ten milliliters of each dilution was prepared from the previous solution.

	Tube #1 1st dilution	Tube #2 2nd dilution	Tube #3 3rd dilution	Tube #4 4th dilution
	5 ml 10% NaCl + 5 ml water	2 ml 1st dilution + 8 ml water	1 ml 2nd dilution + 9 ml water	0.2 ml 3rd dilution + 9.8 ml water
Volume before transfer:	10 ml	10 ml	10 ml	10 ml
Volume after transfer:	8 ml	9 ml	9.8 ml	10 ml
Tube dilution:	1/2 (5/10 = 1/2)	1/5 (2/10 = 1/5)	1/10 (1/10 = 1/10)	1/50 (0.2/10 = 1/50)
Solution dilution:	1/2	1/10 (1/2 × 1/5)	1/100 (1/2 × 1/5 × 1/10)	1/5,000 (1/2 × 1/5 × 1/10 × 1/50)

The solution dilution is simply the cumulative dilutions of a solution in a tube and is found by using the tube dilutions only.

Substance Concentration

The substance concentration of a solution in a series pertains to the *actual concentration* of the original solution being diluted in a particular tube. This is found by multiplying the original concentration times the first tube dilution times the second tube dilution times the third tube dilution, etc. This gives the final concentration of the original substance *in the same form* used for the original concentration.

Original concentration $\times$ 1st tube dilution $\times$ 2nd tube dilution $\times$ 3rd tube dilution . . . = concentration of last dilution.

Sometimes it may be helpful or necessary to know the concentration of one of the intermediate dilutions in a series. This is accomplished in the same manner as finding the concentration of the final solution. One simply stops the calculations with the dilution for which the concentration is desired. Consider the last two examples.

EXAMPLE 5-21: A serum sample is diluted with saline 1/5, rediluted 1/10, and again 1/100. Ten milliliters of the 1/100 dilution was made. What is the substance concentration of each of these solutions?

Remember that the original concentration of serum is considered to be 1/1, so the concentration of the original solution in this example is 1/1.

	Tube #1 1st dilution	Tube #2 2nd dilution	Tube #3 3rd dilution
	1 ml serum + 4 ml saline	1 ml dilution #1 + 9 ml saline	0.1 ml dilution #2 + 9.9 ml saline
Volume before transfer:	5 ml	10 ml	10 ml
Volume after transfer:	4 ml	9.9 ml	10 ml
Tube dilution:	1/5	1/10	1/100
Solution dilution:	1/5	1/50	1/5,000
Solution concentration:	1/5 dilution	1/50 dilution	1/5,000 dilution

The substance concentration of the first dilution can be found by multiplying the concentration of the original substance, 1/1, by the tube dilution of the first tube, 1/5.

$$1/1 \times 1/5 = 1/5 \text{ dilution}$$

Hence, the substance concentration of the first tube is 1/5 dilution.

The substance concentration of the second tube is the product of the original concentration and the first and second tube dilutions.

$$1/1 \times 1/5 \times 1/10 = 1/50 \text{ dilution}$$

The substance concentration of the second tube is 1/50 dilution.

The calculation for the third tube in this example is below.

$$1/1 \times 1/5 \times 1/10 \times 1/100 = 1/5,000 \text{ dilution}$$

In this example the substance concentration of serum in saline in each of these solutions is equal to the solution dilution of the particular solution. This is because the original substance was undiluted serum. For purposes of calculation, the concentration of a pure, undiluted substance, such as concentrated sulfuric acid, absolute alcohol, serum, or urine, is expressed as 1/1. When the original substance is something that can be represented by the notation, 1/1, the solution dilution and the substance concentration are the same.

EXAMPLE 5-22: What is the substance concentration in all tubes of a series resulting from the dilution of a 10% NaCl solution with water 1/2, redilute 1/5, redilute 1/10, and again 1/50? Ten milliliters of each dilution was prepared from the previous dilution.

The concentration of the original solution is 10% NaCl.

	Tube #1 1st dilution	Tube #2 2nd dilution	Tube #3 3rd dilution	Tube #4 4th dilution
	5 ml 10% NaCl + 5 ml water	2 ml 1st dilution + 8 ml water	1 ml 2nd dilution + 9 ml water	0.2 ml 3rd dilution + 9.8 ml water
Volume before transfer:	10 ml	10 ml	10 ml	10 ml
Volume after transfer:	8 ml	9 ml	9.8 ml	10 ml
Tube dilution:	1/2	1/5	1/10	1/50
Solution dilution:	1/2	1/10	1/100	1/5,000
Substance conc.:	5% $(10\% \times 1/2)$	1% $(10\% \times 1/2 \times 1/5)$	0.1% $(10\% \times 1/2 \times 1/5$ $\times 1/10)$	0.002% $(10\% \times 1/2 \times 1/5$ $\times 1/10 \times 1/50)$

In this example the original substance was 10% NaCl in water. The substance concentration of the first solution is:

$$10\% \times 1/2 = 5\%$$

To calculate the substance concentration of the second dilution:

$$10\% \times 1/2 \times 1/5 = 1\%$$

The third dilution:

$$10\% \times 1/2 \times 1/5 \times 1/10 = 0.1\%$$

And the fourth dilution:

$$10\% \times 1/2 \times 1/5 \times 1/10 \times 1/50 = 0.002\%$$

Recall that the **final** answer to a problem is in the same form as the original substance or solution. *This is very important.* The final answer is *always* in the same form as the original concentration. If the original solution was a dilution, the answer is a dilution; if the original substance was mg/ml, the answer is in mg/ml; if the original substance was a percentage, the answer is a percentage, etc.

EXAMPLE 5-23: A 1/10 dilution of a substance is diluted 3/5, rediluted 2/15, and diluted once again 1/2. What is the final concentration?

$$\frac{\text{Original}}{\text{concentration}} \times \frac{\text{1st tube}}{\text{dilution}} \times \frac{\text{2nd tube}}{\text{dilution}} \times \frac{\text{3rd tube}}{\text{dilution}} \ldots = \text{final concentration}$$

$$\text{1/10 dilution} \times \quad 3/5 \quad \times \quad 2/15 \quad \times \quad 1/2 \quad = \frac{\text{6/1,500 dilution or a}}{\text{1/250 dilution}}$$

The tube containing the last dilution (that is, third dilution) has a concentration of 1/250 dilution.

EXAMPLE 5-24: A 6N solution is diluted 1/5, 1/2, 5/15, and 1/3. What is the final concentration?

$$6N \times 1/5 \times 1/2 \times 5/15 \times 1/3 = 30/450N = 1/15N \text{ (or } 0.067N)$$

The tube containing the last dilution (1/3) has a concentration of 1/15N or 0.067N.

EXAMPLE 5-25: A solution that contains 80 mg/100 ml is diluted 1/10 and again 2/20. What is the final concentration?

$$80 \text{ mg/100 ml} \times 1/10 \times 2/20 = 160 \text{ mg/20,000 ml} = 1 \text{ mg/125 ml} = 0.8 \text{ mg/100 ml}$$

The 2/20 dilution has a concentration of 0.8 mg/100 ml.

The calculation of the concentration of a given solution in a series can be made from the closest previous solution in the series for which the concentration is known. It is not necessary to always begin with the first dilution in the series.

EXAMPLE 5-26: A urine sample is diluted 1/2 with distilled water, rediluted 1/4, 1/4, and again 1/4. What is the concentration of the third and fourth dilutions?

One could find the concentration of the third dilution in the usual manner:

$$\frac{\text{Original}}{\text{concentration}} \times \frac{\text{1st tube}}{\text{dilution}} \times \frac{\text{2nd tube}}{\text{dilution}} \times \frac{\text{3rd tube}}{\text{dilution}} = \frac{\text{concentration of solution}}{\text{in the 3rd tube}}$$

$$(1/1) \quad \times \quad 1/2 \quad \times \quad 1/4 \quad \times \quad 1/4 \quad = \text{1/32 dilution}$$

The concentration of the fourth dilution could be obtained in one of two ways:

1. In the usual manner, beginning with the first tube dilution

$$1/1 \times 1/2 \times 1/4 \times 1/4 \times 1/4 = \text{1/128 dilution (concentration in 4th tube)}$$

2. Using the concentration of the preceding solution, the third dilution, whose concentration was 1/32 dilution

$$\frac{\text{Concentration of}}{\text{3rd dilution}} \times \frac{\text{4th tube}}{\text{dilution}} = \text{concentration of solution in 4th tube}$$

$$1/32 \quad \times \quad 1/4 \quad = \frac{\text{1/128 dilution}}{\text{(concentration in 4th tube)}}$$

Study the following example. Be sure all relationships are understood before continuing.

EXAMPLE 5-27: A 5M solution is diluted 1/10 and again 1/5. What is the concentration of each dilution?

	Tube #1	**Tube #2**
	1 ml 5M solution	1 ml solution from Tube #1
	+ 9 ml diluent	+ 4 ml diluent
Volume before transfer:	10 ml	5 ml
Volume after transfer:	9 ml	5 ml
Tube dilution:	1/10	1/5
Solution dilution:	1/10	1/50
Substance conc.:	0.5M	0.1M
	(5M × 1/10 = 0.5M)	(5M × 1/10 × 1/5 = 0.1M)
Tube contains before transfer:	10 ml of a 1/10 dilution of a 5M solution with a concentration of 0.5M	5 ml of a 1/50 dilution of a 5M solution with a concentration of 0.1M
Tube contains after transfer:	9 ml of a 1/10 dilution of a 5M solution with a concentration of 0.5M	5 ml of a 1/50 dilution of a 5M solution with a concentration of 0.1M (there was none transferred)

Those of you who have been working through this with your minds as well as your eyes realize by now that the substance concentration can also be found by multiplying the *concentration of the original substance* by the *solution dilution* of the tube in question. Review the examples in this section to confirm this.

Amount of Original Solution in Each Dilution of a Series

The amount of the original solution in a given volume of a dilution often needs to be known to produce a valid result. To determine such values, one needs to know the *solution dilution and the total volume* in a particular tube. When these two values are known, the actual volume of the original solution can then be calculated by ratio and proportion.

EXAMPLE 5-28: A 1/10 dilution of serum is diluted 1/10 and rediluted 1/100. Ten milliliters total volume is desired for each solution. How much actual serum is present in each tube after transfer?

The original concentration of serum is 1/1.

	Tube #1 **1st dilution**	**Tube #2** **2nd dilution**	**Tube #3** **3rd dilution**
	1 ml serum	1 ml dilution #1	0.1 ml dilution #2
	+ 9 ml saline	+ 9 ml saline	+ 9.9 ml saline
Volume before transfer:	10 ml	10 ml	10 ml
Volume after transfer:	9 ml	9.9 ml	10 ml
Tube dilution:	1/10	1/10	1/100
Solution dilution:	1/10	1/100	1/10,000
Solution concentration:	1/10 dilution	1/100 dilution	1/10,000 dilution
Amount of serum present before transfer:	1 ml ($1/10 × x/10$)	0.1 ml ($1/100 × x/10$)	0.001 ml ($1/10,000 × x/10$)
Amount of serum present after transfer:	0.9 ml ($1/10 × x/9$)	0.099 ml ($1/100 × x/9.9$)	0.001 ml ($1/10,000 × x/10$)

In calculating the volume of serum in the first dilution, remember that there is one part of serum for each 10 parts of total solution in a 1/10 dilution. Use a ratio-proportion procedure. If there was one part in every 10 parts, then there would be x milliliters in the 10 milliliters present before the transfer.

$$\frac{1}{10} = \frac{x}{10}$$

$$10x = 10$$

$$x = 1 \text{ ml}$$

The tube contains 1 ml of serum before any of the dilution is transferred to the next tube.

After transferring 1 ml to the next tube, the total volume is 9 ml. There is still 1 ml of serum in every 10 ml of dilution, but there are only 9 ml total volume. Calculate the amount of serum in this 9 milliliters.

$$\frac{1}{10} = \frac{x}{9}$$

$$10x = 9$$

$$x = 0.9 \text{ ml}$$

In the remaining 9 ml of the first dilution, there are 0.9 ml of serum.

The second dilution consists of 10 ml of a 1/100 dilution. To determine the amount of serum present before transfer, use the same procedure.

$$\frac{1}{100} = \frac{x}{10}$$

$$100x = 10$$

$$x = 0.1$$

The second dilution contains 0.1 ml of serum before transfer. After transfer of 0.1 ml, this 1/100 dilution has a total volume of 9.9 ml. If there was 1 ml of serum in every 100 ml of solution, then there would be x ml of serum in 9.9 ml.

$$\frac{1}{100} = \frac{x}{9.9}$$

$$100x = 9.9$$

$$x = 0.099$$

The second solution contains 0.099 ml of serum after transfer.

The amount of serum in the third solution is calculated in a similar manner.

$$\text{Solution dilution} = 1/10,000$$

$$\text{Volume present} = 10 \text{ ml}$$

There is 1 ml of serum in every 10,000 ml of solution; therefore there are x ml of serum in 10 ml of solution.

$$\frac{1}{10,000} = \frac{x}{10}$$

$$10,000x = 10$$

$$x = 0.001 \text{ ml}$$

There are 0.001 ml of serum present in this 10 ml of solution.

The above example used a dilution as the original substance. The following example uses a percent as the original substance.

EXAMPLE 5-29: Five percent HCl is diluted 1/2, again 2/6, and again 4/12. How much of the 5% HCl is actually present in each tube before transfer?

The original concentration is 5% HCl.

	Tube #1	Tube #2	Tube #3
	1 ml 5% HCl	2 ml from Tube #1	4 ml from Tube #2
	+ 1 ml diluent	+ 4 ml diluent	+ 8 ml diluent
Volume before transfer:	2 ml	6 ml	12 ml
Volume after transfer:	0 ml	2 ml	12 ml
			(none removed)
Tube dilution:	1/2	2/6	4/12
Solution dilution:	1/2	2/12	8/144
Substance concentration:	2.5%	0.83%	0.28%
Amount of 5% HCl in tube before transfer:	In this tube there is 1 ml of 5% HCl ($1/2 \times x/2$)	In this tube there is 1 ml of 5% HCl ($2/12 = x/6$)	In this tube there is 0.67 ml of 5% HCl ($8/144 = x/12$)

Note that the substance concentration is not used in either of these examples. Problems determining the volume of original solution in a given dilution may seem difficult and confusing. However, if one realizes that all one needs to know is the solution dilution and the volume of the solution in question, then the calculations should not seem too hard. It is important in this type of calculation that the worker carefully think through what is being done. No set procedure may suffice in all situations.

SECTION 5.4 DILUTIONS WITH PRESCRIBED CONCENTRATIONS AND/OR VOLUMES

The calculations used to determine the concentration of each solution in a series may be used in reverse to produce a dilution or a dilution series having prescribed concentrations and/or volumes at each step.

EXAMPLE 5-30: Make the following dilutions of serum in buffer: 1/10, 1/100, and 1/500. The serum sample consists of only 1.5 ml.

These are independent dilutions. In each of them the numerator refers to one part of serum and the denominators, 10, 100, and 500, refer to the number of parts of the total solution. One way to satisfy the preceding instructions is to make each dilution separately, always using pure serum and pure buffer. However, that requires 3 ml of serum. The serum sample is of limited volume, so the use of one dilution to make another becomes expedient. To do this, complete the following procedure. Note the reason for each step, and recognize the possibility of adjusting each step to meet some other situation.

1. To make the first dilution, that is, the dilution most concentrated in serum, place 1 ml of serum in a tube and bring the total volume up to 10 ml. This gives 10 ml of a 1/10 dilution of serum in buffer.

2. To make the 1/100 dilution of serum in buffer using the first dilution, determine the tube dilution to be made of the 1/10 dilution needed to yield the desired dilution. Remember, the concentration of each step of a series equals the product of the concentration of each preceding step and the original concentration.

$$\text{Original concentration} \times \frac{\text{1st tube}}{\text{dilution}} \times \frac{\text{2nd tube}}{\text{dilution}} = \frac{\text{Concentration of 2nd}}{\text{dilution}}$$

Known	Known	Unknown	Known
1/1	$\times$ 1/10 dilution $\times$	$\dfrac{\text{2nd tube}}{\text{dilution}}$	= 1/100 dilution
	1/10 $\times$	1/x	= 1/100

$$\frac{1}{10} \times \frac{1}{x} = \frac{1}{100}$$

$$\frac{1}{x} = \frac{1}{100} \times \frac{10}{1}$$

$$\frac{1}{x} = \frac{10}{100}$$

$$\frac{1}{x} = \frac{1}{10}$$

$$x = 10$$

In substituting 10 for *x*, one can see there is a 1/10 tube dilution needed to make the 1/100 dilution. To one part of the 1/10 dilution, add enough buffer to bring the tube dilution up to 10 parts of total volume. This results in 10 ml of a 1/100 dilution.

3. To make the 1/500 dilution of serum in buffer using the 1/100 dilution, follow the same procedure using the 1/100 dilution.

Known	Unknown	Known
1/100 dilution $\times$	3rd tube dilution	= 1/500 solution dilution
1/100 $\times$	1/x	= 1/500

$$\frac{1}{100} \times \frac{1}{x} = \frac{1}{500}$$

$$\frac{1}{x} = \frac{1}{500} \times \frac{100}{1}$$

$$\frac{1}{x} = \frac{100}{500}$$

$$\frac{1}{x} = \frac{1}{5}$$

$$x = 5$$

To make the 1/500 dilution of serum in buffer, bring one part of the 1/100 dilution of serum in buffer up to five parts total volume.

Study the summary of these procedures in table format on p. 111.

	Tube #1 1st dilution	Tube #2 2nd dilution	Tube #3 3rd dilution
	1 ml serum + 9 ml diluent	1 ml dilution #1 + 9 ml diluent	1 ml dilution #2 + 4 ml diluent
Volume before transfer:	10 ml	10 ml	5 ml
Volume after transfer:	9 ml	9 ml	5 ml
Tube dilution:	1/10	1/10	1/5
Solution dilution:	1/10	1/100	1/500
Solution concentration:	1/10 dilution	1/100 dilution	1/500 dilution

EXAMPLE 5-31: Make 100 ml of a 10/1,000 dilution from a 5/50 solution of hydrogen peroxide.

The concentration of the solution used to make the dilution is 5/50 hydrogen peroxide. One hundred milliliters of a 10/1,000 dilution are needed. The volume of the original solution needed to make the new dilution can be calculated using the rule *original concentration times the first tube dilution times the second dilution . . . etc.* to determine the final concentration.

Original concentration $\times$ 1st tube dilution = desired concentration

Known	**Unknown**	**Known**

$$5/50 \text{ dilution} \times \quad x/100 \quad = 10/1,000$$

$$\frac{5}{50} \times \frac{x}{100} = \frac{10}{1,000}$$

$$\frac{5x}{5,000} = \frac{10}{1,000}$$

$$5,000x = 50,000$$

$$x = 10$$

Put 10 in place of the x to find that a 10/100 dilution is needed. Therefore dilute 10 ml of the 5/50 solution up to a total volume of 100 ml to give 100 ml of a 10/1,000 solution.

EXAMPLE 5-32: A 5M HCl solution is on hand. Prepare 50 ml of a 0.25M solution, and from this solution prepare 100 ml of a 0.01M solution?

First, determine what dilution will give 50 ml of the desired 0.25M solution.

$$5\text{M} \times \frac{x}{50} = 0.25\text{M}$$

$$5x = 0.25 \times 50$$

$$5x = 12.5$$

$$x = 2.5$$

A 2.5/50 dilution of the 5M solution yields 50 ml of a 0.25M solution.

Next determine what dilution of the 0.25M solution will give 100 ml of the 0.01M solution.

$$0.25\text{M} \times \frac{x}{100} = 0.01\text{M}$$

$$0.25x = 0.01 \times 100$$

$$0.25x = 1$$

$$x = 4$$

Hence, 4 ml of the 0.25M solution diluted up to 100 ml gives 100 ml of a 0.01M solution.

In table form, Example 5-32 is as follows:

	Tube #1	Tube #2
	2.5 ml of 5M	4 ml from tube #1
	+ 47.5 ml diluent	+ 96 ml diluent
Total volume:	50 ml	100 ml
Tube dilution:	1/20	1/25
Solution dilution:	1/20	1/500
Substance concentration:	0.25M	0.01M
	(5M × 1/20)	(0.25M × 1/25* or 5M × 1/500)

*Notice that the substance concentration may also be found by multiplying the tube dilution of the tube in question by the previous substance concentration.

SECTION 5.5 SERIAL DILUTIONS

Many procedures call for a dilution series in which the magnitude of all dilutions is the same. This type of dilution series is referred to as a **serial dilution.** This procedure is generally used in producing a series of solutions having equal increments of variation. The term **fold** is often used in connection with serial dilutions. For example, a dilution in which each succeeding dilution is twice that of the preceding one is termed a *two-fold dilution* (1/2, 1/4, 1/8, 1/16, 1/32, etc.). Similarly, a series in which each dilution is 4 times that of the preceding one is a fourfold dilution (1/4, 1/16, 1/64, 1/256, etc.), and one whose values are incremented by 10 times is referred to as a tenfold dilution (1/10, 1/100, 1/1,000, 1/10,000, etc.).

Occasionally, the first dilution may be different from the rest. For example, if the first dilution was 1/20 and each succeeding dilution was 1/2, one would have a twofold dilution that started from 20 (that is, 1/20, 1/40, 1/80, 1/160, 1/320, etc.). The first dilution determines the starting point, and the remaining dilutions determine the magnitude of the increase.

The methods and calculations previously discussed for other types of dilution series apply to serial dilutions.

EXAMPLE 5-33: A procedure for the titration of irregular antibodies in maternal serum requires 10 dilutions of serum in saline. An abbreviated procedure of this test is given below.

1. Place ten 12 × 75 mm test tubes in a rack and label them according to the serum dilution: 1, 2, 4, 8. . . . 512.
2. Using a 1-ml pipet, deliver to the bottom of all tubes except the first, 0.1 ml isotonic saline solution.
3. Using a clean pipet, place 0.1 ml of serum into the first two tubes.
4. Mix and transfer 0.1 ml of the dilution in the second tube to the third, thence 0.1 ml of the third to the fourth and so through the series. Discard the last 0.1 milliliter.

Careful study of this procedure will show that each tube except the first will have a 1/2 tube dilution of the previous tube in the series. Additionally, the solution dilution in each tube will be twice the dilution of the previous tube, and the concentration of serum in each tube in the series will be one half that of the previous tube. The following table shows some properties of each tube after this series is made.

Tube #:	1	2	3	4	5	6	7	8	9	10
Serum, ml:	0.1	0.1	No pure serum added to tubes 3 through 10							
Amount transferred, ml:			0.1	0.1	0.1	0.1	0.1	0.1	0.1	0.1
Saline, ml:	0.0	0.1	0.1	0.1	0.1	0.1	0.1	0.1	0.1	0.1
Volume before transfer, ml:	0.1	0.2	0.2	0.2	0.2	0.2	0.2	0.2	0.2	0.2
Volume after transfer, ml:	0.1	0.1	0.1	0.1	0.1	0.1	0.1	0.1	0.1	0.1
Tube dilution:	1/1	1/2	1/2	1/2	1/2	1/2	1/2	1/2	1/2	1/2
Solution dilution:	1/1	1/2	1/4	1/8	1/16	1/32	1/64	1/128	1/256	1/512
Volume of serum after transfer, ml:	0.1	0.05	0.025	0.0125	0.00625	0.00312	0.00156	0.00078	0.00039	0.000195

The above example is a simple twofold serial dilution of serum in saline. All tubes in the series have one-half the concentration of serum as the previous tube. Serial dilutions are often more complicated. Consider the next example.

EXAMPLE 5-34: A serial dilution of serum is made by placing 9 ml diluent in the first tube of a series and 4 ml in each of the remaining four tubes. One milliliter of serum is added to the first tube, and 4 ml from the first tube is transferred to the second tube and then to each succeeding tube. The last 4 ml transferred is discarded. Give:

a. Total volume in each tube before transfer
b. Total volume in each tube remaining after transfer
c. Tube dilution of each tube
d. Solution dilution of each tube
e. Substance concentration of each tube
f. Actual amount of serum present in each tube before transfer
g. Actual amount of serum present in each tube after transfer

If one sets up a systematic table as in the above examples, this type of problem is relatively easy to solve.

Tube #:	1	2	3	4	5
Serum:	1 ml				
Amount transferred:		4 ml	4 ml	4 ml	4 ml
Diluent:	+ 9 ml	+ 4 ml	+ 4 ml	+ 4 ml	+ 4 ml
Volume before transfer:	10 ml	8 ml	8 ml	8 ml	8 ml
Volume after transfer:	6 ml	4 ml	4 ml	4 ml	4 ml
Tube dilution:	1/10	1/2	1/2	1/2	1/2
Solution dilution:	1/10	1/20	1/40	1/80	1/160
Substance concentration:	1/10 dilution	1/20 dilution	1/40 dilution	1/80 dilution	1/160 dilution
Amount of serum before transfer:	1 ml	0.4 ml	0.2 ml	0.1 ml	0.05 ml
Amount of serum after transfer:	0.6 ml	0.2 ml	0.1 ml	0.05 ml	0.025 ml

In this example, the first tube dilution is 1/10, and the other tubes in this series form a twofold serial dilution. Again, careful study is needed to understand the concentrations of serum in each of these tubes.

EXAMPLE 5-35: A serum sample is diluted 1/2 with buffer. A series of five dilutions is made of this first dilution by diluting it 1/10, rediluting 1/10, and then three times more 1/10.

$$1/2 \times 1/10 = 1/20 \times 1/10 = 1/200 \times 1/10 = 1/2,000 \times 1/10 = 1/20,000 \times 1/10 = 1/200,000$$

The concentration of serum in each solution is as follows: 1/2, 1/20, 1/200, 1/2,000, 1/20,000, and 1/200,000.

Study of this example shows that the first dilution was 1/2 dilution and the other dilutions form a tenfold serial dilution.

SECTION 5.6 SPECIAL DILUTION PROBLEMS
Problems Related to Dilution Correction Factors

Occasionally a solution is too strong to be used as it is. For example, when one is performing manual blood counts, the blood contains too many cells to be counted without some dilution. In performing a given test, it may be found that the concentration of the substance being measured is too high for measurement without a dilution. In these cases the original substance or solution on which the test is being performed is altered, and for this change a correction must be made.

The general rule for this type of problem states:

To correct for having used a dilution in a determination other than the concentration or quantity called for, multiply the answer obtained times the reciprocal of the dilution made.

EXAMPLE 5-36: A blood sample is diluted 1/500; 300 cells are counted in the diluted sample. How many cells were there in the blood before the dilution was made?

If a 1/500 dilution of blood was made, the diluted sample would contain only 1/500 as many cells as the undiluted sample, or, stated another way, whole blood would contain 500 times the number of cells as the diluted specimen. Therefore if the number of cells counted in the diluted sample is multiplied times 500 (dilution = 1/500 and reciprocal = 500/1 = 500), one would have the number of cells present in the undiluted specimen.

$$300 \times 500 = 150,000$$

EXAMPLE 5-37: A test on a urine sample is to be run. The concentration of the substance in the urine is too high to be determined with the present procedure. Make a 1/10 dilution of the urine sample and run the test on the diluted solution. The answer obtained is 50 mg/dl. What should be reported?

The 1/10 dilution of urine would contain one-tenth the amount of substance as undiluted sample, or the undiluted sample should contain 10 times the quantity of substance as the diluted solution. Multiply the answer obtained times the reciprocal of the dilution made (dilution = 1/10 and reciprocal = 10).

$$50 \times 10 = 500 \text{ mg/dl}$$

Problems Related to Making Large Dilutions

The instructions indicate that a 1/10,000 dilution of a substance is to be made. This means 1 part of solute (substance being diluted) in a total volume of 10,000 parts. If a 1/10,000 dilution of serum in saline is being made, it could be done by taking 1 milliliter of serum and diluting it up to a total volume of 10,000 milliliters. However, it is rare that this quantity of a solution is needed. If the approximate volume needed is known, a dilution problem procedure may be used to determine how to prepare a smaller quantity or volume of the desired concentration. The preceding dilution of serum could be made in several ways:

1. One could make a 1/10 dilution of serum, redilute 1/10, redilute 1/10, and redilute once more 1/10.

$$1/10 \times 1/10 \times 1/10 \times 1/10 = 1/10,000 \text{ dilution}$$

This would produce 10 ml of a 1/10,000 dilution of serum in saline.

2. One could make a 1/10 dilution of serum, redilute 1/10, and again 1/100.

$$1/10 \times 1/10 \times 1/100 = 1/10,000 \text{ dilution}$$

This would yield 100 ml of a 1/10,000 dilution of serum in saline.

3. One could also make a 1/100 dilution of serum and redilute 1/100.

$$1/100 \times 1/100 = 1/10,000 \text{ dilution}$$

This would give 100 ml of a 1/10,000 dilution of serum in saline.

Any combination of dilutions that yields a final concentration of 1/10,000 may be used. The combination is determined in part by the glassware available and the volume needed. To decide what dilutions to use, one needs to know several things:

1. The original concentration of the substance being diluted
2. The final volume desired
3. The final concentration desired
4. The glassware and equipment available

SECTION 5.7 DILUTIONS AS AN EXPRESSION OF TEST ENDPOINT (TITERS)

Dilution notation is sometimes used to express the endpoint of some test. Usually this method of expressing notation is used in connection with the titer of test solutions. Strictly speaking, titer is the concentration of a solution as determined by titration. Hence the **titer** is the smallest amount or concentration that produces a particular effect or endpoint. Although the test may be reported as the endpoint of the titer, it is usually reported as the reciprocal of the titer.

EXAMPLE 5-40: A series of solutions of serum in saline is prepared in the following dilutions: 1/2, 1/4, 1/8, and 1/16. A test for the presence of an antibody was made on each solution. It was positive for the 1/2 and 1/4 dilutions but negative for the 1/8 and 1/16 dilutions. The titer of the antibody is said to be 1/4, the greatest dilution yielding a positive result, and the test is reported as 4 (reciprocal) or 1/4 (endpoint).

PRACTICE PROBLEMS

Calculate the answer for each problem. Understand each portion of the calculation and determine whether the answer is logical. *Just because an answer can be calculated does not mean that it is reasonable.*

Calculations involving one dilution—introduction

1. There are 8 milliliters of saline in a test tube. You add 2 ml serum. Give the following:
   a. The saline to serum ratio

   b. The saline to total volume ratio
   c. The serum to saline ratio
   d. The total volume to serum ratio
2. Give the serum to saline ratio for the following dilutions:
   a. 1/15
   b. 2/23
   c. 7/9
   d. 30/45
3. Give the part to part ratio of the following dilutions:
   a. 2/30
   b. 6/10
   c. 8/16
4. Give the serum to saline ratio of 3 milliliters of serum diluted with 17 milliliters of water. Give the dilution of the solution.
5. If 20 milliliters of saline is added to 4 milliliters of serum, what is the serum dilution? What is the serum to saline ratio?
6. If you add 30 milliliters of saline to 2 milliliters of serum, what is the serum dilution?
7. If 0.5 ml of serum is obtained and diluted to 1.5 ml, the amount of diluent added is _____ ml.
8. What is the final dilution of an unknown specimen using 0.1 ml of blood with 3.4 ml of water and 1.5 ml of reagents?
9. The following quantities are placed in a test tube: 0.1 ml of sample, 2.9 ml of diluent, 0.5 ml of reagent #1, and 0.5 ml of reagent #2. What is the final dilution of the sample?
10. If a primary serum/saline dilution of 1/100 is chosen, it may be prepared by:
    a. Mixing 1 part of serum with 99 parts of diluent
    b. Mixing 100 parts of diluent with 1 part of serum
    c. Mixing 100 parts of serum with 1 part of diluent
    d. Mixing 1 part of diluent with 99 parts of serum
11. If one has 10 milliliters of urine plus 20 oz. of diluent, what is the urine to diluent ratio? What is the urine to diluent dilution?
12. 0.2 milliliters of serum is obtained and diluted 1/10. The amount of diluent added is _____.
13. Express the dilutions in question 2 as ''1 to something.''
14. Express the dilutions in question 3 as ''1 to something.''
15. Express the following dilutions as ''1 to something.''
    a. 1/5
    b. 6/20
    c. 2/14
16. If 0.5 ml of serum is diluted to 80 milliliters, what is the resulting dilution?
17. 0.25 milliliters is diluted to 20 ml. The resulting dilution is:
    a. 1/20
    b. 1/80
    c. 1/60
    d. 1/40
18. 50 milliliters of H_2SO_4 (specific gravity [sp. gr.] 1.86, 96% assay) is in a total volume of 300 ml. Express as a dilution (expressed as 1 to something).

Calculations involving one dilution—volume

19. A total of 400 ml of a 1/4 dilution is to be prepared. How much of the concentrated solution is to be used?

20. How much 1/10 solution can be made from 5 ml of concentrated solution?
21. How would you make 300 ml of a 2/5 dilution of alcohol?
22. How much serum is present in 25 ml of a 1/5 dilution?
23. Three milliliters of urine make how much of a 2/6 dilution?
24. You have 100 milliliters of a 1/50 dilution of serum in saline. How much serum is present in that 100 milliliters?
25. You want to make 30 milliliters of a 1/500 dilution of urine in water. How much diluent will it take?

Calculations involving one dilution—concentration

26. If 1 milliliter of a 1/4 dilution is further diluted by adding to it 1.5 milliliters of distilled water, the final dilution is:
    a. 1/5
    b. 1/6
    c. 1/10
    d. 1/25
    e. None of these
27. A 1/6 dilution is further diluted by adding 2.5 milliliters of water to 1 ml of the original dilution. What is the concentration of the second solution?
28. If 2 milliliters of a 1/5 dilution is further diluted by adding to it 3.0 ml of distilled water, what would be the final concentration of the resulting solution?
29. How would you dilute a 43% aqueous solution 1/5? What is the concentration of the resulting solution?
30. A 7% solution is diluted 1/100. What is the final concentration?
31. A 20% solution is diluted 1/200. What is the volume and concentration of the final solution?
32. A 20N solution is diluted 1/60. What is the volume and concentration of the final solution?
33. A solution of 10 ml/100 ml is diluted 1/10. What is the final concentration?
34. A stock glucose standard has a concentration of 1,000 mg/dl. A 1/5 dilution of this standard is made. What would be the concentration of the final solution?
35. A glucose standard contains 5 mg/ml of glucose. A 1/10 dilution of this standard would contain how much glucose per milliliter?
36. A glucose standard contains 10 mg/dl of glucose. A 1/50 dilution of this standard would contain how much glucose per milliliter?

Total volume before and after transfer

37. You are asked to make the following dilutions of serum: 2/10, 3/25, and 4/50. If you make them independently and as the dilutions state, what volume would you have of each dilution?
38. If you were asked to dilute a serum sample 2/10, redilute 3/25, and again 4/50, and you made them as stated, what volume would you have of each dilution before and after transfer?
39. If you were asked to dilute a serum sample 2/10, redilute 3/25, and again 4/50, and you were asked to make 100 ml of each dilution, what volume would you have of each dilution before and after transfer?

Tube dilution

40. What would be the tube dilution of each tube in question 37?
41. What would be the tube dilution of each tube in question 38?
42. What would be the tube dilution of each tube in question 39?

Solution dilution

43. What would be the solution dilution of each tube in question 37?
44. What would be the solution dilution of each tube in question 38?
45. What would be the solution dilution of each tube in question 39?
46. Give the solution dilution of each tube in the following:
    a. A 1/3 dilution is diluted 1/6 and again 1/10.
    b. A 4% solution is diluted 2/5, 1/3, and again 1/8.
    c. A 3N solution is diluted 1/4, 1/4, and again 1/4.
47. A 1/10 dilution is diluted 1/100 and again 1/50. What is the final solution dilution?

Substance concentration

48. A 1/10 dilution is diluted 1/5, 1/2, and then 5/10. What is the final concentration?
49. A 5% solution is diluted 1/20 and then rediluted 1/100. What is the final concentration?
50. A 4.1% solution is diluted 1/10 and rediluted 1/25. What is the concentration of the final solution? What is the volume of the final solution?
51. A 4M solution is diluted 1/10, 1/5, and again 4/6. What is the concentration of the final solution?
52. A 6N solution is diluted 1/10, rediluted 1/5, and that solution rediluted 5/50. What is the volume and concentration of the final solution?
53. A 1N solution of NaOH is diluted 4/20, then rediluted 1/50. What is the final normality?
54. A solution containing 10 mg/30 ml is diluted 1/10 and again 1/5. What is the volume of the final solution? What is the concentration of the final solution?
55. A solution contains 45 g/L. It is diluted 1/10 and rediluted 1/10. What is the concentration of the final solution?
56. Give the final volume and concentration of each of the following:
    a. A 1/3 dilution of a substance is diluted 1/6 and again 1/5.
    b. A solution with 80 mg/dl is diluted 1/50.
    c. A 6N solution is diluted 2/10, rediluted 1/3, and again 4/6.
    d. A solution that contains 20 mg in 50 ml is diluted 1/4 and again 3/10.
57. Give the final volume and concentration of each of the following:
    a. A 4M solution is diluted 2/7 and again 6/9.
    b. A 1/5 dilution is rediluted 1/3, 5/15, and 4/9.
    c. A solution with a 300 mg/dl concentration is diluted 20/500.
58. Sixty grams of $CuSO_4$ are dissolved and diluted to 800 ml. This solution is diluted 1/5 and then rediluted 3/100. How many grams of $CuSO_4$ are present in 1 liter of the final solution?
59. Thirty-five grams of NaCl are dissolved and diluted to 750 ml. This solution is diluted 1/10 and rediluted 5/25. How many grams of $CuSO_4$ are present in 1 liter of the final solution?

Amount of original solution present

60. One milliliter of serum is added to a tube containing 9 ml of saline; 1 ml of the resulting solution is diluted 1/50. How much serum is there in the final solution?
61. Five milliliters of urine is diluted up to 100 ml. One milliliter of this solution is diluted 1/10. What is the actual volume of urine in the final solution?
62. If one were asked to take 8.5N NaOH, dilute it 1/10 and redilute it 2/5, and again 4/25:
    a. Exactly what procedure should be followed?
    b. What would be the volume of the final solution?
    c. What would be the concentration of the final solution?
    d. How much 8.5N NaOH would actually be present in the final solution?

63. A 10% solution is diluted 1/10, 1/5, and again 2/6. Give the following:
   a. The concentration of the final solution
   b. The total volume of the final solution present
   c. The volume of 10% solution present in the final solution
64. Five milliliters of 5% alcohol is added to 5 ml of urine. Two milliliters of this solution is diluted to 50 ml with water, and 5 ml of this is used for analysis. How many milliliters of urine are in the analysis sample?
65. You were asked to take 6N NaOH, dilute it 1/5, redilute it 2/3, and again 3/15.
   a. Exactly what would you do?
   b. What would be the volume of the final solution?
   c. What would be the concentration of the final solution?
   d. How much of the original 6N NaOH would actually be present in the final solution?
66. Four milliliters of blood are diluted with 16 ml of water, and 3 ml of this solution is diluted to a final volume of 12 ml with diluent. Give the following:
   a. The final volume of solution
   b. The final concentration of the solution
   c. How much blood is present in the final solution
   d. How much blood is present in 1 ml of the final solution
67. Two milliliters of serum is diluted to 25 ml. One milliliter of this solution is diluted 4/20. How much serum is present in the final solution?

Dilutions with prescribed concentrations and/or volumes

68. You need 50 milliliters of an HCl solution that is 0.02N. You have on hand a 0.5N solution. How would you prepare this solution to give the desired volume and concentration?
69. A 10/1,000 stock solution of boric acid is available, and 30 ounces of a 1/250 solution are needed. How would you make the desired solution?
70. You have a 50/1,000 stock solution of boric acid, and you need 30 ounces of a 1/500 solution. How would you prepare the desired volume and concentration?
71. You need 12 ounces of a 35% solution of phenylephrine. You have a 20% solution. How do you prepare the needed solution?
72. You need 200 ml of a 0.5% solution of iodine. You have a 10% solution. How would you prepare the desired quantity of 0.5% solution?
73. You have a stock standard with a stated concentration of 1000 mg/dl. How would you prepare 50 ml of a 0.5 mg/dl working standard?
74. How would you dilute a solution that contained 20 mg/100 ml so as to obtain a solution with a concentration of 1 mg/50 ml?
75. A stock glucose standard contains 200 grams of glucose/L. What dilution is necessary to prepare a working standard containing 5 mg/100 ml?
   a. 1/500   d. 1/100
   b. 1/1,000   e. 1/400
   c. 1/4,000

Serial dilutions

76. You are given a series of 10 tubes, each of which contains 4 ml of diluent. One milliliter of fluid is added to the first tube, and a dilution using 0.5 ml is carried out in the remaining tubes. What is the dilution of the fluid in tube 5? In tube 10?

77. You are given a series of 10 tubes, each of which contains 5 ml of diluent. To the first tube is added 1 ml of serum, and a serial dilution using 1 ml is carried out in the remaining tubes. What is the serum concentration in tubes 4 and 8?

78. Use the following procedure to make a serial dilution of the patient's serum:
    a. Place 11 tubes in a rack.
    b. Pipette 1.5 ml of saline into the first tube.
    c. Pipette 1 ml of saline into each of the remaining tubes.
    d. Add 0.5 ml of the test serum into the first tube.
    e. Transfer 1.0 ml to the second tube.
    f. Continue transferring 1 ml to the remaining tubes.
    Give for each tube:
    a. Tube dilution
    b. Solution dilution
    c. Substance concentration

79. You have a series of 5 tubes. In the first is placed 5 ml of urine, in the second is placed 9 ml of water, and in the third, fourth, and fifth tubes is placed 5 ml of water. One milliliter of urine is added to tube 2, and 5 ml is carried down to each of tubes 3, 4, and 5. What is the tube dilution in tube 4, and how much urine is present before transfer? What is the tube dilution in tube 1?

80. You are given a series of 10 tubes, each of which contains 4.5 ml of diluent. Half a milliliter of fluid is added to the first tube, and a serial dilution using 1 ml is carried out in the remaining tubes. For each tube give the following:
    a. Total volume in each tube after transfer
    b. Tube dilution
    c. Solution dilution
    d. Amount of specimen in each tube before transfer
    e. Amount of specimen in each tube after transfer

81. You are given a series of 10 tubes, each of which contains 4 milliliters of diluent. To the first tube is added 0.5 ml of serum, and a serial dilution using 1 ml is carried out in the remaining tubes. What is the serum concentration as a dilution, and what is the serum volume in tubes 4 and 8 before transfer?

82. You are given a series of 10 tubes. In the first is placed 9 milliliters of saline. In each of the others is placed 5 ml of saline. One milliliter of serum is added to the first tube. Five milliliters from this tube are transferred to the second tube, and 5 ml are transferred throughout the remaining tubes. Discard the last 5 ml transferred. Give the following:
    a. The tube dilution for tubes 1 and 6
    b. The solution dilution for tubes 1, 4, and 7
    c. The amount of serum actually present in tube 3 after transfer
    d. The serum volume and solution dilution of the last tube after transfer

83. Set up a series of 10 tubes. Into the first tube place 4 milliliters of saline. In tubes 2 through 10, place 2 ml of saline. To the first tube add 1 ml of serum. Transfer 2 ml from tube 1 to tube 2 and do the same throughout the remaining tubes. Discard the last 2 ml transferred. Give the following:
    a. The tube dilution in tubes 1, 3, and 5.
    b. The solution dilution in tubes 1, 2, and 7.
    c. The total volume and solution dilution in tube 10 before transfer
    d. The amount or volume of serum in tube 6 before transfer and after transfer

84. Into a series of six tubes, place 0.9 milliliters of saline in the first tube and 0.5 ml of saline into each of the remaining tubes. Add 0.1 ml of serum to the first tube; mix and carry down

0.5 ml to each succeeding tube. Discard the last 0.5 ml. To each tube add 0.5 ml of sheep blood cells. Give the following:

a. The tube dilution of each tube before the addition of sheep cells
b. The solution dilution of each tube before the addition of sheep cells
c. The amount of serum present in each tube after transfer
d. The solution dilution after the addition of sheep cells

Dilution correction factor

85. Give the dilution factor for the following dilutions:

a. 1/50   d. 1/60
b. 3/45   e. 4/250
c. 2/200   f. 1/3,000

86. You are doing a procedure that calls for 5 ml of undiluted urine. You use 3 ml of a 1/5 dilution of urine instead. The answer obtained is 50 mg/dl. What should be reported?

87. A test procedure calls for 5 ml of undiluted specimen. Two milliliters of a 1/50 dilution is used. The answer obtained is 30 mg/dl. What should be reported?

88. If the result of a bilirubin determination was 4.1 mg/dl and the original specimen had been diluted 1/5, what is the result to be reported?

89. If the result in a serum glucose determination was 56 mg/dl and the original specimen had been diluted 1/10, what is the result to be reported?

90. If the result of a glucose determination was 80 mg/dl and the original specimen had been diluted 1/2 and rediluted 1/10, what is the result to be reported?

91. A procedure indicates that color development should be carried out on a 5-ml aliquot of 1/20 dilution of serum. Because of a laboratory accident, only 4 ml of the well-mixed 1/20 dilution is available for analysis. One milliliter of water is added to the 4 ml of the 1/20 dilution to obtain a volume of 5 ml. This unknown gave an answer of 10 mg/dl. The concentration of the unknown is:

a. 4.0 mg/dl
b. 8.0 mg/dl
c. 12.5 mg/dl
d. 16.0 mg/dl
e. 25.0 mg/dl

92. You are running a urine potassium. The directions say to make a 1/10 dilution and run as serum. Instead you make a 1/50 dilution. The procedure calls for a 0.5 ml sample, but by mistake you use 0.3 ml. The reading is 20 mEq/L. What should be reported?

Making large dilutions

93. Make a 1/100,000 dilution of serum in saline using three tubes or less, but never having more than 100 milliliters total volume in any one tube.

94. How would you make 100 ml of a 1/10,000 dilution of serum in saline if you only had 0.5 ml of serum and the volumetric flasks on hand were 10-ml, 25-ml, 50-ml, and 100-ml sizes?

95. Make the following dilutions using three containers or less and never having more than 100 ml for the total volume.

a. 1/10,000
b. 3/50,000
c. 1/1,000,000
d. 2/600,000

6

Solutions

EDUCATIONAL OBJECTIVES

To have successfully learned the material in this chapter, the student should be able to do the following properly:

- Describe the major types of solutions.
- Describe the types and components of solutions in accepted nomenclature.
- Differentiate among the types of concentration expression used in describing biological solutions.
- Calculate the concentration of a solution, and express this concentration in several ways.
- Calculate the amount of one solution needed to make a solution of lesser concentration.
- Calculate the concentration of a solution resulting from a mixture of two solutions.
- Accommodate various hydrates of a solute in the preparation of solutions of given concentrations.
- Differentiate among parts and percent concentration described in terms of weight per unit weight, weight per unit volume, and volume per unit volume.
- Calculate the molarity of a solution that has a concentration expressed in other ways.
- Differentiate between molarity and molality, and describe where these expressions are used in the chemical or clinical laboratory.
- Determine the gram equivalent weight of ionic substances, and use this result to make a solution of given normality.
- Determine the mass of one osmole of a substance, and describe a procedure to produce a solution of given osmolarity and volume.
- Determine the osmolarity of a solution from its freezing-point depression.
- Determine the concentration of a solution from its density.
- Convert concentration expressions from one form to others.

SECTION 6.1 INTRODUCTION

Solutions are mixtures of substances. The substances in a solution are not in chemical combination with one another, although chemical reactions can occur in solutions. However, the phases of solutions are not combined chemically one with another.

Most solutions can be thought of as having two parts or phases, the dispersed phase and the dispersing phase. The dispersed phase is the substance that is dissolved. This is often called the **solute.** The dispersing phase is the substance that dissolves the other. This material is called the **solvent.** In some solutions the distinction between the solvent and the solute becomes questionable. A one-to-one solution of alcohol in water is an example of such a solution. In such cases the worker will do well not to spend much mental energy trying to designate one as the solvent and the other as the solute.

Solutions found in biology and clinical systems are one of two types, true or colloid. In **true solutions** the particles of the solution are less than 1 nanometer in size. They are usually thought of as being dispersed at the atomic or molecular level. **Colloidal solutions** have solute particles that are between 1 and 200 nanometers in size. Such particles are usually considered to be aggregations of many molecules or atoms. One common exception to this in biology is the large molecules of nucleic acids, proteins, and the other macromolecules of protoplasm. These large molecules confer the properties of colloids on the mixture. Mixtures of materials in which the particles are larger than 200 nanometers are called **suspensions.** These mixtures usually separate unless agitated. The true solutions and colloids remain mixed without any agitation.

Not all substances form solutions with one another. Substances that *will* form solutions are said to be **miscible;** those that *will not* form solutions are said to be **immiscible** with one another. The degree of miscibility varies with environmental factors such as temperature, pressure, and other dissolved materials.

When a solution contains the maximum amount of solute possible at a particular temperature and pressure, the solution is said to be **saturated.** Under some conditions a solution may contain more solute than the normal saturation amount. In such cases the solution is **supersaturated.** Such solutions normally lose the excess solute easily.

Solutions are either uniform or are becoming uniform; that is, all parts of one solution contain equal proportions of all substances involved, or this situation is developing. This is due to the principle of diffusion. **Diffusion** is the physical principle that substances in solution have a tendency to move from regions of their greater concentration to regions of their lesser concentration. All substances in a solution diffuse at their own rates; that is, both solvents and solutes diffuse through a solution independently of each other.

In dealing with solutions, it soon becomes important to know, or be able to measure, the relative amounts of the substances in solution. These relative amounts are referred to as concentration. Concentration may be measured in many ways. In all cases, **concentration** refers to the amount of one substance relative to the amounts of the other substances in the solution. Concentration values are not simply volumes or masses alone, but they always exist in relation to volumes or masses of the other parts of the solution. In some methods of stating concentration values, the amount or proportion of one or more parts of the solution may not be stated but may be implied by the terminology of the concentration statement.

Several methods of stating and manipulating concentration values are discussed in detail in this chapter.

SECTION 6.2 EXPRESSIONS OF CONCENTRATION

There are many ways of expressing the concentration of a solution. All of these express or imply an amount of one ingredient of a mixture relative to an amount of another ingredient. With solutions, this usually involves an amount of solute relative to an amount of solvent. The following are common expressions of solution concentration used in laboratories. Detailed discussions of calculations involving solutions are in later sections of this chapter.

Parts

The term *parts* is sometimes used in descriptions of procedures involving solutions. The use of this term allows discussion of the relationships in a procedure without being limited to any specific unit of measure. Any concentration expression involves a number of parts of one thing relative to a given number of parts of another in the mixture. However, the simple use of *parts* in a description is nebulous and prone to confusion and error. This manner of concentration expression is recommended only for describing solutions in the most general terms and not in specific procedures for solution preparation or description. Use care with this term.

The same unit of measure should be inferred throughout any procedure using parts. For example, if a procedure states, "Mix one part A with two parts B," this can mean mix 1 gram of A with 2 grams of B, or 3 liters of A with 6 liters of B, or 10 pounds of A with 20 pounds of B. In all cases there are twice as many of the same units of B as A. The worker should fully understand the meaning of any expression using parts.

There are expressions of parts concentration in which even the word parts is omitted. Such expressions as *one-to-one, 50-50,* and *two-to-three* indicate situations in which the term *parts* is meant to be understood. Again, approach any use of the term *parts* with caution. Make sure you understand the context in which it is used.

Weight per Unit Weight

In the expression of a solution as weight per unit weight (w/w), the term *weight* really refers to mass. In physics, **mass** is an amount of something, whereas **weight** is the force of gravity on something. This is a picky point in the context of the clinical laboratory. The two terms may be used interchangeably as long as the measurements are made on Earth. Mass is used more often in this context. The worker needs to be aware of this and get on with the work at hand.

Weight per unit weight as an expression of concentration means that there is a number of grams (or other unit of mass) of solute per a given number of grams (or other unit of mass) of solvent. This is the most accurate method of concentration expression. Mass does not vary with temperature or other environmental factors. This expression is used for mixtures involving an amount of solid in an amount of solid or where very precise measurements of concentration are needed.

Weight per Unit Volume

Weight per unit volume (w/v) is the most commonly used expression of concentration in laboratory work. It describes a solution as a number of units of mass of a solute per some number of unit of volume of solvent or solution. It is convenient for work involving the mixing of a solid in a liquid, and it is acceptably accurate within small variations of temperature.

Volume per Unit Volume

Volume per unit volume (v/v) is usually used in the preparation of solutions of a liquid in a liquid. This is the least accurate method to use in expressing concentration, because the volume of both phases of the solution can vary with temperature change. Care should be used to ensure that the amount of variation is acceptable for the particular use of the solution.

Percent

As discussed in Chapter 1, pp. 18-19, **percent** refers to parts per 100. Percent concentration, used correctly, refers to a number of parts in 100 parts of solution. It is used to express concentration in terms of weight per unit weight, weight per unit volume, and volume per unit volume. This is a very flexible form of concentration expression. Concentration values expressed in some manner to refer to parts per 100 are usually considered to be percent concentration values.

Molarity

Molarity is defined as the number of moles of solute per liter of solution. A **mole** is the number of grams of a substance equal to its atomic or molecular weight. This is a weight per unit volume method of expressing concentration that is much used in chemistry laboratories as a way to determine the relative number of reacting atoms and molecules in a solution.

Molality

A more *precise* but less convenient concentration expression similar to molarity is molality. **Molality** is defined as the number of moles of solute per kilogram of solvent. Molality is an expression of concentration in terms of weight per unit weight, and because of this the relative amounts of the components of a molal solution do not change with variations in temperature or pressure.

Normality

Normality is defined as the number of equivalent weights per liter of solution. An **equivalent weight** is defined as that amount of an element or compound that will combine with or replace 1 mole of hydrogen in a chemical reaction. Normality expresses concentration in terms of weight per unit volume.

Osmolarity

Another expression of weight per unit volume is **osmolarity.** This is defined as the number of osmoles of solute per liter of solution. An **osmole** is the amount of a substance that will produce 1 mole of particles having osmotic activity. One osmole of any substance is equal to 1 gram molecular weight (1 mole) of the substance divided by the number of particles formed by the dissociation of the molecules of the substance.

Density

Density is defined as the amount of matter per unit volume of a substance. This is a property of all substances, not just solutions. **Specific gravity** is an expression of density. It is defined as the ratio between the mass of a substance relative to the mass of an equal volume of water.

$$\text{Specific gravity} = \frac{\text{mass of substance}}{\text{mass of equal volume of water}}$$

SECTION 6.3 SOLUTION CALCULATIONS
General Considerations

Solution calculations may or may not involve a change in the concentration of a solution. Those calculations that do not involve a change in the concentration may be done to determine the amount of solute and solvent needed to make a solution or to determine the amount of the components of an existing solution. They are also used to determine the concentration of a solution and to change one expression of concentration to another. Calculations that do involve a change in a solution concentration are used to determine the amount of one solution needed to make another. These two kinds of calculations can all be done using one of three procedures:

1. Ratio and proportion
2. $V_1 \times C_1 = V_2 \times C_2$
3. Use of a specific formula

As with any calculation, one should endeavor to understand the relationship of each step of solution calculations to the entire problem and how the answers relate to the procedure for which they are calculated.

Calculations Not Changing Concentration

The ratio and proportion procedure is most useful for solution calculations in which the concentration is not changed.

Several of the following examples use percent concentration because of the common use of this method in laboratories. Detailed explanation of this expression of concentration is given later in this chapter.

EXAMPLE 6-1: A procedure calls for a mixture of 1 part liquid soap to 5 parts water, v/v. How much soap would need to be added to 250 ml of water?

Since there is not a change in concentration here, the ratio and proportion procedure can easily be used to make this calculation.

$$\frac{1 \text{ part soap}}{5 \text{ parts water}} = \frac{x \text{ ml soap}}{250 \text{ ml water}}$$

$$5x = 250$$

$$x = \frac{250}{5}$$

$$x = 50 \text{ ml soap}$$

Mix 50 ml of liquid soap with 250 ml of water to make a mixture with 1 part soap to 5 parts water.

Because this solution was made by mixing volumes of two liquids, the precision of the proportions is crude. Be sure this is acceptable for the purpose of the mixture.

EXAMPLE 6-2: Make 500 g of a 10%$^{w/w}$ NaCl aqueous solution.

Remember that a percentage indicates a number of parts of something in 100 parts of the mixture. Hence, to prepare a 10% solution, mix 10 g of NaCl with 90 g of water to make a total of 100 g of the 10%$^{w/w}$ salt solution. If more or less total solution is desired, then the mass of both constituent substances needs to be adjusted.

Since 500 g of solution is needed, set up the following ratio and proportion.

$$\frac{10 \text{ g NaCl}}{100 \text{ g H}_2\text{O}} = \frac{x \text{ g NaCl}}{500 \text{ g H}_2\text{O}}$$

$$100x = 10 \times 500$$

$$x = \frac{5,000}{100}$$

$$x = 50 \text{ g NaCl}$$

Since this is a weight per unit weight solution, one would mix 50 g of NaCl with 450 g, not milliliters, of water. The result would be 500 g of 10%$^{w/w}$ NaCl in water.

The weight per unit weight method of determining concentration allows precision, but it is tedious to use. Weight per unit volume is more commonly used in laboratories.

EXAMPLE 6-3: A solution contains 24 g of solute in 300 ml of solution. What is the percent concentration?

The problem states that there are 24 g of solute per 300 ml of solution. Percent concentration is the number of grams of solute per 100 ml of solution. Arrange this information in a ratio and proportion setup.

$$\frac{24 \text{ g}}{300 \text{ ml}} = \frac{x \text{ g}}{100 \text{ ml}}$$

$$300x = 2,400$$

$$x = 8 \text{ g}$$

The solution has a concentration of 8%$^{w/v}$.

EXAMPLE 6-4: How much of a 20%$^{w/v}$ NaCl solution could be made from 50 g of NaCl?

A 20%$^{w/v}$ solution contains 20 g of solute per 100 ml of solution. The problem states that 50 g of solute are to be used.

$$\frac{20 \text{ g}}{100 \text{ ml}} = \frac{50 \text{ g}}{x \text{ ml}}$$

$$20x = 5,000$$

$$x = 250 \text{ ml}$$

Therefore 50 g of NaCl will make 250 ml of 20%$^{w/v}$ NaCl solution.

Calculations Changing Concentration

Often, a solution is made by adding some additional solvent to an existing solution. This results in a new solution having a lesser concentration of solute than the original solution. The relationship between the volume and concentrations of these two solutions can be expressed as:

> The volume of one solution times the concentration of that solution equals the volume of the second solution times the concentration of the second solution.

This relationship is shown by the formula:

$$V_1 \times C_1 = V_2 \times C_2$$

This is called an *inverse* relationship. It is not a ratio and proportion. When the volume of a solution is increased by adding solvent, the amount of the solute remains the same. The same amount of solute is in a greater volume of solution; hence, the concentration of the solute is less. When an amount of one phase of a solution is added to the solution, the concentration of the other phase is decreased. This is an important relationship to understand in working with solutions.

EXAMPLE 6-5: There are 0.8 g of sugar in 20 ml of a 4% sugar solution. How much of a 2% solution can be made with this 20 ml of solution?

Here, one solution is being made from another by adding additional water to the original solution. This results in a change in concentration. The $V_1 \times C_1 = V_2 \times C_2$ method can be used to determine the volume of the second solution. Place all information known about one of the solutions on one side of the equation and the information about the other solution on the other side of the equation.

$$\overbrace{V_1 \times C_1}^{\text{Solution 1}} = \overbrace{V_2 \times C_2}^{\text{Solution 2}}$$

$$20 \text{ ml} \times 4\% = x \text{ ml} \times 2\%$$

$$x = \frac{20 \times 4}{2}$$

$$x = \frac{80}{2}$$

$$x = 40 \text{ ml}$$

Using this method it is found that 20 ml of a 4% solution of sugar will make 40 ml of a 2% solution.

As with ratio and proportion, one needs to know three of the four values to determine the fourth in the $V_1 \times C_1 = V_2 \times C_2$ procedure.

Both solutions contain the same amount of solute but different amounts of solvent. Both solutions contain 0.8 grams of sugar, but the second solution has 20 more milliliters of water. Hence, the concentration of sugar in the second solution is less than that of the first. Also, note that the units of volume and mass and the manner of expressing concentration are the same in both solutions. This is necessary for a correct result. Any proper units of mass or weight, volume, or expression of concentration may be used as long as their use is consistent within one calculation.

EXAMPLE 6-6: How much 30% alcohol is required to make 100 ml of a 3% solution?

Here, one solution is being made from another. The 30% solution is being used to make the 3% solution. The concentration is to be changed by adding a volume of water to an amount of the more concentrated solution. Since the concentration is being changed, the problem cannot be solved with the ratio and proportion procedure. Use the $V_1 \times C_1 = V_2 \times C_2$ procedure.

$$\overbrace{\text{Solution 1}} \quad \overbrace{\text{Solution 2}}$$
$$V_1 \times C_1 = V_2 \times C_2$$
$$100 \text{ ml} \times 3\% = x \text{ ml} \times 30\%$$

Solve for x, in this case the volume of the 30% solution needed to make 100 ml of the 3% solution.

$$30x = 100 \times 3$$
$$x = \frac{100 \times 3}{30}$$
$$x = 10 \text{ ml}$$

Therefore 100 ml of a 3% solution are equivalent to 10 ml of a 30% solution, or if 10 ml of a 30% solution were diluted up to 100 ml, the result would be 100 ml of a 3% solution.

$$(10 \text{ ml of } 30\% \uparrow 100 \text{ ml} \rightarrow 100 \text{ ml of } 3\%)$$

If all of these values are placed in the $V_1 \times C_1 = V_2 \times C_2$ formula, one can see that this is an equality.

$$\overbrace{\text{Solution 1}} \quad \overbrace{\text{Solution 2}}$$
$$V_1 \times C_1 = V_2 \times C_2$$
$$100 \text{ ml} \times 3\% = 10 \text{ ml} \times 30\%$$
$$300 = 300$$

Knowing what an answer means and what to do with it is often the most difficult part of solving problems. Mathematics may be used to produce an answer that is impossible to use in a procedure. For this reason, write out answers in a complete form until the procedure becomes familiar. Understand all of the answer before proceeding.

EXAMPLE 6-7: Ten milliliters of a 6% solution will make how many milliliters of a 10% solution?

$$V_1 \times C_1 = V_2 \times C_2$$
$$10 \text{ ml} \times 6\% = x \text{ ml} \times 10\%$$
$$10x = 60$$
$$x = 6 \text{ ml}$$
$$10 \text{ ml of } 6\% \uparrow 6 \text{ ml} \rightarrow 6 \text{ ml of } 10\%$$

The above calculation produced an answer of 6 milliliters. However, it is impossible to use this result in the procedure. Ten milliliters cannot be diluted *up to* 6 milliliters. The answer to Example 6-7 is "none," since you cannot make a stronger solution from a weaker one. Mathematics can be used to produce nonsensical results if you start with nonsense.

To use the formula, $V_1 \times C_1 = V_2 \times C_2$, the following factors must be considered:
1. The concentration must change. In other words, the solution is different.
2. The concentration expression must be in the same units on both sides of the equation.

3. The volume must be in the same units on both sides of the equation.
4. The two known pieces of information for one solution go on one side of the equation.
5. The other side is filled in appropriately, and the unknown is solved.

Mixed Solutions

> When two or more solutions are mixed together, the product of the volume times the concentration of the final solution is equal to the sum of the products of the volume times the concentration of the solutions that were mixed together.

This can be expressed by the formula:

$$(V_1 \times C_1) + (V_2 \times C_2) + (V_3 \times C_3) \ldots = V_F \times C_F$$

This is a modified $V_1 \times C_1 = V_2 \times C_2$ procedure.

To use this formula fill in the known values and solve for the unknown. The final volume (V_F) will be the sum of the volumes of the solutions mixed together. Remember that all solutions must use the same units of volume and concentration.

EXAMPLE 6-8: What will be the concentration resulting from mixing 20 ml of a 5% NaCl solution with 30 ml of a 10% NaCl solution?

The total volume of these two solutions is 50 ml.

Solve for the final concentration using the above formula.

$$(V_1 \times C_1) + (V_2 \times C_2) = (V_F \times C_F)$$
$$(20 \text{ ml} \times 5\%) + (30 \text{ ml} \times 10\%) = (50 \text{ ml} \times x\%)$$
$$100 + 300 = 50x$$
$$x = \frac{400}{50}$$
$$x = 8\%$$

The concentration of the final solution is 8%.

EXAMPLE 6-9: Ten milliliters of a 2% sugar solution was mixed with 15 ml of a sugar solution of unknown concentration to produce 25 ml of a 5% sugar solution. What was the concentration of the second solution?

Solve for the concentration of the second solution using the formula:

$$(V_1 \times C_1) + (V_2 \times C_2) = (V_F \times C_F)$$
$$(10 \text{ ml} \times 2\%) + (15 \text{ ml} \times x\%) = (25 \text{ ml} \times 5\%)$$
$$20 + 15x = 125$$
$$15x = 125 - 20$$
$$x = \frac{105}{15}$$
$$x = 7\%$$

The concentration of the second solution is 7%.

Hydrates

The molecules of some salts can chemically combine with one or more molecules of water to form **hydrates.** These water molecules must be considered when determining the amount of salt to be used in the preparation of a solution. The water molecules do not have to be present in the molecule, and if not, the salt is said to be the **anhydrous** form. Molecules with one water molecule per molecule of salt are called **monohydrates;** two molecules of water per molecule of salt, **dihydrates;** three molecules, **trihydrates;** and so on.

If a solution is to be made with a salt that has more than one form of hydration, directions for preparing the solution should specify the hydration intended. If this information is not given, assume the most common form to be the one required.

Often a prescribed hydrate of a salt is not readily available, but some other form is. One needs to be able to determine how much of the form available is equivalent to the quantity of the form prescribed. To do this, one must have a basis of comparison. The molecular weights of the substances involved may be used.

The molecular weight of a hydrate can be found in a reference such as the *Handbook of Chemistry and Physics* (1995), or it can be calculated by adding the atomic weights of the constituent atoms of the molecules, including the atoms of hydrogen and oxygen of the water. Hence, the ratio between equivalent amounts of the anhydrous form and the hydrates of a salt is the ratio of the molecular weights of the forms.

EXAMPLE 6-10: A procedure states, "Make a 10% solution of $CuSO_4$." Only $CuSO_4 \cdot H_2O$ is available.

$$10\% = 10 \text{ g/100 ml}$$

How much of the monohydrate is equivalent to the 10 g of the anhydrous form called for in the procedure?

Determine the molecular weight of each form of cupric sulfate.

	$CuSO_4$				$CuSO_4 \cdot H_2O$		
Element	Atomic Weight	Number in Molecule	Weight of Element	Element	Atomic Weight	Number in Molecule	Weight of Element
Cu	64	1	64	Cu	64	1	64
S	32	1	32	S	32	1	32
O	16	4	64	O	16	4	64
	Molecular weight of $CuSO_4$ = 160			H	1	2	2
				O	16	1	16
				Molecular weight of $CuSO_4 \cdot H_2O$ = 178			

The molecular weight of $CuSO_4$ is 160, and the molecular weight of $CuSO_4 \cdot H_2O$ is 178.

$$\frac{160 \text{ anhydrous}}{178 \text{ monohydrate}}$$

Ten grams of anhydrous $CuSO_4$ equal x grams of the monohydrate.

$$\frac{160 \text{ anhydrous}}{178 \text{ monohydrate}} = \frac{10 \text{ g anhydrous}}{x \text{ g monohydrate}}$$

$$\frac{160}{178} = \frac{10}{x}$$

$$160x = 178 \times 10$$

$$x = \frac{1,780}{160}$$

$$x = 11.125 \text{ g } CuSO_4 \cdot H_2O$$

If 11.125 g of the monohydrate ($CuSO_4 \cdot H_2O$) were diluted up to 100 ml, the result would be 11.13% monohydrate $CuSO_4$ solution, but this would be equivalent to the 10% anhydrous $CuSO_4$ solution originally required.

When working with compounds that have more than one hydration, be sure the correct amount is used. Remember the relationship among the amounts of the different hydrations of a compound is the ratio of their molecular weights. Be sure this relationship is thoroughly understood before using different hydrations of compounds in solutions.

SECTION 6.4 PARTS CALCULATIONS

As stated in Section 6.2, the term **parts** is a nonspecific method of stating a concentration. Also, remember that the use of parts as an expression of concentration is discouraged in laboratory work because of the strong possibility of confusion. However, the use of these kinds of expressions of concentration is still fairly common in most laboratories.

A unit of concentration occasionally encountered in laboratory work is **parts per million (ppm).** This unit refers to a number of parts of one substance in one million parts of the solution. Hence, 5 parts per million chlorine means that there are 5 grams of chlorine in one million grams of water or that there are 5 micrograms of chlorine in 1 gram of water, since 1 gram equals one million micrograms.

The term **parts per billion (ppb)** is used less often. This refers to a number of parts of solute in one billion parts of solution.

Fig. 6-1 may be used to convert parts per million to any of the concentrations listed and vice versa.

To use Fig. 6-1 to convert from parts per million to the other concentration units given in the center of the chart, multiply the number of parts per million to be changed by the factor above the concentration unit desired. The answer will be the number of desired concentration units.

EXAMPLE 6-11: Convert 500 ppm to grams per liter.

Locate grams per liter, g/L, on the chart and find above it the figure 0.001. Multiply 500 ppm by 0.001 to obtain the equivalent number of grams per liter.

$$500 \times 0.001 = 0.5$$

Hence, 500 ppm are equal to 0.5 g/L.

	grams				milligrams				micrograms			
×	1	0.001	0.0001	0.000001	1,000	1	0.1	0.001	1,000,000	1,000	100	1
ppm	↓ = g/10^6 ml ↓ ×	↓ = g/L ↓ ×	↓ = g/100 ml (%) ↓ ×	↓ = g/ml ↓ ×	↓ = mg/10^6 ml ↓ ×	↓ = mg/L ↓ ×	↓ = mg/100 ml (mg/dl) ↓ ×	↓ = mg/ml ↓ ×	↓ = μg/10^6 ml ↓ ×	↓ = μg/L ↓ ×	↓ = μg/100 ml ↓ ×	↓ = μg/ml ↓ ×
=	1	1,000	10,000	1,000,000	0.001	1	10	1,000	0.000001	0.001	0.01	1

Fig. 6-1. Parts per million conversion chart.

EXAMPLE 6-12: Convert 3 ppm to milligrams per milliliter (mg/ml), milligrams per 100 milliliters (mg/dl), and milligrams per liter (mg/L).

$$3 \times 0.001 = 0.003 \text{ mg/ml}$$

$$3 \times 0.1 = 0.3 \text{ mg/100 ml (This is also called mg/dl.)}$$

$$3 \times 1 = 3.0 \text{ mg/L}$$

If the conversion from parts per million is to be made to a concentration other than one listed on the chart, make the conversion first to a concentration given on the scale; then use ratio and proportion to convert to the desired concentration.

EXAMPLE 6-13: Convert 500 ppm to nanograms per milliliter.

First convert parts per million to a unit given on the scale, that is, milligrams per milliliter. From the scale find that ppm $\times$ 0.001 = mg/ml.

$$500 \times 0.001 = 0.5 \text{ mg/ml}$$

Now convert milligrams per milliliter to nanograms per milliliter using ratio and proportion or any other proper method.

$$1 \text{ mg} = 1,000,000 \text{ ng}$$

$$\frac{1 \text{ mg}}{1,000,000 \text{ ng}} = \frac{0.5 \text{ mg}}{x \text{ ng}}$$

$$x = 500,000$$

Hence, 500 ppm is equal to 0.5 mg/ml, which is equal to 500,000 ng/ml.

To convert a value in a concentration unit on the chart in Fig. 6.1 to parts per million, multiply the concentration by the factor given below the unit. The answer is the number of parts per million equivalent to the value.

EXAMPLE 6-14: Convert 0.5 g/L to parts per million.

Find grams per liter on the scale and note 1,000 below it. Multiply the number of grams per liter by 1,000 to obtain the equivalent parts per million.

$$0.5 \times 1,000 = 500$$

Hence, 0.5 g/L equals 500 ppm.

If the concentration to be converted to parts per million is one other than one given on the scale, convert the concentration to one of those on the scale by ratio and proportion and proceed as above.

EXAMPLE 6-15: Convert 5 g per 250 ml to parts per million.

1. First convert 5 g per 250 ml to an expression of concentration on the chart. This could be $g/10^6$ ml, g/L, g/100 ml, or g/ml.

Use a ratio and proportion to convert 5 g/250 ml to x g/10^6 ml.

$$\frac{5 \text{ g}}{250 \text{ ml}} = \frac{x \text{ g}}{1,000,000 \text{ ml}}$$

$$250x = 5,000,000$$

$$x = 20,000 \text{ g}$$

From the chart find that g/10^6 ml × 1 = x ppm.

$$20,000 \text{ g}/10^6 \text{ ml} \times 1 = 20,000 \text{ ppm}$$

Therefore 5 g per 250 ml is equal to 20,000 ppm.

2. One could solve this problem by first converting 5 g per 250 ml to g/L and then converting this to parts per million.

$$\frac{5 \text{ g}}{250 \text{ ml}} = \frac{x \text{ g}}{1,000 \text{ ml}}$$
$$250x = 5,000$$
$$x = 20 \text{ g/L}$$

From the chart find that g/L × 1,000 = ppm

Hence, 20 g/L times 1,000 is equal to 20,000 ppm.

Follow this same procedure in converting a concentration expression to any others on the chart to change the concentration to parts per million.

If preferred, the following formulas may be used to convert from a given concentration to parts per million and vice versa. As before, if the conversion answers are not in the exact concentrations desired, these may be found by ratio and proportion.

To convert from a concentration to ppm

When converting from a concentration to parts per million, the ppm is x.

To convert from ppm to another concentration

When converting from parts per million to another concentration, the number of units of the concentration is usually x. In this case, *the number of milliliters must be selected.*

$$\boxed{\frac{\text{g}}{x \text{ ml}} \times 1,000,000 = \text{ppm}}$$

Convert 0.5 g/L to parts per million.

$$\frac{0.5}{1,000} \times 1,000,000 = x$$
$$0.5 \times 1,000,000 = 1,000 \times x$$
$$1,000x = 500,000$$
$$x = 500$$

Hence, 0.5 g/L = 500 ppm.

Convert 500 ppm to g/1,000 ml.

$$\frac{x}{1,000} \times 1,000,000 = 500$$
$$1,000,000 \times x = 1,000 \times 500$$
$$1,000,000x = 500,000$$
$$x = 0.5$$

Hence, 500 ppm = 0.5 g/1,000 ml (0.5 g/L).

$$\boxed{\frac{\text{mg}}{x \text{ ml}} \times 1{,}000 = \text{ppm}}$$

Convert 0.3 mg/100 ml to parts per million.

$$\frac{0.3}{100} \times 1{,}000 = x$$

$$0.3 \times 1{,}000 = x \times 100$$

$$100x = 300$$

$$x = 3$$

Hence, 0.3 mg/100 ml = 3 ppm.

Convert 3 ppm to mg/100 ml.

$$\frac{x}{100} \times 1{,}000 = 3$$

$$x \times 1{,}000 = 3 \times 100$$

$$1{,}000x = 300$$

$$x = 0.3$$

Hence, 3 ppm = 0.3 mg/100 ml.

$$\boxed{\frac{\mu\text{g}}{x \text{ ml}} \times 1 = \text{ppm}}$$

Convert 6μg/10 ml to parts per million.

$$\frac{6}{10} \times 1 = x$$

$$10x = 6$$

$$x = 0.6$$

Hence, 6μg/10 ml = 0.6 ppm.

Convert 0.6 ppm to μg/10 ml.

$$\frac{x}{10} \times 1 = 0.6$$

$$1x = 10 \times 0.6$$

$$x = 6$$

Hence, 0.6 ppm = 6 μg/10 ml.

SECTION 6.5 PERCENT CONCENTRATION

As stated earlier, percent concentration is used with all three types of concentration statements: that is, weight per unit weight, weight per unit volume, and volume per unit volume.

The term **percent** refers to any expression of concentration or other relationship that involves parts per 100. Concentration values expressed in some manner to refer to parts per 100 are considered to be percent concentration values. Such values are usually expressed in a manner involving the term *percent* or the symbol (%).

Weight per Unit Weight (w/w)

Percent concentration involving weight per unit weight is not used very much in the clinical or biological laboratory. This method of expressing concentration is the most accurate type of percent concentration; therefore it is useful in the few incidences in which extraordinary precision is needed.

EXAMPLE 6-16: Make a $10\%^{\text{w/w}}$ NaCl solution.

To make this solution, mix 10 g of NaCl with 90 g of water. This makes a total of 100 g of the $10\%^{\text{w/w}}$ salt solution. If more or less of the total solution is desired, then the mass of each of the constituent substances has to be adjusted. Note that in a weight per unit weight solution, any measurement must be in units of weight or mass.

EXAMPLE 6-17: Make 500 g of a $10\%^{\text{w/w}}$ NaCl aqueous solution.

In this solution, 10% of the mass of the total solution must be NaCl.

$$\frac{10 \text{ g NaCl}}{100 \text{ g solution}} = \frac{x \text{ g NaCl}}{500 \text{ g solution}}$$

$$100x = 10 \times 500$$

$$x = \frac{10 \times 500}{100}$$

$$x = 50 \text{ g NaCl}$$

Hence, to make 500 g of this solution, one would mix 50 g of NaCl with 450 g of water. The total result would be 500 g, not milliliters, of $10\%^{w/w}$ NaCl in water.

Weight per Unit Volume (w/v)

The weight per unit volume system of percent concentration is a frequently used method in the clinical laboratory. This method is almost always used when a solid solute is mixed with a liquid solvent. In the clinical laboratory and related situations, any time a weight per unit volume solution is described by a number followed by a percent symbol and there is nothing between the number and the percent symbol, the concentration of the solution is expressed as *grams per 100 milliliters*.

It is important to note that in the usual method for making a weight per unit volume solution and most volume per unit volume solutions, the desired amount of solute is placed in a vessel, and enough solvent is added to make the desired total volume. The reason for this is that in some situations the volume of the solute plus the volume of the solvent does not always equal the desired volume of the final solution.

This procedure is often referred to as **diluting up** the solute or **bringing up** the solution to some volume. The symbol ↑ is used to mean this in working with solutions. Weight per unit volume is a true percent expression in all respects if the solvent is water. Remember that 1 milliliter of water has a mass of 1 gram under certain conditions; hence, 100 milliliters of water have a mass of 100 grams.

The system of grams per 100 milliliters is also used for other solvents even though a volume of 100 milliliters of these other solvents does not have a mass of 100 grams. In terms of weight per unit volume, this remains a true percent value, although it is not parts per 100 in terms of weight per unit weight.

EXAMPLE 6-18: Make 100 ml of a 10% aqueous solution of KOH.

Since this solution consists of an amount of a solid in an amount of liquid and the 10% expression is not modified in any way, this is understood to be a weight per unit volume solution. Hence, to make this solution, combine 10 g of KOH with enough water to make 100 ml of the final solution.

EXAMPLE 6-19: How much of a 0.9% NaCl solution can be made with 2.5 g of NaCl?

A 0.9% NaCl solution consists of 0.9 g of NaCl in 100 ml of solution. Hence, to determine the amount of solution containing 2.5 g of NaCl, set up a ratio and proportion as follows:

$$\frac{0.9 \text{ g}}{100 \text{ ml}} = \frac{2.5 \text{ g}}{x \text{ ml}}$$

$$0.9x = 100 \times 2.5$$

$$x = 278 \text{ ml}$$

Hence, 2.5 g of NaCl will make 287 ml of 0.9% NaCl.

Weight per unit volume procedures are often used in making solutions that have liquid solutes. In such cases the notation of the concentration value indicates weight per unit volume in some manner, such as $10\%^{w/v}$ HCl, 10 g% HCl, or 10 mg/dl HCl.

Volume per Unit Volume (v/v)

In most laboratory situations when a solution has a liquid solute in a liquid solvent, percent concentration is expressed as volume per unit volume. If a concentration value for a solution with both a liquid solute and solvent is expressed as a percentage and there are no units of measure between the number and the percent sign, the value is assumed to be volume per unit volume. The expression, 10% HCl, should mean 10 milliliters of concentrated HCl in 100 milliliters of solution.

EXAMPLE 6-20: How much ethanol is in 50 ml of a 5% solution of ethanol in water?

A 5% ethanol solution contains 5 ml of ethanol in 100 ml of the solution.

$$\frac{5 \text{ ml ethanol}}{100 \text{ ml solution}} = \frac{x \text{ ml ethanol}}{50 \text{ ml solution}}$$

$$100x = 5 \times 50$$

$$x = 2.5 \text{ ml ethanol}$$

Hence, 50 ml of a 5% ethanol solution contains 2.5 ml of ethanol.

EXAMPLE 6-21: Make 500 ml of 5% HCl.

$$\frac{5 \text{ ml concentrated HCl}}{100 \text{ ml solution}} = \frac{x \text{ ml concentrated HCl}}{500 \text{ ml solution}}$$

$$x = \frac{5 \times 500}{100}$$

$$x = 25 \text{ ml concentrated HCl}$$

To make this solution, place about 300 ml of water in a vessel and add the 25 ml of the concentrated hydrochloric acid. Let it cool, then add enough water to bring the solution up to 500 ml. Remember, it is not very bright to add water to concentrated acids. This can give you a very warm feeling in your eyes.

All the examples in this chapter thus far have been solved using either ratio and proportion or $V_1 \times C_1 = V_2 \times C_2$ and reasoning. These methods produce more understanding of the relationships of the calculations. However, there are people who find understanding drudgerous. For those people there are always formulas. Here are two formulas that can be used in solving percentage problems with little need for thought.

1. To find an amount of solute to make a given amount of solution:

$$\frac{\% \times \text{Desired volume}}{100} = \text{grams (or milliliters) of solute to be diluted up to the desired volume}$$

2. To find the percent concentration of a solution when the amount of solute and solution is known:

$$\frac{\text{Grams (or ml) of solute} \times 100}{\text{Volume of solution}} = \text{Percent concentration of solution}$$

Both of these formulas are a modification of the ratio and proportion procedure discussed previously. The basic ratio and proportion setup for this type of problem consists of the following:

$$\frac{\text{Grams (or ml) of solute per 100 ml}}{100 \text{ ml of solution}} = \frac{\text{grams (or ml) of solute per desired volume}}{\text{desired volume of solution}}$$

To work any problem of this type, one must know any three of the four values. If three values are known, the fourth can be calculated.

SECTION 6.6 MOLARITY

In chemical reactions, atoms and molecules are either combined or separated during the reaction. In other words, chemical reactions take place at the level of the atoms and molecules of the reactants. A method that allows the worker to know the relative number of reactant particles involved in a chemical reaction would be useful. The mole and the molarity measurements of concentration are such methods. A **mole** of a particular substance is the number of grams equal to the atomic or molecular weight of the substance. The atomic (at wt) or molecular weight (mol wt) of a substance is the actual mass of the chemical particle (atom or molecule) relative to the mass of the carbon atom. These values may be found in a handbook of chemistry and physics or in Appendix Z. Another method to determine the molecular weight of a compound is to add the atomic weights of the atoms comprising the molecule.

EXAMPLE 6-22: Find the molecular weight of NaCl.

$$\text{Atomic weight of Na} = 23$$
$$\text{Atomic weight of Cl} = \underline{35.5}$$
$$58.5$$

The atomic weight for sodium (Na) is 23, that for chlorine (Cl) is 35.5; hence, the molecular weight for NaCl is 58.5. One mole of sodium chloride equals 58.5 g. The term **gram molecular weight** is often used as a definition of mole.

EXAMPLE 6-23: Find the molecular weight of H_2SO_4.

$$2 \text{ H} = 1 \times 2 = 2$$
$$1 \text{ S} = 32 \times 1 = 32$$
$$4 \text{ O} = 16 \times 4 = \underline{64}$$
$$\text{mol wt of } H_2SO_4 = 98$$

Therefore 1 gram molecular weight of sulfuric acid equals 1 mole of sulfuric acid, which equals 98 g.

One mole of any substance contains approximately 6.02×10^{23} particles (Avogadro's number). A *1 molar solution* contains 1 mole of solute per liter of solution; that is, 1 mole of solute diluted up to 1,000 milliliters equals a 1 molar solution. The total volume is 1,000 milliliters, since the solute is *diluted up to* 1 liter.

Molarity (M) is a number that expresses the number of moles of substance in 1 liter of solution. In solving molarity problems, there are three main procedures that are commonly used: (1) the use of a formula, (2) ratio and proportion, and (3) $V_1 \times C_1 = V_2 \times C_2$.

Formula Use

The first procedure is based on the following basic formula:

Molecular weight × molarity = grams/liter

This formula is based on the fact that molarity is equal to the number of moles per liter; for example, a 2M solution contains 2 moles per liter, and a 0.5M solution contains 0.5 moles per liter.

The molecular weight of the substance times the molarity of the solution to be made equals the number of grams of solute to dilute up to 1,000 milliliters. This makes 1,000 milliliters of the desired molarity.

Remember this relationship, because most of the formulas used to calculate values relating to molarity, molality, and normality are modifications of it.

EXAMPLE 6-24: Make 1,000 ml of 0.5M NaCl. The molecular weight of NaCl is 58.5.

$$\text{mol wt} \times \text{M} = \text{g/L}$$

$$58.5 \times 0.5 = 29.25 \text{ g/L}$$

$$29.25 \text{ g NaCl} \uparrow 1,000 \text{ ml} \rightarrow 1,000 \text{ ml of } 0.5\text{M NaCl}$$

This formula may also be used to find the molarity of a solution. The formula expressed another way becomes the following:

$$\text{mol wt} \times \text{M} = \text{g/L} \qquad \text{or} \qquad \text{M} = \frac{\text{g/L}}{\text{mol wt}}$$

EXAMPLE 6-25: There are 300 g of NaCl per liter of solution. What is the molarity of the solution?

$$\text{M} = \frac{\text{g/L}}{\text{mol wt}}$$

$$\text{M} = \frac{300}{58.5}$$

$$\text{Molarity} = 5.13$$

The concentration of this solution is 5.13M; that is, it contains 5.13 moles of solute per liter.

Another expression with which one should be familiar is **millimole (mmole).** A milligram molecular weight (that is, the molecular weight expressed in milligrams) is a millimole. In contrast to the molarity (or number of moles per liter), which is:

$$\frac{\text{g/L}}{\text{mol wt}}$$

the number of millimoles per liter is:

$$\frac{\text{mg/L}}{\text{mol wt}}$$

REMEMBER:

1. A millimole is 1/1,000 mole and 1 mole equals 1,000 millimoles.
2. To convert moles to millimoles, multiply the number of moles by 1,000.
3. To convert millimoles to moles, divide the number of millimoles by 1,000.

4. To retain the same concentration when making solutions involving millimoles of solute, divide the volume of the solution by 1,000.
5. Moles/liter = millimoles/milliliter

$$①M = 1 \text{ mol/L}$$
$$= 1,000 \text{ mmol/L}$$
$$= 1,000 \text{ mmol/1,000 ml}$$
$$= ① \text{ mmol/ml}$$

$$⑥M = 6 \text{ mol/L}$$
$$= 6,000 \text{ mmol/L}$$
$$= 6,000 \text{ mmol/1,000 ml}$$
$$= ⑥ \text{ mmol/ml}$$

Therefore if the number of millimoles per milliliters is known, the molarity is known automatically.

EXAMPLE 6-26: A solution contains 3.5 mmol/ml. What is the molarity of the solution?

This may be solved the long way by finding out the number of moles per liter.
1. 3.5 mmol/ml would be 3,500 mmol/1,000 ml.
2. 3,500 mmol/1,000 ml would be 3.5 mol/1,000 ml.
3. 3.5 mol/1,000 ml is 3.5 mol/L.
4. The number of moles per liter *is* the molarity; therefore the molarity is 3.5.

On the other hand, one could simply look at the problem and remember that the number of millimoles per milliliter is numerically equal to the molarity, and the answer 3.5M would be evident.

IN REVIEW:
1. 1 gram molecular weight = 1 mole
2. 1 milligram molecular weight = 1 mmol
3. 1 mole = 1,000 mmol
4. mol wt $\times$ M = g/L

$$M = \frac{g/L}{mol\ wt}$$

5. M = moles/L or mmol/ml

Ratio and Proportion

The second procedure that may be used involves the use of *ratio and proportion*. Unlike percentages, molarity is always based on 1,000. Remember that molarity is based on the number of grams per liter, so always work toward this relationship to help solve problems.

EXAMPLE 6-27: There are 20 g NaCl in 400 ml of solution. What is its molarity?

To solve this problem, first determine the number of grams per 1,000 ml, because molarity equals the number of grams per liter divided by the molecular weight.

$$M = \frac{g/L}{mol\ wt}$$

To find the number of grams in 1,000 ml, use ratio and proportion. That is, 20 g in 400 ml equals x g in 1,000 ml.

$$20 : 400 = x : 1,000$$

$$\frac{20}{400} = \frac{x}{1,000}$$

$$400x = 20,000$$

$$x = 50$$

There would be 50 g in 1,000 ml. Now that the number of grams in 1,000 ml is known, fill in the following formula:

$$\text{M} = \frac{\text{g/L}}{\text{mol wt}}$$

$$\text{M} = \frac{50}{58.5}$$

$$\text{M} = 0.85$$

The concentration of the solution is 0.85M.

EXAMPLE 6-28: Make 300 ml of 6M NaCl.

$$\text{mol wt} \times \text{M} = \text{g/L}$$

$$58.5 \times 6 = 351 \text{ g/L}$$

It would take 351 g of NaCl to make 1 L of 6M solution. However, only 300 ml are to be made; therefore 351 g are to 1,000 ml as x g are to 300 ml.

$$351 : 1,000 = x : 300$$

$$\frac{351}{1,000} = \frac{x}{300}$$

$$1,000x = 105,300$$

$$x = 105.3 \text{ g}$$

$$105.3 \text{ g} \uparrow 300 \text{ ml} \rightarrow 300 \text{ ml of 6M NaCl}$$

IN REVIEW:

1. Molarity is always based on grams per 1,000 milliliters of solution.
2. For any volume other than 1,000 milliliters, use a ratio and proportion procedure to determine the answer.

A combination of these two procedures (formula use and ratio and proportion), plus a little exercise in common sense, will usually solve most problems involving molarity.

$V_1 \times C_1 = V_2 \times C_2$

The third procedure is the use of the $V_1 \times C_1 = V_2 \times C_2$ method. The product of the volume and concentration of one solution equals the product of the volume and concentration of a related solution.

EXAMPLE 6-29: How much of a 0.5M solution can be made from 25 ml of a 4M solution?

$$V_1 \times C_1 = V_2 \times C_2$$

$$x \text{ ml} \times 0.5\text{M} = 25 \text{ ml} \times 4\text{M}$$

$$x = \frac{25 \times 4}{0.5}$$

$$x = 200 \text{ ml}$$

This shows that 200 ml of 0.5M solution can be made from 25 ml of 4M solution.

EXAMPLE 6-30: What is the molar concentration of the solution resulting from the mixing of 50 ml of a 1M solution and 120 ml of a 3M solution?

Refer to Mixing Solutions in Section 6.3, p. 130 and find the formula:

$$(V_1 \times C_1) + (V_2 \times C_2) + \ldots = V_F \times C_F$$

Insert the data and solve for the final concentration.

$$(V_1 \times C_1) + \qquad (V_2 \times C_2) = \qquad (V_F \times C_F)$$

$$(50 \text{ ml} \times 1\text{M}) + (120 \text{ ml} \times 3\text{M}) = (50 \text{ ml} + 120 \text{ ml}) \times x\text{M}$$

$$170x = 50 + 360$$

$$x = \frac{410}{170}$$

$$x = 2.41\text{M}$$

The concentration of the final solution resulting from mixing the two solutions is 2.41M.

The use of these three procedures, either alone or in combination, and common sense will solve almost all problems involving molar concentration.

SECTION 6.7 MOLALITY

As stated in Section 6.2, **molality** is the number of moles of a solute per 1 kilogram of solvent. This is a weight per unit weight type of concentration expression and is not affected by variation in temperature or pressure. Molality is thought of as the most precise expression of concentration in chemistry.

Molal concentration does not involve any consideration of volume; therefore the relative amounts of solute and solvent are not affected by variation in the temperature of the solution, the density of the materials, or the interaction of the molecules of the components of the solution.

Molal solutions are made by placing a number of moles of something in a given number of kilograms of something else. The molality of the solution is equal to the number of moles of one component in one kilogram of something else. Usually this is a number of moles of solute per kilogram of solvent.

EXAMPLE 6-31: Make a 1 molal solution of NaCl in water.

The molecular weight of NaCl is 58.5, so to make a 1 molal solution, add 58.5 g of NaCl (1 mol) to 1 kg of water. The resulting solution weighs 1,058.5 g. The volume is not determined.

EXAMPLE 6-32: How many grams of NaCl would be in 100 g of a 1 molal solution?

As seen in Example 6-31, a 1 molal solution of NaCl in water would have a ratio of 58.5 g of NaCl to 1,058.5 g of solution. Hence,

$$\frac{x \text{ g NaCl}}{100 \text{ g solution}} = \frac{58.5 \text{ g NaCl}}{1,058.5 \text{ g solution}}$$

$$x = \frac{100 \times 58.5}{1,058.5}$$

$$x = 5.53 \text{ g NaCl}$$

In 100 g of a 1 molal solution there would be 5.53 g of NaCl.

The calculations of molal solutions are similar to molar solutions. The difference is that molal calculations do not involve volumes.

SECTION 6.8 NORMALITY

If the mechanisms of molarity are understood, there should be no difficulty in understanding normality; normality and molarity are based on the same principles with one major change. Molarity is based on molecular weight (mol wt); normality is based on *equivalent weight (eq wt)*. By definition, a **gram equivalent weight** of an element or compound is the mass that will combine with or replace 1 mole of hydrogen.

The materials used to make normal solutions dissociate or separate into positive or negative ions. Normality considers the ability of the ions to combine with other ions. For example, potassium hydroxide, KOH, dissociates into one potassium ion (K^+) and one hydroxyl ion (OH^-). Sulfuric acid, H_2SO_4, dissociates into two hydrogen ions (H^+) and one sulfate ion ($SO_4^=$). One mole of K^+ will replace 1 mole of H^- in a chemical reaction; hence, KOH has an equivalent weight equal to 1 mole of KOH. Consider the combining ability of the sulfate ion, $SO_4^=$. One mole of this ion will combine with 2 moles of H^+. Since 1 gram equivalent weight of an element or compound is the mass that will combine with 1 mole of H^+, then 1 gram equivalent weight of H_2SO_4 equals 0.5 mole, because two H^+ ions will combine with one $SO_4^=$ ion. For purposes of this book, the gram equivalent weight of a compound or element may be considered to be equal to the gram molecular weight divided by the total positive valence of the constituent ions of the material considered.

One very common exception to this rule is the situation found in oxidation-reduction reactions. The calculations for this type of chemical reaction are performed rarely in the medical laboratory. For this reason, these reactions are not considered in this book.

As a general rule, the equivalent weight of an element or compound is equal to the molecular weight divided by the valence.

It should be clear from this rule that for monovalent ions the equivalent weight is equal to the molecular weight, but for polyvalent ions the equivalent weight becomes smaller than the molecular weight. Therefore *equivalent weight is always equal to or less than molecular weight.* (This rule will be restated and used later in this chapter.)

One limitation to the normality system is that, depending on the reaction in which it is used, a given solution may have more than one normality because it may have more than one equivalent weight. However, the molarity of a solution is fixed, since there is only *one* molecular weight of any given substance.

Why then is normality considered more important in chemical reactions? Substances react together on the basis of an equal number of chemically active particles. Because equal weights of different substances contain a different number of chemically active particles, equal gram concentrations of elements or compounds cannot be indiscriminately added together. However, when gram units are converted to equivalents, the concentrations of elements or compounds are expressed in terms of their *combining weights;* that is, they may be freely added together without regard to the nature of the substance, since one equivalent of any substance always contains the same number of chemically active particles as one equivalent of any other substance. For example, 1 equivalent of Na = 1 equivalent H_2SO_4 = 1 equivalent $CaCl_2$. A 1 gram equivalent weight (the equivalent weight expressed in grams) equals 1 equivalent.

A **1 normal** (N) solution contains 1 gram equivalent (or 1 eq) of solute in 1,000 ml of solution.

$$1 \text{ gram equivalent weight} \uparrow 1,000 \text{ milliliters} \rightarrow 1\text{N solution}$$

Therefore **normality** is a number that represents the *number* of equivalent weights (or equivalents) of solute in 1 liter of solution. A 1N solution = 1 eq/L, 6N = 6 eq/L, and 0.3N = 0.3 equivalent per liter.

A term with which one should become familiar before proceeding is **milliequivalent** (mEq). This has the same relation to equivalent as millimole has to mole.

1. milligram equivalent weight (the equivalent weight in milligrams) = 1 mEq
2. $\dfrac{mg}{eq\ wt} = mEq$
3. 1 eq = 1,000 mEq
4. 1 mEq = $\dfrac{1}{1,000}$ eq

The three procedures usually used for solving normality problems are the same as those used for solving molarity, except the equivalent weight is used in the formula instead of the molecular weight.

Formula Use

Molarity (M)	Normality (N)
mol wt × M = g/L	eq wt × N = g/L

The equivalent weight for the substance times the desired normality equals the number of grams of solute to dilute with enough solvent to make 1 liter of solution with the desired normality. If any two of the values are known, solve for the third.

EXAMPLE 6-33: Make 6N NaCl.

$$mol\ wt = 58.5$$
$$eq\ wt = 58.5$$
$$eq\ wt \times N = g/L$$
$$58.5 \times 6 = 351.0\ g/L$$
$$351.0\ g\ NaCl \uparrow 1,000\ ml \rightarrow 1\ L\ of\ 6\text{N NaCl}$$

EXAMPLE 6-34: What is the normality of an NaOH solution containing 200 g of NaOH/L?

$$eq\ wt \times N = g/L$$
$$N = \frac{g/L}{eq\ wt}$$

$$N = \frac{200}{40}$$
$$N = 5$$

As with molarity, an easy way to find normality is to remember that the number of mEq/ml is numerically equal to normality.

①N = 1 eq/L
= 1,000 mEq/L
= 1,000 mEq/1,000 ml
= ① mEq/ml

⓪.3 N = 0.3 eq/L
= 300 mEq/L
= 300 mEq/1,000 ml
= ⓪.3 mEq/ml

IN REVIEW:
1. 1 gram equivalent weight = 1 equivalent
2. 1 milligram equivalent weight = 1 milliequivalent
3. 1 eq = 1,000 mEq
4. Normality of a solution is a number expressing the number of equivalents per liter.
5. eq wt × N = g/L
6. eq wt = $\frac{\text{mol wt}}{\text{valence}}$
7. Equivalent weight is always equal to or less than molecular weight.
8. The number of milliequivalents per milliliter is numerically equal to the normality.
9. 1 eq of any substance = 1 eq of any other substance
10. 1 mEq of any substance = 1 mEq of any other substance

Ratio-Proportion Setup

Like molarity, normality is based on grams per 1,000 milliliters.

$$\text{eq wt} \times N = \text{g/L}$$

First determine this figure (g/L); then complete the solution.

EXAMPLE 6-35: Make 300 ml of a 0.4N NaOH solution.

mol wt of NaOH = 40
eq wt = 40
eq wt × N = g/L
40 × 0.4 = 16.0 g/L

It would take 16 g of NaOH to make 1 L of solution. However, only 300 ml is required; therefore use ratio and proportion as follows: 16 is to 1,000 as x is to 300.

$$\frac{16}{1,000} = \frac{x}{300}$$
$$1,000x = 4,800$$
$$x = 4.8$$

Therefore 4.8 g of NaOH ↑ 300 ml → 300 ml of a 0.4N NaOH solution.

EXAMPLE 6-36: There are 80 g of NaOH in 400 ml of solution. What is the normality?

Eighty grams are to 400 ml as x g are to 1,000 ml.

$$\frac{80}{400} = \frac{x}{1,000}$$

$$400x = 80,000$$

$$x = 200 \text{ g/L}$$

$$N = \frac{\text{g/L}}{\text{eq wt}}$$

$$N = \frac{200}{40}$$

$$N = 5$$

$V_1 \times C_1 = V_2 \times C_2$

As stated earlier, when using $V_1 \times C_1 = V_2 \times C_2$, one may state the concentration in percent, molarity, or normality. When the two concentrations are in different units, it is necessary to change one unit to match the other. It usually does not matter which unit is changed as long as the units are the same. However, there is one exception. If the problem states *neutralize, react with,* or *equal,* then both the units must be in normality, because only in normality does 1 milliliter of a given normality equal 1 milliliter of the same normality of another substance. (Recall that 1 equivalent of a substance equals 1 equivalent of any other substance and that normality is the number of equivalents per liter.)

IN REVIEW:

1. Normality is always based on grams per 1,000 milliliters of solution.
2. For any volume other than 1,000 milliliters, use a ratio-proportion setup to determine the answer. Perhaps a word should be said about the different ways that normality and molarity may be written or expressed when the normality and molarity are fractions with the numeral 1 as the numerator. A solution with a normality of $\frac{1}{10}$ may be written $\frac{1}{10}$N, 0.1N, or $\frac{N}{10}$ (the N taking the place of the 1 in the numerator); $\frac{1}{5}$N may be expressed $\frac{1}{5}$N, 0.2N, or $\frac{N}{5}$.

SECTION 6.9 OSMOLARITY

Still another measure of concentration is **osmolarity.** This value provides an estimate of the osmotic activity of the solution by indicating the relative number of particles dissolved in the solution. In general, the osmotic activity is more or less directly proportional to the number of free particles in a given amount of solution. In most biological fluids the charge of the particles does not greatly affect the osmotic potential. Hence the concentration of separate particles in such solutions determines the osmotic activity.

One **osmole (osmol)** of any substance is equal to 1 gram molecular weight divided by the number of particles formed by the dissociation of the molecules. For those materials that do not ionize, 1 osmole is equal to 1 mole. For example, 1 osmole of glucose is equal to 1 mole of glucose (180 grams). Glucose does not dissociate in aqueous solutions. However, a molecule of sodium chloride does completely ionize in water. It forms one sodium and one chloride ion. One osmole of NaCl is equal to 1 gram molecular weight divided by the number of particles formed upon dissociation. The molecular weight of NaCl is 58.5; hence,

$$1 \text{ osmol} = \frac{1 \text{ mol}}{\text{particles per mole}}$$

$$1 \text{ osmol NaCl} = \frac{58.5}{2} = 29.25 \text{ g}$$

The osmolarity of any solution is dependent only on the number, not the nature, of particles in solution. The osmolarity of a solution of a given substance may be found by multiplying the molar concentration by the number of particles per mole resulting from ionization. The term *osmolality* is sometimes used. This is related to osmolarity in the same way that molality is related to molarity. Osmolarity measurements vary with temperature and are not as accurate as osmolality. However, at the concentration of the solutes of the body fluids there is little difference between the osmolarity and the osmolality of a solution, and the two are often used interchangeably.

Osmolarity (osmol/L) = molarity × number of particles per molecule resulting from ionization

This assumes 100% ionization because the degree of ionization affects the osmolarity of a solution. However, the most common solutions for which osmolarity is determined are biological fluids. Since the concentration of electrolytes in these fluids is so low, complete dissociation is usually assumed.

Because of these low concentrations, it is usually more convenient to measure osmolarity in terms of milliosmoles. One milliosmole (mOsmol) equals 1/1,000 osmole.

$$1 \text{ mOsmol} = \frac{1 \text{ mmol}}{\text{particles per molecule on dissociation}}$$

$$\text{mOsmol/L} = \text{mmol/L} \times \text{particles per molecule resulting from ionization}$$

EXAMPLE 6-37: A NaCl solution contains 50 mmol/L; what is its concentration in milliosmoles per liter?

$$\text{mOsmol/L} = 50 \times 2$$
$$\text{mOsmol/L} = 100$$

In physiological fluids such as plasma and urine, the osmotic activity is due to the combined osmotic activity of the substances that are dissolved in them. Therefore to obtain the osmolarity, it is necessary to calculate it from the concentration and degree of ionization of each constituent in the mixture. The osmolarity of such fluids is therefore most easily determined by measuring the **freezing point depression.** The freezing point of water is depressed 1.86°C when solute is added to make a 1 osmolal (1 osmole per kilogram) solution; therefore 1 osmole of any solute is the amount that will depress the freezing point of 1 kilogram of water by 1.86°C. One milliosmole of osmotic activity per liter is equivalent to the depression in the freezing point of a solution 0.00186°C below that of water (taken at 0°C); hence,

$$1 \text{ osmol} = \Delta 1.86°C$$

$$1 \text{ mOsmol} = \Delta 0.00186°C$$

EXAMPLE 6-38: The freezing point of a sample of human plasma was found to be $-0.62°C$. What is the milliosmolarity?

1 mOsmol gives $\Delta 0.00186$; therefore x mOsmol would give $\Delta 0.62$.

$$\frac{1}{0.00186} = \frac{x}{0.62}$$

$$0.00186x = 0.62$$

$$x = 333.3$$

$$\Delta 0.62 = 333.3 \text{ mOsmol/L}$$

SECTION 6.10 DENSITY

Specific gravity (sp gr) is a method of measuring density. **Density** is the amount of matter in a given volume. In other words, density is the mass per unit volume. **Specific gravity** is a ratio between the mass of a substance and the mass of an equal volume of pure water at 4°C.

$$\text{Specific gravity} = \frac{\text{weight of solid or liquid}}{\text{weight of equal volume of water at 4°C}}$$

Since 1 milliliter of water has a mass of 1 gram, specific gravity is equal to the mass in grams of 1 milliliter of any substance. Materials less dense than water have a specific gravity of less than 1, whereas materials more dense than water have a specific gravity greater than 1.

One use of specific gravity values in the clinical laboratory is in working with concentrated commercial liquids. Often a bottle label shows the specific gravity and a value called either *assay* or *percent purity*. These values indicate the mass of 1 milliliter of the solution and the proportion of the solution by weight that is the substance desired. Using these values, one can determine the actual amount of the substance in a given volume of the supply solution.

Specific gravity $\times$ % assay = g/ml

EXAMPLE 6-39: The values listed on the label of a bottle of nitric acid are sp gr 1.42 and assay 70%. What do these values mean?

These values mean that 1 ml of the solution has the mass of 1.42 g and that 70% of this mass is HNO_3.

To find how much HNO_3 is in 1 ml of the supply solution, multiply the specific gravity by the assay percentage. The answer is the number of grams of HNO_3 per milliliter of the solution.

$$\text{sp gr} \times \text{\% assay} = \text{g/ml}$$

$$1.42 \times 0.70 = 0.9940 \text{ g } HNO_3/\text{ml}$$

Hence, there are 0.994 g HNO_3 per milliliter of solution. This information is used in making other solutions from concentrated solutions.

EXAMPLE 6-40: Make 1 L of 10%$^{w/v}$ HNO$_3$ solution.

Use the information from the preceding example (a nitric acid supply with a specific gravity of 1.42 and an assay of 70%; hence a supply solution containing 0.994 g of nitric acid per milliliter).

The instructions call for 1 L (or 1,000 ml) of a 10%$^{w/v}$ HNO$_3$ solution. The solution should contain 10 g HNO$_3$ per 100 ml of solution. Find how much nitric acid should be in 1,000 ml of this solution by using ratio and proportion.

$$\frac{10 \text{ g}}{100 \text{ ml}} = \frac{x \text{ g}}{1,000 \text{ ml}}$$

$$100x = 10,000$$

$$x = 100$$

One liter of 10%$^{w/v}$ HNO$_3$ solution will contain 100 g of HNO$_3$.

The next part of the problem is to determine how much of the supply solution will contain 100 g of nitric acid. Since each milliliter of the solution contains 0.994 g of HNO$_3$, a ratio-proportion setup can be used to determine the volume of the supply solution containing 100 g of HNO$_3$.

$$\frac{0.994 \text{ g}}{1.0 \text{ ml}} = \frac{100 \text{g}}{x \text{ ml}}$$

$$0.994x = 100$$

$$x = 100.6 \text{ ml}$$

Therefore 100 g of pure nitric acid would be contained in 100.6 ml of solution. This 100.6 ml of the concentrated HNO$_3$ ↑ 1,000 ml would give 1,000 ml of a 10.06%$^{v/v}$ solution of the supply solution that would also be the 10%$^{w/v}$ HNO$_3$ solution called for in the problem.

This is not actually a weight per unit volume solution, since the nitric acid was not measured by weight but by volume. However, because water and solutions of water vary little in volume at the temperatures of the laboratory, the use of volume does not produce a degree of variation great enough to warrant the inconvenience of weighing highly corrosive liquids.

Two more examples of this type problem are given showing a greater variation in the values.

EXAMPLE 6-41: Make 250 ml of a 20%$^{w/v}$ HCl solution.

The supply of concentrated HCl has a specific gravity of 1.19 and an assay of 38%. Find the amount of HCl per milliliter of supply solution.

$$\text{sp gr} \times \% \text{ assay} = \text{g/ml}$$

$$1.19 \times \quad 0.38 \quad = 0.4522$$

There are 0.4522 g HCl/ml of solution.

Next determine how much HCl is needed to produce 250 ml of a 20%$^{w/v}$ solution using ratio and proportion.

$$\frac{20 \text{ g}}{100 \text{ ml}} = \frac{x \text{ g}}{250 \text{ ml}}$$

$$100x = 5{,}000$$

$$x = 50$$

Therefore 50 g of HCl is needed in 250 ml of 20%$^{w/v}$ solution of HCl.

Now, how much supply solution is needed to yield 50 g of the desired material?

$$\frac{0.4522 \text{ g}}{1 \text{ ml}} = \frac{50 \text{ g}}{x \text{ ml}}$$

$$0.4522x = 50$$

$$x = 110.6 \text{ ml}$$

110.6 ml of the supply solution contains 50 g HCl.

Therefore 110.6 ml HCl ↑ 250 ml → 250 ml of 20%$^{w/v}$ solution.

From the preceding calculations it is known that 110.6 milliliters of the supply solution diluted up to 250 milliliters will give a 20%$^{w/v}$ solution; remember that the *weight* was based on a volume measure. This would be a 44.24%$^{v/v}$ solution of HCl. Try to calculate this.

EXAMPLE 6-42: Make a 0.5N HCl solution using the preceding supply of concentrated HCl.

To make a normal solution, the equivalent weight of the solute has to be known. In the case of HCl the equivalent weight equals 1 mol. The molecular weight of HCl is 36.5; hence 1 mol of HCl equals 36.5 g and 1 equivalent weight equals 36.5 g. A 1N solution would have the concentration of 1 eq wt/L of solution. In this case, 36.5 g of HCl/L would be a 1N solution, and 1 L of a 0.5N HCl solution would contain one half of a mole.

$$\text{eq wt} \times \text{N} = \text{g/L}$$

$$36.5 \times 0.5 = 18.25 \text{ g/L}$$

How much of the supply solution of HCl would contain 18.25 g? From calculations in the last problem, it was determined that the supply solution contained 0.4522 g HCl/ml. To determine how much solution is needed to contain 18.25 g of HCl, use a ratio-proportion setup.

$$\frac{0.4522 \text{ g}}{1 \text{ ml}} = \frac{18.25 \text{ g}}{x \text{ ml}}$$

$$0.4522x = 18.25$$

$$x = 40.4 \text{ ml}$$

Hence, 40.4 ml of supply solution ↑ 1,000 ml equals a 0.5N HCl solution.

SECTION 6.11 CONVERSION FROM ONE EXPRESSION OF CONCENTRATION TO ANOTHER

There are several instances in which the form a concentration value is expressed in is not the form desired. Consider the following examples:

1. A procedure may call for 0.5M NaOH, and all that is on hand is 10% NaOH.
2. A problem may ask how much 5M HCl would be neutralized by a certain amount of 10N NaOH.

3. An answer in a given test procedure may be in milligrams per deciliter, and the physician wants it in milliequivalents per liter.

The relationship between these various units and how to convert them should present no problem if the worker understands the material covered in this chapter.

This discussion concerns some methods to use in converting one type of concentration to another.

% ⇄ N, M

Consider the conversion of percent concentration to molarity or normality and vice versa. Remember two basic facts: (1) percent, unless stated otherwise, is grams per 100 milliliters, and (2) molarity and normality are based on grams per liter.

Recall the basic molarity and normality formulas:

$$\text{mol wt} \times \text{M} = \text{g/L} \qquad\qquad \text{eq wt} \times \text{N} = \text{g/L}$$

$$\text{M} = \frac{\text{g/L}}{\text{mol wt}} \qquad\qquad \text{N} = \frac{\text{g/L}}{\text{eq wt}}$$

If the grams per liter and the molecular or equivalent weights are known, one can find molarity and normality. The percentage equals the number of grams per 100 milliliters; therefore multiply the percent value by 10 to get the number of grams per liter. One point about percentages needs to be brought out here. Since molarity and normality are based on grams (weight) per liter, the percent value used in these formulas *must* be a weight per unit volume concentration (g/100 ml). A volume per unit volume concentration *cannot* be used unless it is first converted to a weight per unit volume concentration. Consider a 10% NaCl solution. This solution contains 10 grams of NaCl per 100 milliliters of solution. Multiply the 10 grams in 100 milliliters by 10 to get the number of grams in 1,000 milliliters (10 × 10 = 100 g/1,000 ml). Using this information, one may derive the formula for converting percent concentration to molarity or normality, or vice versa.

$$\text{mol wt} \times \text{M} = \text{g/L} \qquad\qquad \text{eq wt} \times \text{N} = \text{g/L}$$

$$\text{M} = \frac{\text{g/L}}{\text{mol wt}} \qquad\qquad \text{N} = \frac{\text{g/L}}{\text{eq wt}}$$

$$\text{M} = \frac{\text{g/100 ml} \times 10}{\text{mol wt}} \qquad\qquad \text{N} = \frac{\text{g/100 ml} \times 10}{\text{eq wt}}$$

$$\text{M} = \frac{\% \times 10}{\text{mol wt}} \qquad\qquad \text{N} = \frac{\% \times 10}{\text{eq wt}}$$

The only difference between converting percent concentration to molarity or normality is the use of molecular weight for molarity and equivalent weight for normality.

These formulas may be used to convert from a percentage to molarity or normality or to convert from molarity and normality to a percentage. Fill in all known quantities and solve for *x*. There is no need to memorize them. If one remembers the basic formulas (mol wt × M = g/L; eq wt × N = g/L) and understands them, the conversion formula can be figured out when it is needed.

EXAMPLE 6-43: Convert 30% NaCl to molarity.

$$M = \frac{\% \times 10}{\text{mol wt}}$$

$$M = \frac{30 \times 10}{58.5}$$

$$M = \frac{300}{58.5}$$

$$M = 5.13$$

$$30\% \text{ NaCl} = 5.13\text{M NaCl}$$

EXAMPLE 6-44: Convert 6M NaOH to a percentage.

$$M = \frac{\% \times 10}{\text{mol wt}}$$

$$6 = \frac{\% \times 10}{40}$$

$$6 \times 40 = \% \times 10$$

$$\% \times 10 = 240$$

$$\% = 24$$

$$6\text{M NaOH} = 24\%^{w/v} \text{ NaOH}$$

EXAMPLE 6-45: Convert 3N H_2SO_4 to a percentage.

$$\text{mol wt of } H_2SO_4 = 98$$

$$\text{eq wt of } H_2SO_4 = 49$$

$$N = \frac{\% \times 10}{\text{eq wt}}$$

$$3 = \frac{\% \times 10}{49}$$

$$3 \times 49 = \% \times 10$$

$$\% \times 10 = 147$$

$$\% = 14.7$$

$$3\text{N } H_2SO_4 = 14.7\%^{w/v} H_2SO_4$$

mg/dl ⇄ mEq/L

Another type of conversion problem involves the conversion of milligrams per deciliter to milliequivalents per liter, or vice versa.

REMEMBER:

$$\text{eq wt} \times N = \text{g/L}$$

$$N \text{ (or eq/L)} = \frac{\text{g/L}}{\text{eq wt}}$$

$$\text{mEq/L} = \frac{\text{mg/L}}{\text{eq wt}}$$

Recall that mg/dl means mg/100 ml; as with a percentage, multiply the number of mg/100 ml by 10 to get the number of mg/1,000 ml. Therefore

$$\text{mEq/L} = \frac{\text{mg/L}}{\text{eq wt}}$$

$$\text{mEq/L} = \frac{\text{mg/100 ml} \times 10}{\text{eq wt}}$$

$$\text{mEq/L} = \frac{\text{mg/dl} \times 10}{\text{eq wt}}$$

EXAMPLE 6-46: Express 300 mg/dl Cl as mEq/L Cl.

$$mEq/L = \frac{300 \times 10}{35.5}$$

$$mEq/L = \frac{3,000}{35.5}$$

$$mEq/L = 84.51$$

300 mg/dl Cl = 84.51 mEq/L Cl

EXAMPLE 6-47: Express 150 mEq/L NaCl as mg/dl NaCl.

$$mEq/L = \frac{mg/dl \times 10}{eq\ wt}$$

$$150 = \frac{mg/dl \times 10}{58.5}$$

$$mg/dl \times 10 = 150 \times 58.5$$

$$mg/dl \times 10 = 8,775$$

$$mg/dl = 877.5$$

150 mEq/L NaCl = 877.5 mg/dl NaCl

Notice in the two previous examples that Cl has been converted to Cl and NaCl to NaCl. Suppose one were asked not only to change concentration units, but to change the values to the concentration of another substance as well.

EXAMPLE 6-48: Express 700 mg/dl NaCl as mEq/L Cl.

There are two main ways to solve this problem; use whichever makes the most sense to you.

1. First change mg/dl NaCl to mg/dl Cl by ratio and proportion using the molecular weights; then convert mg/dl Cl to mEq/L Cl.

2. Recall that 1 mEq of any substance equals 1 mEq of any other substance; therefore the number of mEq/L NaCl equals the number of mEq/L of Cl.

Compare the above problem worked both ways

$$\frac{35.5}{58.5} = \frac{x}{700}$$

$$58.5x = 700 \times 35.5$$

$$58.5x = 24,850$$

$$x = 424.8$$

700 mg/dl NaCl = 424.8 mg/dl Cl

$$mEq/L\ Cl = \frac{424.8 \times 10}{35.5}$$

$$mEq/L = \frac{4248}{35.5}$$

$$mEq/L = 119.66$$

424.8 mg/dl Cl = 119.66 mEq/L Cl

$$mEq/L\ NaCl = \frac{mg/dl \times 10}{eq\ wt}$$

$$mEq/L\ NaCl = \frac{700 \times 10}{58.5}$$

$$mEq/L\ NaCl = \frac{7,000}{58.5}$$

$$mEq/L\ NaCl = 119.66$$

119.66 mEq/L NaCl = 119.66 mEq/L Cl

The preceding is true because of the relationship between the two. In the first method, 700 mg/dl NaCl = 424.8 mg/dl Cl. If these two figures are converted to mEq/L, the result is the following:

$$mEq/L\ NaCl = \frac{700 \times 10}{58.5}$$

mEq/L NaCl = 119.66

$$mEq/L\ Cl = \frac{424.8 \times 10}{35.5}$$

mEq/L Cl = 119.66

When converting mg/dl NaCl to mEq/L, use the equivalent weight of NaCl (58.5), and when converting mg/dl Cl to mEq/L, use the equivalent weight of Cl (35.5).

Do the same problem in reverse

Convert 119.66 mEq/L Cl to mg/dl NaCl

Convert 119.66 mEq/L Cl to mg/dl Cl and then ratio-proportion mg/dl Cl to mg/dl NaCl.

$$119.66 = \frac{x \times 10}{35.5}$$

$$10x = 119.66 \times 35.5$$

$$10x = 4{,}247.9$$

$$x = 424.8 \text{ mg/dl Cl}$$

$$\frac{35.5}{58.5} = \frac{424.8}{x}$$

$$35.5x = 58.5 \times 424.8$$

$$35.5x = 24{,}850.8$$

$$x = 700 \text{ mg/dl NaCl}$$

$$424.8 \text{ mg/dl Cl} = 700 \text{ mg/dl NaCl}$$

$$\boxed{119.66 \text{ mEq/L Cl} = 700 \text{ mg/dl NaCl}}$$

The 119.66 mEq/L Cl is also equal to 119.66 mEq/L NaCl, so convert 119.66 mEq/L NaCl to mg/dl NaCl.

$$119.66 = \frac{x \times 10}{58.5}$$

$$10x = 119.66 \times 58.5$$

$$10x = 7{,}000.1$$

$$x = 700 \text{ mg/dl NaCl}$$

$$\boxed{119.66 \text{ mEq/L Cl} = 700 \text{ mg/dl NaCl}}$$

REMEMBER:

1. 1 milliequivalent of any substance equals 1 milliequivalent of any other substance.
2. To change one substance to equivalent milligrams of another substance, use *ratio and proportion and milligrams* (not milliequivalents).

M ⇄ N

One should now be able to convert a percentage (w/v) to molarity and normality and vice versa, and mEq/L to mg/dl and vice versa. Another important category to consider is how to convert molarity to normality and normality to molarity.

The following are the formulas for these conversions:

$$\text{N} = \text{M} \times \text{Valence}$$

$$\text{M} = \frac{\text{N}}{\text{Valence}}$$

Recall that the normality of a solution must always equal or be greater than the molarity of the same solution, the reason being that normality is based on equivalent weight and molarity is based on molecular weight. To arrive at the equivalent weight, divide the molecular weight by the valence; therefore the equivalent weight is always equal to or less than the molecular weight.

$$H_2SO_4 \text{ mol wt} = 98$$

$$\text{eq wt} = \frac{98}{2} = 49$$

A molecular weight may contain two or more equivalent weights. If this is the case and if a solution contains one molecular weight, it would contain two or more equivalent weights, and since molarity is the number of moles (molecular weights) per liter and normality is the number of equivalents (equivalent weights) per liter, the molarity of that solution would be 1 and the normality would be 2 or more.

$$H_2SO_4 \text{ molecular weight} = 98$$

$$98 = 1 \text{ mol wt} = 1\text{M}$$

$$98 = 2 \text{ eq wt} = 2\text{N}$$

EXAMPLE 6-49: Convert 6N NaOH to molarity.

The valence of NaOH is 1; therefore the normality and the molarity are the same.

$$\text{M} = \frac{\text{N}}{\text{Valence}}$$

$$\text{M} = \frac{6}{1}$$

$$\text{M} = 6$$

$$6\text{N NaOH} = 6\text{M NaOH}$$

EXAMPLE 6-50: Convert 10M H_2SO_4 to normality.

$$\text{N} = \text{M} \times \text{Valence}$$

$$\text{N} = 10 \times 2$$

$$\text{N} = 20$$

$$10\text{M } H_2SO_4 = 20\text{N } H_2SO_4$$

EXAMPLE 6-51: Express 0.6N H_3PO_4 as molarity.

$$\text{M} = \frac{\text{N}}{\text{Valence}}$$

$$\text{M} = \frac{0.6}{3}$$

$$\text{M} = 0.2$$

$$0.6\text{N } H_3PO_4 = 0.2\text{M } H_3PO_4$$

Notice that in each case the normality is equal to or greater than the molarity.

IN REVIEW:

1. $\text{M} = \dfrac{\% \times 10}{\text{mol wt}}$

2. $\text{N} = \dfrac{\% \times 10}{\text{eq wt}}$

3. $\text{mEq/L} = \dfrac{\text{mg/dl} \times 10}{\text{eq wt}}$

4. $N = M \times \text{Valence}$

5. $M = \dfrac{N}{\text{Valence}}$

Conversion of Volume Percent CO_2 to Millimoles per Liter

A rather specialized concentration conversion is the changing of the concentration expression of carbon dioxide from milliliters per 100 milliliters of serum to millimoles per liter.

Under standard conditions of temperature and pressure, 1 mole (1,000 millimoles) of a perfect gas occupies 22.4 liters of space. However, carbon dioxide is not a perfect gas. One mole of this gas occupies 22.260 liters (22,260 milliliters) under standard conditions. Carbon dioxide determinations are occasionally reported as volume percent (milliliters per 100 milliliters of serum). Most people prefer to have the CO_2 concentration in millimoles per liter. Since 1,000 millimoles of CO_2 occupy 22,260 milliliters of space, 22.26 milliliters CO_2 equals 1 millimole. Thus the number of milliliters of CO_2 divided by 22.26 will give the number of millimoles.

The number of milliliters of CO_2 per 100 milliliters of serum can be converted to the number of millimoles per liter in the following manner:

$$\text{vol\%} = \text{ml } CO_2/100 \text{ ml serum}$$

$$\frac{\text{vol\%}}{22.26} = \text{mmol}/100 \text{ ml}$$

$$\frac{\text{vol\%} \times 10}{22.26} = \text{mmol/L}$$

$$\frac{\text{vol\%}}{2.226} = \text{mmol/L}$$

Or:

$$\text{vol\%} \times \frac{1}{2.226} = \text{mmol/L}$$

Thus to convert vol% to mmol/L:

$$\text{vol\%} \times 0.45 = \text{mmol/L}$$

Recall:

$$\frac{\text{vol\%}}{2.226} = \text{mmol/L}$$

Thus to convert mmol/L to vol%:

$$\text{vol\%} = \text{mmol/L} \times 2.226$$

The equivalent weight of CO_2 is the same as the molecular weight. Therefore mmol/L are equal to mEq/L.

Conversion of Complex Metric Units

Values often have a combination of units used together to form the actual unit. The unit for speed in the SI system is meters per second (m/s). Here, the units meter and second are used together to form one unit of measure for the property *speed*. In most laboratory work the most common of these complex units are used for expressions of concentration. Units of concentration usually involve a number of units of one thing per some number of another unit; for example, grams of salt per liter of water or moles of solute per kilogram of solvent. The conversion of a concentration in one unit to the equivalent concentration in another unit involves the two units written in the form of common fractions. For example, if there is a need to change milligrams per deciliter to micrograms per milliliter or grams per liter to milligrams per microliter, the following formula can be used.

$$\text{Desired units} = \text{original units} \times \frac{\text{power of 10 to convert the top unit}}{\text{power of 10 to convert the bottom unit}}$$

EXAMPLE 6-52: Express 130 mg/dl as micrograms per milliliter.

$$\frac{\text{mg}}{\text{dl}} \rightarrow \frac{\mu\text{g}}{\text{ml}}$$

On the top it is desired to change milli- to micro-. The power of 10 to accomplish this is 10^3. On the bottom it is desired to convert deci- to milli-. The power of 10 to accomplish this is 10^2.

Place this information in the formula:

$$\frac{x\ \mu\text{g}}{1\ \text{ml}} = \frac{130\ \text{mg}}{1\ \text{dl}} \times \frac{10^3}{10^2}$$

$$x = 130 \times 10$$

$$x = 1,300$$

Hence, 130 mg/dl = 1,300 μg/ml.

Ratio and proportion may be used as well.

$$130\ \text{mg}/100\ \text{ml} = 130,000\ \mu\text{g}/100\ \text{ml}$$

$$\frac{130,000\ \mu\text{g}}{100\ \text{ml}} = \frac{x}{1}$$

$$100x = 130,000$$

$$x = 1,300$$

EXAMPLE 6-53: Express 21 g/L as milligrams per microliter.

$$\frac{\text{g}}{\text{L}} \rightarrow \frac{\text{mg}}{\mu\text{l}} = \frac{10^3}{10^6}$$

Using the formula:

$$x\ \text{mg}/\mu\text{l} = 21\ \text{g/L} \times \frac{10^3}{10^6}$$

$$x = 21 \times 10^{-3}$$

$$x = 0.021$$

21 g/L is equal to 0.021 mg/μl.

EXAMPLE 6-54: Express 316 μg/ml as milligrams per deciliter.

$$\frac{\mu g}{ml} \to \frac{mg}{dl} = \frac{10^{-3}}{10^{-2}}$$

$$x \text{ mg/dl} = 316 \ \mu g/ml \times \frac{10^{-3}}{10^{-2}}$$

$$x = 316 \times 10^{-1}$$

$$x = 31.6$$

316 μg/ml is equal to 31.6 mg/dl.

Conversion of Metric Units to SI Units

There has been some effort to adapt the units used in medical laboratories to a convenient adaptation of the SI system. Appendix X lists most of the recommended units of this adaptation.

This generally involves the steps given above with one extra step. Since most SI units in the laboratory involve moles per some unit, division by the molecular weight must be added to the calculations. Conversion to moles is discussed in Section 6.6, pp. 138 in this chapter.

EXAMPLE 6-55: Convert 1 g of sodium per milliliter to the SI unit picomoles per liter.

First convert grams per milliliter to picograms per liter.

$$1 \text{ g} = 10^{12} \text{ pg}$$
$$1 \text{ ml} = 10^{-3} \text{ L}$$

Hence,

$$\frac{1 \text{ g}}{1 \text{ ml}} = \frac{10^{12} \text{ pg}}{10^{-3} \text{ L}}$$

$$x \text{ pg/L} = 1 \text{ g/ml} \times \frac{10^{12}}{10^{-3}}$$

$$x = 1 \times 10^{15} \text{ pg/L}$$

1 g/ml is equal to 1×10^{15} pg/L.

Divide the number of picograms by the atomic or molecular weight of the substance to determine the equivalent number of picomoles.

The atomic weight of sodium is about 23.

$$\frac{1 \times 10^{15}}{23} = 4.35 \times 10^{13}$$

Hence, 1 g of sodium per milliliter is equal to 4.35×10^{13} picomoles per liter.

APPENDIXES RELATED TO THIS CHAPTER

I   Symbols of Units of Measure
K   Conversion Factors for Units of Measure
L   Conversion Factors for the More Common Electrolytes
Q   Formulas Presented in This Book

T   Conversions Among Metric Prefixes
U   Conversions Among Square Metric Units
V   Conversions Among Cubic Metric Units
W   Conversions Between Liter Units and Cubic Metric Units
X   Conversions Between Conventional and SI Units
Y   Periodic Chart of the Elements
Z   Atomic Weights
BB Concentration of Acids and Bases—Common Commercial Strengths
DD Clinical Tests With Units, Normal Values, and Conversion Factors

PRACTICE PROBLEMS

Calculate the answer for each problem. Understand each portion of the calculation and determine whether the answer is logical. *Just because an answer can be calculated does not mean that it is reasonable.*

Parts

Convert to ppm:
1. 320 mg/dl
2. 2.6 g/dl
3. 4.52 g/L
4. 0.07%
5. 16 ng/ml
6. 320 μg/L
7. 20%
8. 16,200 mg/ml

9. 320 ng/dl
10. 63 pg/ml
11. 796 mg/L
12. 1,000 μg/dl
13. 1,000 μg/ml
14. 14 g/2,000 ml
15. 16 dg/ml

Convert to the indicated units:
16. 1 ppm to milligrams per deciliter
17. 155 ppm to nanograms per milliliter
18. 3.6 ppm to grams per liter
19. 20,100 ppm to micrograms per deciliter
20. 0.01 ppm to decigrams per milliliter
21. 22 ppm to nanograms per deciliter
22. 979 ppm to grams per milliliter
23. 1.06 ppm to milligrams per liter
24. 0.001 ppm to milligrams per milliliter
25. 0.30 ppm to micrograms per milliliter
26. 555 ppm to grams per deciliter
27. 10 ppm to picograms per liter
28. 1,353 ppm to picograms per milliliter
29. 0.09 ppm to nanograms per liter
30. 193 ppm to micrograms per liter

31. A technologist wishes to prepare 1 L of a stock standard solution for a calcium determination with a concentration of 200 ppm calcium. The weight of $CaCO_3$ required for preparation of the solution is:
    a. 100 mg   c. 250 mg
    b. 150 mg   d. 500 mg

Percentages

Indicate whether the following are w/w, w/v, or v/v:

32. 10 g in 100 g of solution
33. 10 ml in 100 ml of solution

34. 31 g in 100 ml of solution

State the following as percentage w/w, w/v, or v/v:

35. 3 g in 100 g of solution
36. 12 ml in 100 ml of solution
37. 6.3 g in 100 ml of solution
38. 0.06 mg in 100 ml of solution
39. 32 mg in 50 ml of solution

40. 3.5 g in 40 ml of solution
41. 10 g in 80 g of solution
42. 6 g + 70 g of solution
43. 28 g + 60 g of solution
44. 150 mg in 80 ml of solution

State how you would prepare the following:

45. 400 ml of 6%$^{w/v}$ NaCl
46. 30 ml of 20%$^{v/v}$ HCl
47. 1,200 ml of 5%$^{w/v}$ HCl

48. 350 g of 1.6%$^{w/w}$ NaOH
49. 3 L of 40%$^{w/v}$ H_2SO_4
50. 500 ml of 0.06%$^{v/v}$ HNO_3

Give the percentages and state whether the following are w/w, w/v, or v/v:

51. 12 g of NaCl ↑ 200 ml
52. 1.3 ml of HCl ↑ 40 ml
53. 1,300 mg of NaOH ↑ 2 L
54. 130 mg of HCl + 90 g H_2O
55. 0.05 ml of H_2SO_4 ↑ 20 ml

56. 1.6 ml of HNO_3 ↑ 2.5 L
57. 60 g of urea ↑ 180 g
58. 0.21 mg + 20 g H_2O
59. 152 g of NaCl ↑ 400 ml
60. 10 g of NaOH + 90 g solvent

Tell how much solution can be made from the following:

61. 40 g of NaCl: Make 25%.
62. 0.6 g of NaOH: Make 0.6%.
63. 1.32 g of HCl: Make 5%.

64. 53 g of NaCl: Make 15%.
65. 4 g of NaOH: Make 0.005%.

For the following quantities and percentages, tell how much substance would be present in each:

66. 300 ml of 8%$^{w/v}$
67. 10 ml of 0.6%$^{w/v}$
68. 3 L of 30%$^{v/v}$

69. 5 ml of 25%$^{w/v}$
70. 1.8 L of 0.09%$^{v/v}$
71. 120 ml of 90%$^{w/v}$

72. Thirty grams of NaCl would make 200 ml of what percentage Cl?
73. A 10% $(NH_4)_2SO_4$ standard is needed. How much $(NH_4)_2SO_4$ would be needed to make 50 ml?
74. A solution of 20% KCl is on hand. What percentage K would that be?
75. How much KCl would be required to make 100 ml of 1.5% Cl solution?
76. How many grams of sodium chloride are contained in 300 ml of an 8% solution?
77. How many milliliters of glacial acetic acid are contained in 150 ml of a 40% solution of acetic acid?
78. How many grams of salt are present in 500 ml of physiological saline?
79. How would you make 2,000 ml of 40%$^{v/v}$ HCl?
80. Place 0.5 ml packed sheep blood cells in a 30 ml centrifuge tube. How much saline has to be added to obtain a 2% suspension? A 3% suspension?
81. How would you make 300 ml of a 5% NaCl solution?
82. How much NaCl is actually present in 5 ml of a 50% NaCl solution?
83. How would you make 2,000 ml of a 6.2%$^{w/v}$ HCl solution?
84. If you had 4 g of NaOH in 20 ml of H_2O, what would be the percent concentration? What would be the mg% concentration?

85. How would you make a 100 mg% NaCl standard?
86. Make 650 ml of a 20% NaCl solution.
87. You have 50 g of NaOH and you need to make a 10% solution. How much can you make?
88. Convert 16% to grams per liter.
89. There are 25 g in 200 ml of solution. What is its percent concentration?
90. Convert 3.8% to milligrams per liter and then to grams per liter.
91. How much 20% solution can be made from 45 g of NaCl?
92. A sodium concentration is reported as 323 mg%. What is the concentration in milligrams per liter?
93. You have 10 g of substance. It takes 2 g to make 10 ml of solution. The 10 g will make _____ ml of solution. What will be the percent concentration?
94. If there are 30 g in 100 ml, how many grams would be in 20 ml?
95. How would you make 135 ml of 6% NaCl?
96. How much NaOH would be present in 300 ml of a 10% solution?
97. How would you make 50 ml of a 0.9% NaCl solution?
98. There are 25 g in 300 ml of solution. What is its percent concentration?
99. Twenty grams of NaOH will make 500 ml of what percentage?
100. You have 10 g of NaCl. You need to make a 4% solution. How much 4% solution could be made from the 10 g?
101. There are 32 g in 800 ml of solution. What is its percent concentration?
102. How much NaCl would be required to make 300 ml of a 16.6% solution?
103. You have 50 ml of a 2% NaOH solution. How much NaOH is present in those 50 ml?
104. You have 3 g of NaCl. You need to make a 0.5% solution. How much could you make with those 3 g?
105. There are 2.3 g of NaOH in 275 ml. What is its percent concentration?
106. If 0.5 of Töpfer's reagent is dissolved in 100 cc of 95% alcohol, this is approximately:
    a. a 0.5% solution   c. an 80% solution
    b. a 1% solution   d. a 95% solution
107. How many grams of sodium chloride are there in 1.5 L of a 5% solution?
108. A 0.1% solution is made by diluting _____ to 1 L with distilled water:
    a. 0.1 g   c. 100 mg
    b. 1.0 g   d. 1 mg
109. How many grams of a salt would be required to make each of the following solutions?
    a. 100 ml of a 12% solution   c. 75 ml of a 2% solution
    b. 400 ml of a 6% solution
110. What is the concentration expressed in a percent value (w/v) of each of the following solutions?
    a. 1 g of $CuSO_4$ in 25 ml   c. 2 g of $AgNO_3$ in 400 ml
    b. 55 g of $CaCl_2$ in 120 ml   d. 280 g of KCl in 600 ml
111. What amount of NaOH is needed to make 50 ml of a 30% solution?
112. A _____ percent solution is made with 5 g of NaCl in 95 ml of water.
113. How many grams of sodium chloride are there in 2.6 L of a 0.3% solution?

$$V_1 \times C_1 = V_2 \times C_2$$

114. Will 5 ml of 1N H_2SO_4 exactly neutralize 5 ml of 1N NaOH?
115. It required 20 ml of 0.1N NaOH to neutralize 10 ml of HCl. What is the normality of the HCl?
116. It required 4.2 ml of NaOH to neutralize 15 ml of 0.2N oxalic acid. What is the normality of the NaOH?

117. You use 9.1 ml of NaOH to neutralize 20 ml of 0.8N oxalic acid. What is the normality of the NaOH?

118. You have 1.01N NaOH and you wish to make 3,000 ml of 1N NaOH. How much of the 1.01N solution do you need?

119. You need 11.0 ml of 3N NaOH to neutralize 4 ml of H_2SO_4. What is the normality of the sulfuric acid?

120. You have 2.1N H_2SO_4 and wish to make 200 ml of 2N. How much water would be required?

121. If 20.00 ml of a 1.000N solution of HCl required 19.50 ml of a solution of sodium hydroxide for neutralization using phenolphthalein as an indicator, the normality of the sodium hydroxide solution is:
    a. 0.975
    b. 1.026
    c. unable to be sure because phenolphthalein is the wrong indicator to use
    d. 2.0

122. How many milliliters of a 2% solution will 20 ml of a 10% solution make?

123. How much water would be needed to make 50 ml of 5% from 25%?

124. If you mix 10 ml of a 6N solution of HCl and 20 ml of a 3N HCl solution, what would be the concentration of the resulting solution?

125. How much 1N NaOH and 5N NaOH must be mixed together to make 500 ml of a 4N NaOH?

126. How much 75% alcohol is needed to make 500 ml of 60% alcohol?

127. How much 0.3M solution can be made from 50 ml of a 2M solution?

128. How would you make 1 L of a 0.04N solution from a 0.6N solution?

129. A total of 2.7 ml of base is needed to neutralize 10 ml of 0.04N acid. What is the normality of the base?

130. How much 0.4N acid is needed to neutralize 50 ml of 0.9N base?

131. How many milliliters of 0.1N NaOH will 10 ml of 1N HCl neutralize?

132. The normality of an HCl solution is 4.5N. How much water must be added to 25 ml of this solution to make a 1.8N solution?

133. You have on hand 250 ml of a stock solution of H_2SO_4. You discover that 30 ml of this stock solution is neutralized by 30.25 ml of 1N NaOH. How much water must be added to the remainder of the stock H_2SO_4 to make it 1N?

134. How much 30% NaOH can be made from 6 ml of 50% NaCl?

135. How much 0.05N NaOH can be made with 5 ml of 200N NaOH?

136. You could make 60 ml of 20% from 30 ml of what percentage?

137. How much water would be needed to make 30 ml of a 0.6% NaCl from 10%?

138. You would use 20 cc 0.1N HCl to neutralize 40 cc NaOH of what normality?

139. You mix 30 ml of 6N and 70 ml of 4N NaOH in a flask. What is the concentration of the final solution?

140. Given: 5 L of approximately 0.5N HCl. Wanted: exactly 0.5N HCl. If 25 ml of this solution was titrated and found to be 0.6N, how would you make the 0.5N desired?

141. If you mixed 20 ml of a 6N NaOH and 80 ml of 0.6N NaOH together, what would be the normality of the resulting solution?

142. You could make 30 ml of 10% from how much 6%?

143. You could make 150 ml of 0.2% from 3 ml of what percentage?

144. You have 5M NaOH. You need 100 ml of 1M solution. How much 5M would be required?

145. Make 100 ml of 4% NaCl from 9%.

146. How much 10% is needed to make 69 ml of 9%?

147. You could make 150 ml of 0.2% from 5 ml of what percentage?

148. How much 15% alcohol can be made from 30 ml of 10% alcohol?

149. How much 4% H_2SO_4 would be required to make 750 ml of 0.6% H_2SO_4?

150. How much 25% can be made from 1.5 ml of 75%?
151. How much 20% solution is required to make 200 ml of 3% solution?
152. You could make 5 ml of 6% from 3 ml of what percentage?
153. You could make 2,000 ml of what percentage from 250 ml of 10%?
154. Add 20 ml of 6% plus 3 ml of 2%. What percentage is produced?
155. How much 15% HCl must be mixed with 4% HCl to produce 40 ml of 10%?
156. How much 3% solution would need to be mixed with a 40% solution to produce a 15% solution?
157. On hand you have 50% HNO_3. The procedure calls for 5 ml per test of freshly made 0.4%. You have one blank, two controls, and six patients' samples. How would you prepare the dilute solution, and how much would you make?

Hydrates

158. a. What is the molecular weight of $CuSO_4$?
     b. What is the molecular weight of $CuSO_4 \cdot H_2O$?
159. You have $CuSO_4 \cdot 10\ H_2O$. You need to make 400 ml of a 5% $CuSO_4$ solution. How would you do it?
160. You need 450 ml of a 10% $Na_2SO_4 \cdot 10\ H_2O$ solution. Carry out the steps involved in making the required 10% solution using Na_2SO_4.
161. Calcium chloride ($CaCl_2$) is available; the procedure calls for an 8% $CaCl_2 \cdot 10\ H_2O$ solution. What would be the procedure for making 2,000 ml of the desired concentration?
162. How many grams of $CuSO_4 \cdot 5\ H_2O$ are needed to make 1 L of a 1% solution of $CuSO_4$?
163. How many grams of $Co(NO_3)_2 \cdot 6\ H_2O$ are needed in preparing 400 ml of a 0.02% solution of $Co(NO_3)_2$?
164. A 9% $CuSO_4$ (anhydrous) solution is made up by dissolving 9 g of anhydrous $CuSO_4$ in 100 ml of solution. How is a 9% $CuSO_4 \cdot 5\ H_2O$ solution made?
165. a. Do a 6% $CuSO_4$ solution and a 6% $CuSO_4 \cdot 5\ H_2O$ solution contain the same quantities of $CuSO_4$?
     b. If not, which one has more?
     c. How much more does it have?
166. How many grams are required to make 60 ml of a 2% solution of $CuSO_4$? $CuSO_4 \cdot 5\ H_2O$?
167. What volume of 23% $CaCl_2$ can be prepared from 500 g of $CaCl_2 \cdot 10\ H_2O$?
168. A 7.5 g%$^{(w/v)}$ sodium acetate solution (anhydrous) is to be prepared in 130 ml from $CH_3COONa \cdot 3\ H_2O$. How much of the hydrated compound will be needed?

Molarity

169. The molarity of a solution prepared by diluting 100 g of NaH_2PO_4 to 1 L is:
     a. 0.833   d. 1.67
     b. 1.20   e. 2.82
     c. 1.41
170. What weight of NaOH would be required to prepare 3,000 ml of a 2.5M solution?
171. If you had 6 mol in 600 ml of solution, what would be the molarity?
172. A solution contains 100 g NaCl/L. What is its molarity?
173. There are 200 mmol NaOH/400 ml. What is the molarity of the solution?
174. There are 140 g of H_2SO_4 in 400 ml of solution. What is the molarity of the solution?
175. How would you make 300 ml of 6M NaOH?
176. You could make 180 ml of what molar with 30 ml of 4M?
177. There are 200 g of NaCl per 300 ml of solution. What is the molarity?
178. How much 7.5M NaOH solution can be made with 40 g of NaOH?

179. What is the molecular weight of NaCl?
180. In a solution of NaCl containing 400 mmol in 150 ml, what is the molarity?
181. What is the molecular weight of H_3PO_4?
182. If one has a 15 g/400 ml solution that is 12M, what is the molecular weight of the substance?
183. What is the molecular weight of $Ca_3(PO_4)_2$?
184. To make a solution of $CaCl_2$ that contains ⅕ gm mol/L, how much $CaCl_2$ would be needed?
185. What are the molecular and gram molecular weights of Na_2SO_4?
186. How many grams of NaOH are present in 80 ml of a 7M solution of sodium hydroxide?
187. How many moles are in 336 g of $NaHCO_3$?
188. How much sodium hydroxide would be present in 1 L of 0.0014M KOH?
189. How many grams of NaCl does 600 ml of a 1M NaCl solution contain?
190. How much 0.09M can be made from 10 ml of 4M HCl?
191. How many grams does 1 L of a 0.3M solution of NaCl contain?
192. How many grams of NaCl are required to make 250 ml of a 0.4M solution?
193. How many grams of NaCl are required to make 50 ml of a 0.3M solution?
194. How many grams of HCl are required to make 1,200 ml of 0.03M solution?
195. What is the molarity of a solution of Na_2SO_4 in which 284.2 g of this salt are placed in a 1 L volumetric flask and made up to volume with water?
196. Describe fully how you would prepare a 1M solution of Na_2SO_4.
197. How many grams of each of the following are necessary to make 200 ml of a 2M solution:
    a. H_3PO_4 c. $CaCl_2$
    b. NaOH   d. H_2SO_4
198. Outline the steps you would use in preparing 500 ml of a 0.6M $NaHCO_3$ solution.
199. What is the molar concentration of each of the following:
    a. 60 g of NaOH in a total volume of 300 ml
    b. 112 g of $BaSO_4$ in 700 ml
    c. 38 g of $BaCl_2$ diluted to 200 ml
200. How many grams of solute does 1,300 ml of a 0.15M H_3PO_4 solution contain?
201. Make 800 ml of a ⁵⁄₁₅ KOH.
202. What weight of NaOH would be required to prepare 2,300 ml of a 1.5M solution?
203. A solution contains 300 g of NaCl/L. What is its molarity?
204. How much 4M NaOH solution can be made with 40 g of NaOH?
205. How many nanograms of NaCl would 800 ml of a 1×10^{-9}M solution contain?
206. A solution contains 1.9 g of HCl in 1 L. How many millimoles of HCl does it contain? How many micromoles would be in 250 ml of solution?
207. The gram molecular weight of $(C_4H_9)_2NH$ is _____.
208. What weight of H_2SO_4 is required to prepare 400 ml of a 3M solution?
209. How many grams of HCl would be required to prepare 500 ml of a 1×10^{-3}M solution?
210. What weight of NaOH is required to prepare 3,000 ml of a 0.7M solution?
211. How many micrograms of NaCl would 350 ml of a 1×10^{-6}M solution contain?
212. A solution contains 4.8 g of HCl in 1 L. How many millimoles does it contain?
213. Do a 6M $CuSO_4$ solution and a 6M $CuSO_4 \cdot 5 H_2O$ solution contain the same quantities of $CuSO_4$? If no, why? If yes, why?
214. How many grams of each of the following are required to make 1 L of a 0.8M solution?
    a. $CuSO_4$ c. $CuSO_4 \cdot 5 H_2O$
    b. $CuSO_4 \cdot H_2O$

Osmolarity

215. If a substance has a concentration of 85 mmol/L and gives three particles on ionization, what would be its concentration in milliosmoles per liter?

216. A solution contains 6.2 mol/L of a substance that yields three ions on dissociation. What is the concentration in osmoles per liter?

217. A certain substance has a freezing point of $-0.16°C$. What would be its concentration in milliosmoles per liter?

218. A solution of a substance that does not ionize has a concentration of 60 mmol/L. What is its concentration in milliosmoles per liter?

219. A solution contains 3 mol/L of a substance that yields three ions on dissociation. What is its concentration in osmoles per liter?

220. A NaCl solution contains 430 mg NaCl/700 ml of solution. What is its concentration in milliosmoles per liter?

221. A urine sample has a freezing point of $-0.52°C$. What is its concentration in milliosmoles per liter?

222. A urine sample has a freezing point of $-0.69°C$. What is its concentration in milliosmoles per liter?

223. A substance has a concentration of 30 mmol/L. On dissociation it produces two particles. What is its milliosmoles-per-liter concentration?

224. A solution contains 25 mOsmol/L of NaCl and 135 mOsmol/L of glucose. What would be its freezing point?

225. A substance has a freezing point depression of $\Delta-0.80°C$. What is its concentration in milliosmoles per liter?

226. A solution of NaCl and glucose gives a freezing point of $-0.95°C$. It contains 140 mOsmol glucose/L. Give the concentration of NaCl in milliosmoles per liter and molarity.

227. A solution contains 24 mmol NaCl/L. Give its concentration in milliosmoles per liter.

228. A plasma sample gives a freezing point reading of $-0.70°C$. Give its concentration in milliosmoles per liter.

229. If a substance has a concentration of 85 mmol/L and gives three particles on ionization, what would be its concentration in milliosmoles per liter?

230. A certain substance has a freezing point of $-0.35°C$. What would be its concentration in milliosmoles per liter?

Normality

231. How many equivalent weights of NaOH are there in 3 L of 0.6N NaOH?

232. Make 500 ml of 4N H_3PO_4.

233. How many equivalent weights of sulfuric acid are there in 1 L of 1.3N H_2SO_4?

234. A 7.2N $CaCl_2 \cdot 10\ H_2O$ solution is needed. If $CaCl_2$ is available, how would one make the needed solution?

235. The molecular weight of H_2SO_4 is 98. A 2N solution of H_2SO_4 contains:
    a. 196 g in 100 ml   d. 98 g in 100 ml
    b. 49 g in 1,000 ml   e. 196 g in 1,000 ml
    c. 98 g in 1,000 ml

236. Given: 4 L of approximately 0.7N HCl. Wanted: exactly 0.7N HCl. When titrated, 50 ml of the solution was found to be 0.65N. How much water should be added to make the 0.7N solution desired?

237. Calculate the chloride concentration in milliequivalents per liter of a solution prepared by diluting 20 g of barium chloride to 1 L:
    a. 96 mEq/L   d. 1,480 mEq/L
    b. 192 mEq/L   e. 2,817 mEq/L
    c. 1,040 mEq/L

238. What would be the normality of 38 g of NaOH in 600 ml of solution?

239. How many milliliters of 0.1N NaOH are required to react with 100 mEq of H_2SO_4?
   a. 1 ml   d. 100 ml
   b. 5 ml   e. 1,000 ml
   c. 50 ml
240. How much 8N HCl will be required to neutralize 50 ml of 0.5N NaOH?
241. How would you make 3 L of 3N H_3PO_4?
242. You could convert 15 ml of $^N/_{10}$ solution to $^N/_{100}$ by adding water to make a total of how many milliliters?
243. There are 20 mEq NaOH/400 ml. What is the normality?
244. Make 7,500 ml of $^N/_8$ HCl.
245. Make 200 ml of $^N/_6$ NaOH.
246. In a titration procedure 15 ml of 1.2N solution was required to titrate 4 ml of an unknown solution. What is the normality of the unknown solution?
247. In a calcium procedure 1 ml of $KMnO_4$ equals 0.05 mg of Ca. What is the normality of the $KMnO_4$ solution?
248. How many grams of NaCl will be in 50 ml of a 25N solution?
249. You need to make some $Hg(NO_3)_2$ for a chloride procedure. You want 1 ml of the $Hg(NO_3)_2$ to equal 5 mg of Cl. What normality would you make?
250. How would one make 2.3 L of 4N H_3PO_4?
251. In a calcium procedure one uses a 0.04N $KMnO_4$ solution for titration. How much Ca would 1 ml of this solution equal?
252. How many milliequivalents of $Ba(OH)_2$ are there in 300 ml of 0.6N $Ba(OH)_2$?
253. In HCl chloride is monovalent. In $CaCl_2$ the calcium is divalent. In K_3PO_4, what valence does K possess?
254. Make 150 ml of $^N/_5$ $BaCl_2$.
255. What is the molecular weight of NaCl? What is the equivalent weight of NaCl?
256. There are 10 mEq in 200 ml of a NaOH solution. What is the normality?
257. What is the molecular weight of H_2SO_4? What is the equivalent weight of H_2SO_4?
258. How would one prepare 300 ml of 0.03N $BaSO_4$?
259. What is the molecular weight of H_3PO_4? What is the equivalent weight of H_3PO_4?
260. How many milliliters of a 3N solution can be made from 60 g of $CaCl_2$?
261. How many grams of solute per liter does a 10N HCl solution contain?
262. If 200 ml of a 15N $CaCl_2$ solution is desired and $CaCl_2 \cdot 10\ H_2O$ is on hand how should one proceed?
263. How many grams of solute does 1 L of a 2.5N Na_2CO_3 solution contain?
264. Make 1,800 ml of 20N H_2SO_4.
265. How many grams of solute does 1 L of a 0.15M H_3PO_4 solution contain?
266. A procedure calls for 15 ml of 3N $AgNO_3$ for each test. Five tests and two controls per day, 7 days a week, are averaged. The solution is stable for 3 months. Pure $AgNO_3$ is ordered in 1.5-lb jars. It costs 10 cents/oz. How much should be ordered for a 6-month supply, and how much will it cost?
267. Calculate the amount of $CaCl_2 \cdot 2\ H_2O$ necessary to prepare 700 ml of a 0.4N solution of $CaCl_2$.
268. There are 400 mEq in 40 ml of a solution. What is its normality?
269. How many grams of each of these substances are needed to make a liter of a 6.1N solution?
   a. $AgNO_3$ c. NH_4OH
   b. Na_2CO_3 d. H_3PO_4
270. If 25 ml of 3N NaOH and 90 ml of 0.6N NaOH are mixed together, what would be the normality of the resulting solution?
271. How many milliequivalents are in 1 L of a 4.5N HCl solution?

272. How many milliliters of 12N solution can be made from 30 ml of 18N?
273. How many milliequivalents are there in 284 mg of Na_2SO_4?
274. A solution contains 7.5 g eq/L. What is its normality?
275. How many milliequivalents are contained in 0.284 g of Na_2SO_4?
276. How much 1.5N HCl and 7.5N HCl must be mixed together to make 3 L of 5N solution?
277. If you have 50 mg of NaCl in 400 ml, what normality would you have?
278. A procedure calls for 60 ml of a 0.4N NaOH. If 8N NaOH is on hand, how would one make 100 ml of 0.4N?
279. You want to set up a chloride procedure using mercuric nitrate. You want 0.5 ml of the $Hg(NO_3)_2$ to equal 2.5 mg of NaCl. What normality must you make?
280. An $Hg(NO_3)_2$ solution to use in a titration chloride procedure is desired. What normality would one have to make so that each milliliter of the solution would be equal to 2.0 mg of chloride?
281. If you had 40 g of NaOH in 400 ml of solution, what would be the normality?
282. In a chloride procedure 1 ml of $Hg(NO_3)_2$ solution equals 0.1 mg of chloride. What is the normality of the titrating solution?
283. How many gram equivalent weights of solute are contained in:
    a. 1 L of 3N solution   c. 500 ml of 2N solution
    b. 2 L of 0.5N solution
284. How many grams of HNO_3 will be contained in 500 ml of a 2N solution?
285. You want to set up a calcium procedure so that 1 ml of $KMnO_4$ equals 3 mg of Ca. What normality would you have to make?
286. If there are 3 g of $BaCl_2$ in 30 ml of solution, what would be the normality?
287. Make 200 ml of ⅚% $CaCl_2$.
288. There are 20 mEq in 200 ml of a NaOH solution. What is the normality?
289. How many molecular weights of H_2SO_4 does 100 ml of 2N H_2SO_4 contain?
290. A solution that contains 1 eq wt of hydrogen ion/500 ml of solution is of what normality?
291. What normality is a solution of NaOH if it contains 16 g of solute per 80 ml of solution?
292. A solution of barium chloride is made with 18 g in 800 ml of water. The milliequivalents per liter of chloride in this solution are _____.
293. One gram equivalent weight of K_3PO_4 is _____.
294. The label on a bottle of sodium hydroxide states 75.0%. How many grams of chemical dissolved in 400 ml of water are needed to prepare a 1.6N solution of NaOH?
295. You need 100 ml of a 5N $CaCl_2 \cdot 10\ H_2O$ solution. You have available $CaCl_2$. How would you make the needed solution?
296. How many grams of $CuSO_4$, $CuSO_4 \cdot H_2O$, and $CuSO_4 \cdot 10\ H_2O$ are required to make:
    a. 500 ml of a 3% solution of each of these salts
    b. 500 ml of a 3N solution of each of these salts

Specific gravity

297. How would you prepare 200 ml of a 25%$^{w/v}$ H_2SO_4 solution? (sp gr 1.84, 97% assay)?
298. How many grams of HCl (sp gr 1.36, 42% assay) are in 250 ml of concentrated acid?
299. Make 3,000 ml of a 0.6N HNO_3 solution (sp gr 1.4, 70% assay).
300. How many milliliters of H_2SO_4 (sp gr 1.84, 97% assay) would be required to make 200 ml of a 6M solution?
301. If you have 100 ml of concentrated H_2SO_4 (sp gr 1.8, 95% assay) in a total volume of 600 ml of solution, give:
    a. %$^{v/v}$ c. molarity
    b. %$^{w/v}$ d. normality

302. Given 15 ml of concentrated H_2SO_4 diluted up to 400 ml, what would be the percentage v/v and w/v? (sp gr 1.82, 96% assay)?

303. You have a $20\%^{v/v}$ solution of HNO_3. How much concentrated HNO_3 (sp gr 1.49, 72% assay) would need to be added to 100 ml of the 20% solution to make 500 ml of 5M HNO_3?

304. How would one make 1,000 of ml of 8N HNO_3? (sp gr 1.39, 71% assay)?

305. A commercial solution of concentrated nitric acid has a density of 1.48 and contains 75% HNO_3. What is the molarity of the acid?

306. What is the molarity of a commercial solution of H_2SO_4 having a density of 1.86 and containing 96% H_2SO_4?

307. What is the normality of a commercial H_3PO_4 solution having a density of 1.8 and containing 80% H_3PO_4?

308. Make 700 ml of 0.3N H_3PO_4 (sp gr 1.16, 40% pure).

309. How many milliliters of concentrated H_2SO_4 (sp gr 1.85, 93% assay) would be required to make 400 ml of a 4M solution?

310. How would you make 1,000 ml of 6N HNO_3? (sp gr 1.42, 73% assay)

311. How many milliliters of concentrated HCl (sp gr 1.19, 37.5% assay) would be required to prepare 18 L of 0.1M acid?

312. You have 30 ml of H_2SO_4 (sp gr 1.84, 95.5% assay) diluted up to 500 ml. Give the following:
    a. $\%^{v/v}$ c. molarity
    b. $\%^{w/v}$ d. normality

313. A $68\%^{v/v}$ H_2SO_4 solution has a specific gravity of 1.21. Give the following (assume 100% purity):
    a. molarity   c. weight of 500 ml of acid
    b. normality

314. Give the specific gravity of a solution if 4.0 ml weighs 3.4 g.

315. You know that 200 ml of a urine specimen weighs 310.0 g. What is the specific gravity of the specimen?

316. What would be the volume of 6 kg of a solution that had a specific gravity of 0.92?

317. You have 250 ml of a liquid that weighs 325 g. What is the specific gravity of the liquid?

318. What is the concentration of 300 ml of $10\%^{v/v}$ HCl in terms of molarity and normality? (concentrated acid sp gr 1.18, 34% assay)

319. A bottle of concentrated hydrochloric acid has a specific gravity of 1.37 and is 36% HCl. What is the normality of the concentrated acid?

320. A $73\%^{v/v}$ H_3PO_4 solution has a specific gravity of 1.06 (100% H_3PO_4). What is its molarity, normality, and how much does 110 ml of the acid weigh?

321. A concentrated HCl solution contains 37.5% HCl by weight and has a specific gravity of 1.19. Calculate the weight of HCl in 50.0 ml of concentrated acid.

322. Find the specific gravity of ethyl alcohol if 10.0 ml weighs 8.4 g.

323. A volume of urine (400 ml) weighs 430.0 g. What is the specific gravity of the urine specimen?

324. What would be the volume of 15 kg of a glycerol solution that had a specific gravity of 1.51?

325. A small volume, 50 ml, of a heavy liquid weighs 316 g. What is the specific gravity of the liquid?

326. Concentrated HCl contains 36.5% HCl by weight and has a specific gravity of 1.18. Calculate the weight of HCl in 25.0 ml of concentrated acid.

327. How much $4\%^{w/v}$ H_2SO_4 would be required to make 750 ml of $0.6\%^{v/v}$?

Concentration relationships

Use the following information if needed for the problems in this section.

	Specific gravity	Percent purity
HCl	1.19	37
H_2SO_4	1.84	97
HNO_3	1.4	70
H_3PO_4	1.8	80

328. Convert $3\%^{w/v}$ H_2SO_4 to normality.
329. Express 600 mg of NaCl/dl as milliequivalents of Cl per liter.
330. The magnesium concentration of a serum sample was reported as 4.2 mg/dl. The magnesium concentration expressed as milliequivalents per liter would be _____.
331. Express 80 mEq/L Na as milligrams of NaCl per deciliter.
332. Convert $20\%^{v/v}$ HCl to normality.
333. How much 5N HCl could be made from 10 ml of 14M HCl?
334. Convert $10\%^{w/v}$ H_2SO_4 to normality.
335. How much 2M H_2SO_4 can be made from 100 ml of 7N H_2SO_4?
336. Convert 700 mg/dl NaCl to milliequivalents Cl per liter.
337. 40 ml of 0.4N H_2SO_4 will make how much $20\%^{w/v}$ H_2SO_4?
338. Convert 6M NaOH to a percentage.
339. 8N HCl is equal to what $\%^{w/v}$ HCl?
340. How much 6N HCl will be needed to neutralize 3 ml of a 3M NaOH solution?
341. If you had $70\%^{w/v}$ HNO_3, it would equal what normal and what molar HNO_3?
342. Express 30 mg/dl Ca as milliequivalents of Ca per liter.
343. Express the following as milliequivalents per liter:
    a. 11 mg Ca/dl   c. 12 mg K/dl
    b. 600 mg NaCl/dl
344. What molarity equals 10% NaCl?
345. What normality is 0.15% saline?
246. What is the normality of a 0.2M H_3PO_4?
347. Express the following as milligrams per deciliter:
    a. 134 mEq Na/L   c. 6 mEq K/L
    b. 6 mEq Ca/L
348. What is the molarity of a 0.2N H_2SO_4 solution?
349. If you had 30 ml of 2N H_2SO_4, it would react with how many milliliters of 15% NaOH?
350. Express the following in terms of normality:
    a. 0.6M NaOH   c. 0.6M H_3PO_4
    b. 0.6M NaCl   d. 0.6M $CuSO_4$
351. If you had 100 ml of 3N NaOH, it would neutralize how many milliliters of $30\%^{v/v}$ HCl?
352. Express the following in terms of molarity:
    a. 0.4N NaOH   c. 0.6N H_3PO_4
    b. 0.2N NaCl   d. 0.3N $CuSO_4$
353. What normality is equal to 45% NaOH?
354. A sodium concentration reported is 323 mg/dl. What is the concentration in mEq/L?

355. Give the percentage $1.06M$ HNO_3 is equal to as:
    a. w/v   b. v/v
356. A magnesium concentration is reported as 2.7 mEq/L. What is its concentration in milligrams per deciliter?
357. How much $3M$ NaOH can be prepared from 100 ml of $8N$ NaOH?
358. Express an 8% NaCl solution in terms of molarity and normality.
359. What molarity is equal to $6N$ H_2SO_4?
360. What is the molarity of a 12% KCN solution?
361. What normality is equal to $7.3M$ H_3PO_4?
362. What is the normality of a 3% K_2CO_3 solution?
363. What is the concentration of 400 ml of 0.9% NaCl in terms of molarity and normality?
364. What is the normality of a $0.01M$ H_2SO_4 solution?
365. What is the molarity of a $4N$ H_3PO_4 solution?
366. Express 0.5% $CaCl_2$ in terms of molarity and normality.
367. Express the following in terms of milliequivalents per liter:
    a. 315 mg NaCl/dl   c. 315 mg Na/dl
    b. 30 mg K/dl
368. Express the following in mg/dl:
    a. 145 mEq Cl/L   b. 2.6 mEq Mg/L
369. How many cubic centimeters of $5M$ H_2SO_4 will 15 cc of $2N$ NaOH neutralize?
370. Convert 7 mEq Ca/L to mg/dl.
371. Convert 180 mg/dl Na to milliequivalents NaCl per liter.
372. Make 350 ml of $6N$ HCl from $30\%^{w/v}$.
373. If you have 30% NaOH, what normality would you have?
374. Express 90 mEq Na/L as milligrams of NaCl per deciliter.
375. How much $6N$ HCl could be made from 20 ml of $12M$ HCl?
376. To what percent (w/v) HCl is $3N$ HCl equal?
377. Express as milliequivalents per liter:
    a. 10 mg Ca/dl   c. 14 mg K/dl
    b. 700 mg NaCl/dl
378. Express as milligrams per deciliter:
    a. 140 mEq Na/L   c. 5 mEq K/L
    b. 5 mEq Ca/L
379. To what molarity is $5N$ H_2SO_4 equal?
380. To what normality is $3M$ H_3PO_4 equal?
381. What amount of $24.5\%^{(v/v)}$ H_2SO_4, when diluted to 1,800 ml, will give you $5/12$ H_2SO_4?
382. A divalent substance is $20N$. How many milliliters are required to make 1 L of $0.1M$ solution?
383. Determine the amount of chloride (in mg/dl) in a 24-hour urine specimen with a total volume of 1,020 ml if the chloride concentration is known to be 103 mEq/L.
384. How much $2M$ H_2SO_4 can be made from 10 ml of $6N$ H_2SO_4?
385. If 30 ml of concentrated HCl were diluted up to 650 ml, give the following:
    a. $\%^{v/v}$ c. molarity
    b. $\%^{w/v}$ d. normality
386. How much $20\%^{w/v}$ H_2SO_4 can be made with 60 ml of $6.2N$ H_2SO_4?
387. To what normality is $60\%^{w/v}$ HNO_3 equal? What molarity?
388. Express the following in terms of molarity:
    a. $0.06N$ $AgNO_3$ c. $5N$ H_2SO_4
    b. $1.3N$ $CaCl_2$ d. $2N$ NaOH

389. Express the following in terms of normality:
    a. 0.01M $CaCl_2$ c. 0.4M $CuSO_4$
    b. 2M H_2SO_4 d. 6M NaOH

390. Of 15 g of NaOH are diluted to 600 ml, what is the concentration in terms of:
    a. molarity   c. $\%^{w/v}$
    b. normality   d. ppm

391. What volume of 36N H_2SO_4 is required to make 2L of 2.6M H_2SO_4?

392. If 4 g of sodium chloride are added to enough water to make 250 ml of solution, give the concentration in:
    a. %   d. ppm
    b. N   e. SI units
    c. M

393. Express 3,500 mg/dl NaCl in:
    a. %   e. N
    b. mEq Na/L   f. M
    c. mEq Cl/L   g. ppm
    d. mEq NaCl/L   h. SI units

394. In a quantitative test for potassium, 800 mEq K/L were found in a 24-hour urine specimen with a total volume of 2,400 ml. Express in:
    a. mg/dl   d. SI units
    b. g/24 hr   e. ppm
    c. mg/24 hr

395. What is the concentration of 300 ml of 0.9% saline in terms of:
    a. molarity   d. mg/dl
    b. normality   e. ppm
    c. mEq/L

396. A $34\%^{v/v}$ solution of HCl is available. How much concentrated acid must be added to 750 ml of this 34% solution to make 1,500 ml of 6.5N HCl?

397. To what percent (w/v) is $12\%^{v/v}$ H_2SO_4 equal?

398. To make 65 ml of $5\%^{v/v}$ HCl from $5\%^{w/v}$, how much water must be added?

399. To make 65 ml of $5\%^{w/v}$ HCl from $5\%^{v/v}$, how much water must be added?

400. Give the factors to convert the following:
    a. mg Ca/dl to mEq Ca/L   i. mg K/dl to mEq K/L
    b. mEq Ca/L to g Ca/L   j. mEq K/L to mg K/dl
    c. mEq Ca/L to mg Ca/dl   k. mEq K/L to g KCl/L
    d. mg Cl/dl to mEq Cl/L   l. mg Na/dl to mEq Na/L
    e. mg Cl/dl to mEq NaCl/L   m. mg Na/dl to mEq NaCl/L
    f. mEq Cl/L to mg Cl/dl   n. mEq Na/L to mg Na/dl
    g. mEq Cl/L to mg NaCl/dl   o. mEq Na/L to mg NaCl/dl
    h. mEq Cl/L to g NaCl/L   p. mEq Na/L to g NaCl/L

Volume percent CO_2 to millimoles per liter

401. A technologist reported the CO_2 content of a serum sample as 75 ml CO_2/100 ml. The CO_2 content expressed as millimoles per liter is _____.

402. If you convert 65 vol% of carbon dioxide to millimoles per liter, the answer is _____.

403. If you convert 25.4 mmol/L of CO_2 to vol%, the answer is _____.

404. The normal CO_2 combining power in the adult is 53 to 76 vol%. Express this in millimoles per liter.

405. Give the factors to convert the following:
     a. vol% CO_2 to mmol/L   b. mmol/L CO_2 to vol%

Complex metric conversions

Convert the following.

406. 5 mg/ml to μg/dl

407. 15,250 pg/L to g/ml

408. 10 dg/μl to mg/ml

409. 500 ng/μl to μg/L

410. 2 g/L to ng/μl

SI system

Convert to SI units:

411. 4.6 g/dl albumin as grams per liter

412. 62 μg/dl NH_3 as micromoles per liter

413. 1.8 mg/dl bilirubin as micromoles per liter

414. 11.0 mg/dl Ca as millimoles per liter

415. 4.8 mEq/L Ca as millimoles per liter

416. 40 mm Hg P_{CO_2} as kPa

417. 300 mg/dl serum Cl as millimoles per liter

418. 108 mEq/L serum Cl as millimoles per liter

419. 145 mg/dl cholesterol as millimoles per liter

420. 0.06 mg/dl serum creatinine as millimoles per liter

421. 55 mg/dl haptoglobin as micromoles per liter

422. 100 mg/dl serum glucose as millimoles per liter

423. 0.4 g/d urine glucose as millimoles per day

424. 6.0 mg/d 17-ketosteroids as micromoles per day

425. 6.9 μg/dl iodine as micromoles per liter

Convert from SI units to conventional units:

426. 3.5 g/L serum lipids to milligrams per deciliter

427. 3.2 mmol/L magnesium to milligrams per deciliter

428. 1.9 mmol/L magnesium to milliequivalents per liter

429. 0.99 mmol/L serum phosphate to milligrams per deciliter

430. 20 mmol/d urine phosphate to grams per day

431. 35 mmol/d urine potassium to milligrams per day

432. 35 mmol/d urine potassium to milliequivalents per day

433. 70 g/L serum protein to grams per deciliter

434. 200 mmol/L serum sodium to milligrams per deciliter

435. 200 mmol/L serum sodium to milliequivalents per liter

436. 0.10 mmol/L serum uric acid to milligrams per deciliter

437. 2.59 mmol/L serum urea to milligrams per deciliter

438. 2.59 mmol/L urea nitrogen to milligrams per deciliter

439. 73 kPa O_2 to mm Hg

440. 80 cH to pH

7

Logarithms

EDUCATIONAL OBJECTIVES

To have successfully learned the material in this chapter, the student should be able to do the following properly:

- Describe the relationship between a logarithm and a complete number.
- Differentiate between Briggs (common) and Naperian (natural) logarithms.
- Convert Naperian logarithms to Briggs logarithms.
- Identify the characteristic and mantissa of a logarithm.
- Determine the common logarithm of a number using a table of mantissas.
- Determine the antilogarithm of both positive and negative logarithms using a table of mantissas.
- Multiply numbers using logarithms.
- Divide numbers using logarithms.

SECTION 7.1 INTRODUCTION

Logarithms are a part of mathematics developed to make calculations involving very large or very small numbers more manageable. Many laboratory procedures were developed using logarithms. With the advent of cheap computers and calculators, the need for logarithmic calculations was generally eliminated in the laboratory. However, competent workers should know what their machines are doing. This chapter is presented to aid in the understanding of logarithmic calculations done with the computers of any reasonably modern laboratory. If a worker wishes to remain ignorant and has no professional curiosity, this chapter is not needed.

Logarithms are used to indicate very wide ranges of values and to simplify calculations involving very large and very small numbers. The "p" scales such as pH and pK are logarithmic scales. Additionally, some standard curves are based on logarithmic scales. Other uses of logarithms are found here and there in laboratory work. The use of electronic calculators and computers has reduced the use and need for logarithms in laboratory mathematics; however, because of their traditional use, the competent laboratory worker needs some familiarization with logarithms.

A logarithm is not a number. It is thought of as a number, but it is really only *part* of a number, an exponent. The rest of the number is called the **base.** Hence, an exponent and its base form a number. When a logarithm is written, only the exponent is shown; the base is understood.

In working with logarithm calculations, it is important to properly indicate which numbers are logarithms and which are the numbers corresponding to logarithms. The abbreviation **log** is generally written instead of *"the logarithm of."* The abbreviation "log" is neither capitalized nor followed by a period and should be used with care. Since log is the abbreviation for "the logarithm of," it is to be written *only* before the number for which the logarithm either is known or is to be found. It is *never* written before the logarithm itself. This point should be thoroughly understood. For example, the logarithm of 25 is 1.3979; therefore write, "log 25 = 1.3979", because 1.3979 is the logarithm of 25. It would be incorrect to write "25 = log 1.3979", because 25 is not the logarithm of 1.3979.

There are two main systems of logarithms, base 10 and base *e*. The number 10 is used as the base for one system, and all logarithms of this system are exponents of the number 10. Logarithms to the base 10 are called *common* or *Briggs (Briggsian)* logarithms.

In certain special computations, a system of logarithms is used in which the base is the number 2.718281828+. This number is generally denoted by *e*. Logarithms to the base *e* are known as *natural* or *Naperian* logarithms. Logarithms in this system are generally designated by the subscript *e* after the abbreviation "log." When no base is designated, common logarithms are usually meant. For example, "$\log_e 5$" means the natural logarithm of 5, and "log 5" means the common logarithm of 5.

There are tables for each system of logarithms. However, one type may be determined from the other by the use of conversion factors.

EXAMPLE 7-1: $20 = 10^{1.30103} = e^{2.99573}$

$$\log 20 = 1.30103$$

$$\log_e 20 = 2.99573$$

$$\frac{\log_e 20}{\log 20} = \frac{2.99573}{1.30103} = 2.303$$

$$\frac{\log 20}{\log_e 20} = \frac{1.30103}{2.99573} = 0.4343$$

These *ratios* always hold true; therefore:

> To convert common logarithms to natural logarithms, multiply the common logarithm by 2.303. To convert natural logarithms to common logarithms, multiply the natural logarithm by 0.4343.

In this book, we will use common logarithms because these are the ones generally used in laboratory work. It was stated earlier that a logarithm is the exponent of a number called a base. Therefore the logarithm of a number is the power to which the base must be raised to give that number. Examine the following:

$$1 = 10^{0.0000} \qquad \log 1 = 0.0000$$
$$2 = 10^{0.3010} \qquad \log 2 = 0.3010$$
$$5 = 10^{0.6990} \qquad \log 5 = 0.6990$$
$$9 = 10^{0.9542} \qquad \log 9 = 0.9542$$
$$10 = 10^{1.0000} \qquad \log 10 = 1.0000$$
$$100 = 10^{2.0000} \qquad \log 100 = 2.0000$$
$$1,000 = 10^{3.0000} \qquad \log 1,000 = 3.0000$$
$$0.1 = 10^{-1} \qquad \log 0.1 = \bar{1}.0000$$
$$0.01 = 10^{-2} \qquad \log 0.01 = \bar{2}.0000$$

The logarithm of any number between 1 and 10 is zero plus a decimal, because the logarithm is greater than 0 but less than 1. Similarly, the logarithm of any number between 10 and 100 is 1 plus a decimal, because the logarithm is greater than 1 but less than 2. The logarithm of any number between 100 and 1,000 is 2 plus a decimal. Likewise, since log 1 is 0 and log 0.1 is −1, the logarithm of any decimal number between 0.1 and 1 is −1 plus a decimal. The log of 0.01 is −2; therefore the logarithm of any number between 0.01 and 0.1 is −2 plus a decimal. Following this logic, it can be stated that, in general, the logarithm of a number consists of two parts: (1) a whole number, called the **characteristic,** and (2) a decimal fraction, called the **mantissa.** The characteristic of the logarithm may be either positive or negative, depending on whether the number it represents is greater or less than 1. However, *the mantissa is always positive!*

NOTE: Logarithms can be used only with positive numbers. There are no logarithms for negative numbers. The reasons for this involve somewhat complex mathematics beyond the scope of this book.

SECTION 7.2 DETERMINING THE CHARACTERISTIC
Numbers Greater Than 1

The characteristic for any number, 1 or greater, is *always zero or a positive number*. The characteristic's value depends on the location of the decimal point in the original number and is always one less than the number of digits to the left of the decimal point.

EXAMPLE 7-2: Note the characteristic for the following:

$$2.57 = 0$$
$$25.7 = 1$$
$$257 = 2$$
$$2,570 = 3$$

Note that the characteristic is obtained by visual inspection of the original number, does not come from a table, and depends solely on the location of the decimal point in the original number.

Numbers Less Than 1

The characteristic of the logarithm of any number less than 1 is *negative* and is numerically 1 more than the number of zeroes *immediately* following the decimal point in the original number. In other words, the negative characteristic is equal to 1 plus the number of decimal places to the first nonzero digit in the fraction. The fact that the characteristic is negative even though the mantissa is positive may be indicated by the following two means:

1. Writing a minus sign *over* the characteristic indicates that the characteristic is negative and the mantissa is positive.

EXAMPLE 7-3: $\bar{1}.3010$ is the logarithm of 0.2.

This means that the characteristic is −1 and the mantissa is +.3010. For the present it may be stated that it would be incorrect to place a minus sign in front of the characteristic (−1.3010), because this would indicate that both the characteristic and the mantissa are negative; this cannot be correct because the mantissa is *always* positive. (Expressing logarithms in a negative manner is discussed on pp. 182.)

Note the characteristics for the following:

$$0.1206 = -1$$
$$0.01206 = -2$$
$$0.0001206 = -4$$
$$0.000001206 = -6$$

Whereas

$$\log 0.1206 = \bar{1}.0813$$
$$\log 0.01206 = \bar{2}.0813$$
$$\log 0.0001206 = \bar{4}.0813$$
$$\log 0.000001206 = \bar{6}.0813$$

(The source of the mantissa, .0813, is explained on pp. 175-178.)

2. A logarithm with a negative characteristic may be changed to a positive form by adding 10 to the characteristic and adding -10 after the mantissa. This allows some calculations to be more easily completed.

EXAMPLE 7-4: Change the characteristic of $\bar{1}.3010$ to a positive form.

Add 10 to the characteristic.

$$10 + (-1) = 9; \quad 9.3010$$

Then add -10 after the mantissa.

$$9.3010 - 10$$
$$\bar{1}.3010 = 9.3010 - 10$$

Since 10 is both added and subtracted, the value for the logarithm is not affected. In the logarithm $9.3010 - 10$, the characteristic has two parts: (1) the positive part, 9, which precedes the mantissa, and (2) the negative part, -10, which follows the mantissa.

The positive part of the characteristic of the logarithm of a decimal number may also be obtained by subtracting the number of zeros between the decimal point and the first significant figure from 9. This number is the positive part of the characteristic. Place -10 after the mantissa. This is the negative part of the characteristic.

EXAMPLE 7-5: Find the characteristic for 0.00306.

There are two zeros between the decimal point and the first significant figure, 3. Subtract 2 from 9 and make this the positive part of the characteristic: 7._____. Add -10. 7._____ -10.

Note the characteristic of the following:

$$\log 0.4320 = \bar{1} \text{ or } 9.\underline{\qquad} - 10$$
$$\log 0.00432 = \bar{3} \text{ or } 7.\underline{\qquad} - 10$$
$$\log 0.000432 = \bar{4} \text{ or } 6.\underline{\qquad} - 10$$

In summary, for numbers less than 1, the negative characteristic may be expressed two ways.
1. Add 1 to the number of zeros between the decimal point and the first significant figure. This will be a negative number.
2. To change this characteristic to a positive form, add 10 and -10 to the logarithm, or subtract the number of zeros between the decimal point and the first significant figure in the number from 9 and add -10 after the mantissa.

Notice again that the characteristic is found by visual inspection of the number. It does not come from a table and depends entirely on the position of the decimal point in the original number.

SECTION 7.3 DETERMINING THE MANTISSA

As discussed earlier, the mantissa is the decimal part of the logarithm and is *always* positive. The mantissa cannot be found by visual inspection of the original number. It must be found from a logarithm table and has nothing whatever to do with the position of the decimal in the original number. Although tables given in various texts are called tables of logarithms, they are actually tables of mantissas. The mantissa must be found from the table and then added to the characteristic to form the complete logarithm. Notice that the mantissas given in such tables are usually not preceded by decimal points, because when determining mantissas by means of a table, it is convenient to treat them as whole numbers. However, it should be remembered that a mantissa is entirely decimal and that when used in a logarithm, the mantissa should be preceded by a decimal point and a characteristic.

Appendix F is a table of four-place logarithms. Tables of logarithms of more than four places exist. These can be used to increase the precision of calculations if desired. The mantissa of any number from 1 to 9,999 can be found by using this table. Numbers with more than four significant figures are rounded off to four figures. In determining the number to be used in obtaining a mantissa, do not consider the decimal point. Do not consider zeros at the beginning or end of the number, with one exception. This exception is that to find a mantissa in the table, the number for which a mantissa is desired must contain at least three digits, the last two of which may be zero. For numbers with less than three digits, simply add enough zeros to the end to produce a three digit number. *Hence, the number used for obtaining a mantissa is always three or four digits long, begins with a figure other than zero, and does not contain a decimal point.*

Examine Fig. 7-1 on p. 180. This is a portion of the table of four-place logarithms in Appendix F. This table consists of a series of vertical columns and horizontal rows. The first two digits of the number for which a logarithm is desired are found in the first column directly under *N*. The third digit of the number is found in the row directly to the right of N, and the last digit is found in that portion of the table entitled *Proportional Parts.*

To determine the mantissa of a number:
1. Find the first two digits of the number in the left column (N column) of the table.
2. Move across this row to the column headed by the third digit of the number.
3. In logarithms for numbers with less than four digits, record this value as the mantissa of the logarithm.

4. If the number has four digits, record the value found in the column and row of the first three digits of the number and continue to move to the right in the same row to the column of the proportional parts headed by the fourth digit of the number.
5. Add the value found here to the value for the first three figures of the number. This sum is the mantissa of the four-digit number.

Use Fig. 7-1 on p. 180 to follow the next three examples.

EXAMPLE 7-6: Consider the following numbers: 2, 20, 0.002, 200.0, and 0.2.

If the decimal point and all preceding and ending zeros are ignored, the number remaining is 2. Add two zeros to make this a three-digit number, that is, 200. Note that the values in the N column range from 10 to 99. Hence, move down this column to 20. Now move across this row to the column headed by 0. Note the value 3010 at this point in the table. This is the mantissa of log 2, log 20, log 0.002, and so on. Each number containing 200 as the significant digits will have a characteristic, which is determined by the position of the decimal point, and a mantissa of .3010.

$$\log 2 = 0.3010$$
$$\log 20 = 1.3010$$
$$\log 0.002 = \overline{3}.3010 \text{ or } 7.3010 - 10$$
$$\log 200 = 2.3010$$
$$\log 0.2 = \overline{1}.3010 \text{ or } 9.3010 - 10$$

EXAMPLE 7-7: Consider the following numbers: 306, 3.06, 0.00306, and 3,060.

If the decimal point and the beginning and ending zeros are ignored, the figure 306 is present. The first two digits of the number (30) are found in the N column, and the digit (6) is found in the top row. Move down the column headed by 6 to the row directly to the right of 30. Find the number 4857. Hence, the mantissa for 306 is .4857.

$$\log 306 = 2.4857$$
$$\log 3.06 = 0.4857$$
$$\log 0.00306 = \overline{3}.4857 \text{ or } 7.4857 - 10$$
$$\log 3,060 = 3.4857$$

EXAMPLE 7-8: Consider the following numbers: 47,950, 47.95, 0.4795, and 0.004795.

Following the instructions for obtaining a mantissa, one should realize that the number to use with each of the above values is 4795. Move down the N column to 47. Move across this row to the column headed by 9. The value at this point in the table is 6803. Continuing in the same row, move to the proportional parts column headed by 5 and find the value 5. Add this to the value for the first three digits of the number.

$$6803 + 5 = 6808$$

Hence the mantissa for 4795 is .6808. Combine this with the proper characteristic for each number.

$$\log 47,950 = 4.6808$$
$$\log 47.95 = 1.6808$$
$$\log 0.4795 = \overline{1}.6808 \text{ or } 9.6808 - 10$$
$$\log 0.004795 = \overline{3}.6808 \text{ or } 7.6808 - 10$$

SECTION 7.4 DETERMINING ANTILOGARITHMS

An **antilogarithm** is the number corresponding to a given logarithm. It is the number for which a logarithm is found. The term *antilogarithm of* can be abbreviated **antilog.**

EXAMPLE 7-9: log 2 = 0.3010 (the logarithm of 2 = 0.3010)

The number that gives this logarithm (0.3010) is 2; therefore 2 is the antilogarithm of 0.3010.

An antilogarithm may be determined from the logarithm in two ways. One method is to use the logarithm table in reverse order. The second method is to use an antilogarithm table. In both cases the logarithm is divided into the characteristic and the mantissa.

To determine the antilogarithm of the logarithm 0.3010 using the logarithm table (see Fig. 7-1):

1. Find the mantissa .3010 in the mantissa columns. The two figures from the N column that correspond to it are 20.
2. The column heading at the top of the page in the same column with the mantissa is 0. Therefore the digits that correspond to the mantissa, 3010, are 2, 0, and 0 in this order. Now determine the position of the decimal point in the number.
3. This is done by the consideration of the characteristic of the logarithm. In this case the characteristic is 0. The number of places to the left of the decimal point is one more than the characteristic. One more than 0 is 1. Place the decimal point between the 2 and the first 0. The antilog of 0.3010 is 2.00.

EXAMPLE 7-10: Find the antilog of $\overline{3}$.4857.

Locate the value in the body of the mantissa table that is closest to but does not exceed the mantissa, .4857. The exact mantissa is found. Move to the left side of this row to the N column and find the number 30, which is the first two digits of the antilogarithm. Note the number at the head of the column containing 4857. This is the third digit of the antilogarithm. The number at the head of this column is 6. Hence, the *digits* of the antilogarithm of $\overline{3}$.4857 are 306. The characteristic of the logarithm is $\overline{3}$. This indicates that the decimal should be placed two places to the left, 0.00306. Hence the antilog of $\overline{3}$.4857 is 0.00306.

In the event that the exact mantissa value is not in the table, find the closest mantissa in the columns; that is, find the closest tabular mantissa value, without exceeding the value of the mantissa being considered. Now move directly to the right and find the value of proportional parts in the same row that when added to the tabular value, most closely corresponds to the value for which the antilogarithm is being sought. Read the first two digits of the antilogarithm from the left most column (N), the third digit from the top row, and the fourth digit from the head of the column containing the proportional part used.

EXAMPLE 7-11: Find the antilog of 1.6808.

Locate the value in the mantissa table that is closest to but does not exceed the mantissa, .6808. The closest value in the table (without exceeding the mantissa) is 6803. This figure is found in the 47 (N) row and column headed by 9. Hence, the first three digits of the antilogarithm are 479. Move to the right in this same row in which 6803 is found to the proportional parts section of the table. Find the number that when added to 6803 will give 6808. This number is 5. The number 5 is found in the column headed by 5. Hence, 5 is the fourth digit of the antilogarithm, that is, 4795.

	N	0	1	2	3	4	5	6	7	8	9	Proportional Parts* 1	2	3	4	5	6	7	8	9
	10	0000	0043	0086	0128	0170	0212	0253	0294	0334	0374	4	8	12	17	21	25	29	33	37
	11	0414	0453	0492	0531	0569	0607	0645	0682	0719	0755	4	8	11	15	19	23	26	30	34
	12	0792	0828	0864	0899	0934	0969	1004	1038	1072	1106	3	7	10	14	17	21	24	28	31
	13	1139	1173	1206	1239	1271	1303	1335	1367	1399	1430	3	6	10	13	16	19	23	26	29
	14	1461	1492	1523	1553	1584	1614	1644	1673	1703	1732	3	6	9	12	15	18	21	24	27
	15	1761	1790	1818	1847	1875	1903	1931	1959	1987	2014	3	6	8	11	14	17	20	22	25
	16	2041	2068	2095	2122	2148	2175	2201	2227	2253	2279	3	5	8	11	13	16	18	21	24
	17	2304	2330	2355	2380	2405	2430	2455	2480	2504	2529	2	5	7	10	12	15	17	20	22
	18	2553	2577	2601	2625	2648	2672	2695	2718	2742	2765	2	5	7	9	12	14	16	19	21
	19	2788	2810	2833	2856	2878	2900	2923	2945	2967	2989	2	4	7	9	11	13	16	18	20
Ex. 7-6	20	3010	3032	3054	3075	3096	3118	3139	3160	3181	3201	2	4	6	8	11	13	15	17	19
	21	3222	3243	3263	3284	3304	3324	3345	3365	3385	3404	2	4	6	8	10	12	14	16	18
	22	3424	3444	3464	3483	3502	3522	3541	3560	3579	3598	2	4	6	8	10	12	14	15	17
	23	3617	3636	3655	3674	3692	3711	3729	3747	3766	3784	2	4	6	7	9	11	13	15	17
	24	3802	3820	3838	3856	3874	3892	3909	3927	3945	3962	2	4	5	7	9	11	12	14	16
	25	3979	3997	4014	4031	4048	4065	4082	4099	4116	4133	2	3	5	7	9	10	12	14	15
	26	4150	4166	4183	4200	4216	4232	4249	4265	4281	4298	2	3	5	7	8	10	11	13	15
	27	4314	4330	4346	4362	4378	4393	4409	4425	4440	4456	2	3	5	6	8	9	11	13	14
	28	4472	4487	4502	4518	4533	4548	4564	4579	4594	4609	2	3	5	6	8	9	11	12	14
	29	4624	4639	4654	4669	4683	4698	4713	4728	4742	4757	1	3	4	6	7	9	10	12	13
Ex. 7-7	30	4771	4786	4800	4814	4829	4843	4857	4871	4886	4900	1	3	4	6	7	9	10	11	13
	31	4914	4928	4942	4955	4969	4983	4997	5011	5024	5038	1	3	4	6	7	8	10	11	12
	32	5051	5065	5079	5092	5105	5119	5132	5145	5159	5172	1	3	4	5	7	8	9	11	12
	33	5185	5198	5211	5224	5237	5250	5263	5276	5289	5302	1	3	4	5	6	8	9	10	12
	34	5315	5328	5340	5353	5366	5378	5391	5403	5416	5428	1	3	4	5	6	8	9	10	11
	35	5441	5453	5465	5478	5490	5502	5514	5527	5539	5551	1	2	4	5	6	7	9	10	11
	36	5563	5575	5587	5599	5611	5623	5635	5647	5658	5670	1	2	4	5	6	7	8	10	11
	37	5682	5694	5705	5717	5729	5740	5752	5763	5775	5786	1	2	3	5	6	7	8	9	10
	38	5798	5809	5821	5832	5843	5855	5866	5877	5888	5899	1	2	3	5	6	7	8	9	10
	39	5911	5922	5933	5944	5955	5966	5977	5988	5999	6010	1	2	3	4	5	7	8	9	10
	40	6021	6031	6042	6053	6064	6075	6085	6096	6107	6117	1	2	3	4	5	6	8	9	10
	41	6128	6138	6149	6160	6170	6180	6191	6201	6212	6222	1	2	3	4	5	6	7	8	9
	42	6232	6243	6253	6263	6274	6284	6294	6304	6314	6325	1	2	3	4	5	6	7	8	9
	43	6335	6345	6355	6365	6375	6385	6395	6405	6415	6425	1	2	3	4	5	6	7	8	9
	44	6435	6444	6454	6464	6474	6484	6493	6503	6513	6522	1	2	3	4	5	6	7	8	9
	45	6532	6542	6551	6561	6571	6580	6590	6599	6609	6618	1	2	3	4	5	6	7	8	9
	46	6628	6637	6646	6656	6665	6675	6684	6693	6702	6712	1	2	3	4	5	6	7	7	8
Ex. 7-8	47	6721	6730	6739	6749	6758	6767	6776	6785	6794	6803	1	2	3	4	5	5	6	7	8
	48	6812	6821	6830	6839	6848	6857	6866	6875	6884	6893	1	2	3	4	4	5	6	7	8
	49	6902	6911	6920	6928	6937	6946	6955	6964	6972	6981	1	2	3	4	4	5	6	7	8
	50	6990	6998	7007	7016	7024	7033	7042	7050	7059	7067	1	2	3	3	4	5	6	7	8
	51	7076	7084	7093	7101	7110	7118	7126	7135	7143	7152	1	2	3	3	4	5	6	7	8
	52	7160	7168	7177	7185	7193	7202	7210	7218	7226	7235	1	2	2	3	4	5	6	7	7
	53	7243	7251	7259	7267	7275	7284	7292	7300	7308	7316	1	2	2	3	4	5	6	6	7
	54	7324	7332	7340	7348	7356	7364	7372	7380	7388	7396	1	2	2	3	4	5	6	6	7
	N	0	1	2	3	4	5	6	7	8	9	1	2	3	4	5	6	7	8	9

*Interpolation in this section of the table may not be accurate.

Fig. 7-1. Determining the mantissa from a four-place logarithm table. From Appendix F.

N	0	1	2	3	4	5	6	7	8	9	Proportional Parts* 1 2 3 4 5 6 7 8 9
.00	1000	1002	1005	1007	1009	1012	1014	1016	1019	1021	0 0 1 1 1 1 2 2 2
.01	1023	1026	1028	1030	1033	1035	1038	1040	1042	1045	0 0 1 1 1 1 2 2 2
.02	1047	1050	1052	1054	1057	1059	1062	1064	1067	1069	0 0 1 1 1 1 2 2 2
.03	1072	1074	1076	1079	1081	1084	1086	1089	1091	1094	0 0 1 1 1 1 2 2 2
.04	1096	1099	1102	1104	1107	1109	1112	1114	1117	1119	0 1 1 1 1 2 2 2 2
.05	1122	1125	1127	1130	1132	1135	1138	1140	1143	1146	0 1 1 1 1 2 2 2 2
.06	1148	1151	1153	1156	1159	1161	1164	1167	1169	1172	0 1 1 1 1 2 2 2 2
.07	1175	1178	1180	1183	1186	1189	1191	1194	1197	1199	0 1 1 1 1 2 2 2 2
.08	1202	1205	1208	1211	1213	1216	1219	1222	1225	1227	0 1 1 1 1 2 2 2 3
.09	1230	1233	1236	1239	1242	1245	1247	1250	1253	1256	0 1 1 1 1 2 2 2 3
.10	1259	1262	1265	1268	1271	1274	1276	1279	1282	1285	0 1 1 1 1 2 2 2 3
.11	1288	1291	1294	1297	1300	1303	1306	1309	1312	1315	0 1 1 1 2 2 2 3 3
.12	1318	1321	1324	1327	1330	1334	1337	1340	1343	1346	0 1 1 1 2 2 2 3 3
.13	1349	1352	1355	1358	1361	1365	1368	1371	1374	1377	0 1 1 1 2 2 2 3 3
.14	1380	1384	1387	1390	1393	1396	1400	1403	1406	1409	0 1 1 1 2 2 2 3 3
.15	1413	1416	1419	1422	1426	1429	1432	1435	1439	1442	0 1 1 1 2 2 2 3 3
.16	1445	1449	1452	1455	1459	1462	1466	1469	1472	1476	0 1 1 1 2 2 2 3 3
.17	1479	1483	1486	1489	1493	1496	1500	1503	1507	1510	0 1 1 1 2 2 2 3 3
.18	1514	1517	1521	1524	1528	1531	1535	1538	1542	1545	0 1 1 1 2 2 2 3 3
.19	1549	1552	1556	1560	1563	1567	1570	1574	1578	1581	0 1 1 1 2 2 3 3 3
.20	1585	1589	1592	1596	1600	1603	1607	1611	1614	1618	0 1 1 1 2 2 3 3 3
.21	1622	1626	1629	1633	1637	1641	1644	1648	1652	1656	0 1 1 2 2 2 3 3 3
.22	1660	1663	1667	1671	1675	1679	1683	1687	1690	1694	0 1 1 2 2 2 3 3 3
.23	1698	1702	1706	1710	1714	1718	1722	1726	1730	1734	0 1 1 2 2 2 3 3 4
.24	1738	1742	1746	1750	1754	1758	1762	1766	1770	1774	0 1 1 2 2 2 3 3 4
.25	1778	1782	1786	1791	1795	1799	1803	1807	1811	1816	0 1 1 2 2 2 3 3 4
.26	1820	1824	1828	1832	1837	1841	1845	1849	1854	1858	0 1 1 2 2 3 3 3 4
.27	1862	1866	1871	1875	1879	1884	1888	1892	1897	1901	0 1 1 2 2 3 3 3 4
.28	1905	1910	1914	1919	1923	1928	1932	1936	1941	1945	0 1 1 2 2 3 3 4 4
.29	1950	1954	1959	1963	1968	1972	1977	1982	1986	1991	0 1 1 2 2 3 3 4 4
.30	1995	2000	2004	2009	2014	2018	2023	2028	2032	2037	0 1 1 2 2 3 3 4 4
.31	2042	2046	2051	2056	2061	2065	2070	2075	2080	2084	0 1 1 2 2 3 3 4 4
.32	2089	2094	2099	2104	2109	2113	2118	2123	2128	2133	0 1 1 2 2 3 3 4 4
.33	2138	2143	2148	2153	2158	2163	2168	2173	2178	2183	0 1 1 2 2 3 3 4 4
.34	2188	2193	2198	2203	2208	2213	2218	2223	2228	2234	1 1 2 2 3 3 4 4 5
.35	2239	2244	2249	2254	2259	2265	2270	2275	2280	2286	1 1 2 2 3 3 4 4 5
.36	2291	2296	2301	2307	2312	2317	2323	2328	2333	2339	1 1 2 2 3 3 4 4 5
.37	2344	2350	2355	2360	2366	2371	2377	2382	2388	2393	1 1 2 2 3 3 4 4 5
.38	2399	2404	2410	2415	2421	2427	2432	2438	2443	2449	1 1 2 2 3 3 4 4 5
.39	2455	2460	2466	2472	2477	2483	2489	2495	2500	2506	1 1 2 2 3 3 4 5 5
.40	2512	2518	2523	2529	2535	2541	2547	2553	2559	2564	1 1 2 2 3 4 4 5 5
.41	2570	2576	2582	2588	2594	2600	2606	2612	2618	2624	1 1 2 2 3 4 4 5 5
.42	2630	2636	2642	2649	2655	2661	2667	2673	2679	2685	1 1 2 2 3 4 4 5 6
.43	2692	2698	2704	2710	2716	2723	2729	2735	2742	2748	1 1 2 3 3 4 4 5 6
.44	2754	2761	2767	2773	2780	2786	2793	2799	2805	2812	1 1 2 3 3 4 4 5 6
.45	2818	2825	2831	2838	2844	2851	2858	2864	2871	2877	1 1 2 3 3 4 5 5 6
.46	2884	2891	2897	2904	2911	2917	2924	2931	2938	2944	1 1 2 3 3 4 5 5 6
.47	2951	2958	2965	2972	2979	2985	2992	2999	3006	3018	1 1 2 3 3 4 5 5 6
.48	3020	3027	3034	3041	3048	3055	3062	3069	3076	3083	1 1 2 3 4 4 5 6 6
.49	3090	3097	3105	3112	3119	3126	3133	3141	3148	3155	1 1 2 3 4 4 5 6 6
N	0	1	2	3	4	5	6	7	8	9	1 2 3 4 5 6 7 8 9

*Interpolation in this section of the table may not be accurate.

Fig. 7-2. Determining the antilogarithm from a four-place antilogarithm table. From Appendix G.

The characteristic of the logarithm is 1. This indicates the position of the decimal point in the digits.

Hence the antilog of 1.6808 is 47.95.

To find the antilogarithm using a table of antilogarithms (Appendix G), use the same method as for logarithms.

1. Move down the left-most column of the table to the first two digits of the mantissa in question.
2. Move across this row until the column headed by the third digit of the mantissa is reached, and record this value.
3. Continue to the right in the same row to the column in the Proportional Parts portion of the table headed by the fourth digit of the mantissa.
4. Add the value of the proportional part to the antilogarithm of the first three digits. This sum contains the digits of the four place antilogarithm of the logarithm.

EXAMPLE 7-12: Find the antilogarithm of the logarithm 0.3010 using the antilogarithm table in Fig. 7-2.

Move down the left column to .30. Move to the right in this row to the column headed by 1. Record 2000. This is the antilogarithm (minus the decimal point) of the mantissa, .3010.

The characteristic defines the decimal point. The characteristic is zero. Recall that a positive characteristic is found by subtracting 1 from the number of digits to the left of the decimal point. Thus a characteristic of 0 would mean that there was one digit to the left of the decimal point. Therefore put down the number 2000, and put in the decimal point so there is one digit to the left of it; the figure should be 2.000.

EXAMPLE 7-13: Using two methods, find the antilog of the following logarithms: 3.5453 and $\overline{2}$.4116.

Logarithm	Mantissa	Value from tables	Characteristic	Antilogarithm
3.5453	.5453	3510	3	3510
$\overline{2}$.4116	.4116	2580	$\overline{2}$	0.0258

SECTION 7.5 NEGATIVE LOGARITHMS

Sometimes a procedure considers negative logarithms. The most common use of negative logarithms in laboratory calculations is with pH and pK values.

Remember that common logarithms are exponents of 10. An exponent with its base is equivalent to an ordinary number. There is an understood base of 10 with a common logarithm. When a logarithm is written as a negative number, it indicates a number between zero and 1. Such logarithms are the algebraic sum of a negative characteristic and a positive mantissa. Calculators show this form of negative logarithms. If 0.05 is entered on most calculators and the log button is pressed, the number -1.3010 is displayed. This is the power of 10 equivalent to 0.05.

$$0.05 = 10^{-1.3010}$$

This is also the sum of a negative characteristic, -2, and a positive mantissa, .6990.

$$\begin{array}{r} -2 \\ + \quad +\ .6990 \\ \hline -1.3010 \end{array}$$

To find logarithms or antilogarithms using calculators, follow the procedure for the particular calculator. However, finding the antilogarithm of a negative logarithm using a log table requires that the logarithm be converted to a negative characteristic and a positive mantissa. Remember that a logarithm consists of two parts, the characteristic and the mantissa. In negative logarithms these two parts have been added together. The positive mantissa of this logarithm has to be recovered to find it on the log table.

Use the following procedure to determine the antilogarithm of a negative logarithm using a log table.

1. Recover the mantissa by adding the next highest whole number above the characteristic to the entire negative number. This will always result in a positive decimal fraction and will be the positive mantissa.

$$\begin{array}{r} -1.3030 \\ + \quad +2 \\ \hline \end{array}$$

$$\begin{array}{r} +2 \\ + \quad -1.3030 \\ \hline +0.6990 \end{array}$$

The recovered mantissa is .6990.

2. Now use the negative form of the whole number, which was added, as the characteristic of the corrected logarithm. Indicate its sign with a bar over the number rather than the minus sign in front to show a negative characteristic and a positive mantissa.

$$\bar{2}.6990$$

3. Find the mantissa on the log table and note the digits in the N column and at the top of the table.

50 and 0;   500

4. Place the decimal point the number of places to the left of these digits equal to one less than the negative characteristic.

0.0500

You should understand the following relationships before continuing.

$$0.05 = 10^{-1.3010}$$

$$\log 0.05 = -1.3010 = \bar{2}.6990$$

SECTION 7.6 CALCULATIONS USING LOGARITHMS

Logarithms can be used for the easy multiplication and division of very large and very small numbers. Since logarithms are exponents, the rules of exponents apply. However, because they are exponents, logarithms cannot be used to add and subtract numbers.

$$a^b \times a^c = a^{b+c}$$

$$\frac{a^b}{a^c} = a^{b-c}$$

When logarithms are used in calculations, remember that the more they are rounded off, the less precision can be obtained from the calculations.

Multiplication Using Logarithms

To multiply two or more numbers by using logarithms, add the logarithms of the given numbers, then find the antilogarithm for the resulting sum.

$$3 \times 3$$

$$\log (3 \times 3)$$

$$\log 3 + \log 3$$

$$\log 3 = 0.4771$$

$$(+) \log 3 = \underline{0.4771}$$

Sum of logarithms = 0.9542 = logarithm of product

antilog 0.9542 = 9.0

$$3 \times 3 = 9.0$$

If a number to be multiplied is wholly decimal, the logarithm has a negative characteristic. This should be converted to the positive form by the addition and subtraction of 10 as described on p. 176. The sum of the minus tens must be included as part of the sum of the logarithm. Whenever the negative part of the sum is smaller than the positive part, the indicated subtraction is actually performed to have the logarithm in its simplest form.

EXAMPLE 7-14: Find the product of 52.17, 0.0143, and 0.52.

$$\log 52.17 = 1.7174$$

$$\log 0.0143 = 8.1553 - 10$$

$$\log 15 = 1.1761$$

$$\log 0.52 = \underline{9.7160 - 10}$$

Sum of logarithms = 20.7648 − 20 = logarithm of product

20.7648

$$- \underline{20 }$$

0.7648

antilog 0.7648 = 5.818

However, if the negative part of the logarithm is the larger part and is more than 10, it is reduced to 10 by subtracting the necessary number from it and from the positive part of the logarithm.

EXAMPLE 7-15: Find the product of 5.13, 0.0167, 0.91, and 0.00416.

$$\log 5.13 = \quad 0.7101$$
$$\log 0.0167 = \quad 8.2227 - 10$$
$$\log 0.91 = \quad 9.9590 - 10$$
$$\log 0.00416 = \quad \underline{7.6191 - 10}$$

Sum of logarithms $= 26.5109 - 30 =$ logarithm of product

$$26.5109 - 30$$
$$\underline{-20 \qquad -20}$$
$$6.5109 - 10 = \overline{4}.5109 = \text{logarithm of product}$$

antilog $\overline{4}.5109 = 0.0003243$

Division Using Logarithms

To divide one number by another using logarithms, first subtract the logarithm of the divisor from the logarithm of the dividend, then find the antilogarithm for the calculated value.

The logarithm of the dividend should be written first, and below it should be written the logarithm of the divisor. In simple cases, the logarithm of the divisor can be subtracted from the logarithm of the dividend without changing the form of either.

$$12 \div 3$$
$$\log (12 \div 3)$$
$$\log 12 - \log 3$$

$$\log 12 = 1.0792$$
$$\underline{- \log 3 = 0.4771}$$

Difference of logarithms $= 0.6021 =$ logarithm of quotient

$$\text{antilog } 0.6021 = 4.0$$
$$12 \div 3 = 4.0$$

Sometimes it is necessary to change the form of the logarithm of the dividend to obtain the log quotient in a suitable form. The reason for this will become obvious in studying the first setup of the following problem.

EXAMPLE 7-16: Divide 4.72 by 16.6.

$$\log 4.72 = 0.6739$$
$$\log 16.6 = 1.2201$$

Before subtracting 1.2201 from 0.6739, it is necessary to add 10 to the 0.6739 and to write $- 10$ after the mantissa to obtain the log quotient in a positive form.

$$\log 4.72 = 10.6739 - 10$$
$$\underline{- \log 16.6 = \quad 1.2201 \qquad}$$

Difference of logarithms $= 9.4538 - 10 =$ logarithm of quotient

$$9.4538 - 10 = \overline{1}.4538$$

$$\text{antilog } \overline{1}.4538 = 0.2843$$

APPENDIXES RELATED TO THIS CHAPTER

F Four-Place Logarithms
G Antilogarithms

PRACTICE PROBLEMS

Calculate the answer for each problem. Understand each portion of the calculation and determine whether the answer is logical. *Just because an answer can be calculated does not mean that it is reasonable.*

Give the logarithm that corresponds to the following:

1. $10^{0.0128}$
2. $10^{0.9832}$
3. $10^{0.4014}$
4. $10^{0.3010}$

5. $10^{1.6232}$
6. $10^{3.5623}$
7. 10^{-4}

8. 10^{-6}
9. 10^{-1}
10. 10^{-10}

Determining the characteristic and mantissa

Give the characteristics of the following:

11. 1.39
12. 1,390.0
13. 38
14. 4.9278
15. 100.1

16. 29,673
17. 15.49
18. 0.00013
19. 0.1967
20. 0.013

21. 0.000000013
22. 0.193463
23. 0.0010061
24. 0.100000008

25. Find the mantissa for questions 11 to 24.
26. Give the whole logarithm for questions 11 to 24.

Determining antilogarithms

Give the antilogarithm of the following:

27. Questions 1 to 10
28. 1.6990
29. 3.6990
30. 5.6990
31. 3.0000
32. 0.6990
33. 8.6990 − 10

34. $\overline{5}.3010$
35. 4.3979
36. 1.6503
37. 8.6990
38. $\overline{5}.7926$
39. 9.0000
40. 4.5328

Negative logarithms

Give the negative logarithm that corresponds to the following:

41. $10^{-1.0129}$
42. $10^{-0.3420}$
43. $10^{-3.1900}$
44. $10^{-0.0021}$
45. $10^{-2.0160}$

46. Express numbers 41 through 45 in the tabular form (that is, negative characteristic and positive mantissa).

Give the antilogarithm of the following:

47. −3.6911
48. 0.0000
49. −1.0000
50. −5.0070

Express the following logarithms (questions 51-55) as:
   a. Negative characteristic and positive mantissa
   b. Negative logarithm
   c. Antilogarithm

51. 7.3118 − 10
52. 8.9907 − 10
53. 4.3879 − 10
54. 1.0207 − 10
55. 9.0003 − 10

Calculations using logarithms

Perform the following using logarithms:

56. 32 + 761 + 1,000,000
57. 42,673 + 72,981 + 29,799
58. 281 − 762 − 506

Multiply the following using logarithms:

59. 33 × 2.1 × 6,207
60. 33,721 × 2,000,618 × 3,971
61. 12 × 7.2 × 5,991
62. 87.16 × 0.0273 × −0.91 × 0.00621
63. 31.96 × 0.0722 × 13 × 0.77
64. 0.0093 × 13,672 × 6 × 0.000096

Divide the following using logarithms:

65. 43 ÷ 6.1
66. 4,321 ÷ 29
67. 400 ÷ 0.6
68. −18 ÷ 29
69. 1.09 ÷ 42
70. 0.061 ÷ 0.00072

Give the logarithm of the following numbers three different ways:

71. 0.002134
72. 0.9342
73. 0.01016
74. 0.000003987
75. 0.0007366
76. 0.00000008541
77. 0.00006923
78. 0.0000004796

8

Ionic Solutions

EDUCATIONAL OBJECTIVES

To have successfully learned the material in this chapter, the student should be able to do the following properly:

- ◆ Define acid, bases, and salts.
- ◆ Describe the major concepts of the Sørensen pH and pOH scales, and relate this to the dissociation of water as $[H^+] \times [OH^-] = 1 \times 10^{-14}$.
- ◆ Convert molar concentration of free hydrogen ions in an aqueous solution to pH.
- ◆ Calculate the pH of ionic solutions from concentrations and dissociation or ionization constants of solutes.
- ◆ Describe a procedure to produce a solution of given pH and volume.
- ◆ Calculate total CO_2 from the pH and PCO_2 of a solution.
- ◆ Convert pH to cH using an electronic calculator.
- ◆ Calculate the pH of a buffered solution.

SECTION 8.1 INTRODUCTION

Many chemical reactions result from an interaction of charged particles. The charged particles are either atoms or molecules in which the total number of protons does not equal the number of electrons. Such particles of matter are called **ions.** Ions having more protons than electrons have a positive charge and are called **cations.** Ions having more electrons than protons have a negative charge and are called **anions.** Cations are attracted to anions by the electromagnetic forces associated with atoms and molecules. The attraction of two oppositely charged ions forms bonds between the particles. Such bonds are called **ionic bonds.** A molecule formed from ions is stable if the positive charges equal the negative charges. When such compounds are not in solution, the molecules remain intact. Often, many of these molecules form interconnecting bonds to form crystals, which may be quite large.

When ionically bonded molecules are dissolved in a solvent having ionic bonds, the ions separate. Such separation is called **dissociation** or **ionization.** The most common solvent in which ions dissociate is water. Water itself ionizes to some degree. Two kinds of ions are formed from the ionization of water: hydrogen cations, H^+, and hydroxyl anions, OH^-.

The hydrogen ion is a hydrogen atom that has lost its electron. Since a hydrogen atom consists of one proton and one electron, a hydrogen ion consists of one free proton. Such protons are highly reactive ions. Unless they can combine with another ion, they combine with a water atom to form a hydronium ion (H_3O^+). Hydronium ions dissociate to release the extra proton quite easily, so for all practical purposes a hydronium ion acts as a free proton.

In a particular water solution, different compounds dissociate to varying extents. The extent of dissociation of the substance determines what reactions will occur and the speed of those reactions. The rates of dissociation are influenced by the total complement of the ionic substances in the solution.

Three general types of ionic compounds exist: acids, bases, and salts. Stated simply and incompletely, **acids** are compounds that contribute hydrogen ions (free protons) to a solution, **bases** are compounds that accept protons from the solution, and **salts** are ionic compounds that yield neither hydrogen nor hydroxyl ions to the solution. An acid solution has more dissociated or free hydrogen ions than hydroxyl ions. A basic or alkaline solution has more free hydroxyl ions than free hydrogen ions. Those solutions in which the number of free hydroxyl ions is equal to the number of free hydrogen ions are said to be **neutral solutions.** All aqueous (water) solutions contain H^+ and OH^- ions. The degree of acidity or basicity (alkalinity) of a particular solution depends on the relative concentration of the hydrogen and hydroxyl ions. Other ions only affect this indirectly. The acidity or basicity has a profound effect on the chemical reactions that occur in a solution. This effect involves the kinds of reactions and the speed of the reactions. Because of this, it is important to know the relative concentrations of the hydrogen and hydroxyl ions in a solution. One property of aqueous solutions is a great help in determining the concentration of ions.

In all aqueous solutions, whether they are acid, basic, or neutral, the molar concentration of the hydrogen ions (designed $[H^+]$) multiplied by the molar concentration of the hydroxyl ions ($[OH^-]$) is always 1×10^{-14}.

This fact shows that the concentration of hydrogen ions in a solution indicates the concentration of hydroxyl ions in the solution and vice versa. Hence, to indicate the degree of acidity or basicity of a solution, one needs only to determine the concentration of either the dissociated hydrogen or hydroxyl ions. It is not necessary to determine both. In discussions of the degree of ionization of a solution, the concentration of the hydrogen ions is used for the measure. The probable reason for this is that 1 mole of hydrogen ions equals 1 gram. Hence, the molar concentration of a hydrogen ion solution is equal to the grams per liter of hydrogen.

$$[H^+] \times [OH^-] = 1 \times 10^{-14}$$

The H^+ concentration depends on the degree of dissociation or ionization; therefore the degree of dissociation into ions determines the relative strength of an acid or basic solution. The following formula may be used to determine the hydrogen ion concentration (in grams per liter or molarity) when the normality and percent ionization (expressed as a decimal) are known.

$$\text{N} \times \% \text{ ionization} = [H^+]$$

Hydrogen chlorine is called a strong acid because it dissociates completely into H^+ and Cl^- in a dilute solution. The preceding formula could be used to the find the H^+ concentration of a 0.1N HCl solution.

$$\text{N} \times \% \text{ ionization} = [\text{H}^+]$$

$$0.1 \times 1.0 \ (100\%) \ = 0.1 \text{ g } \text{H}^+/\text{L}$$

Acetic acid is called a weak acid because it dissociates only slightly, about 1%, into hydrogen and acetate (CH_3COO^-) ions. For a 0.1N solution the H^+ concentration would be:

$$\text{N} \times \% \text{ ionization} = [\text{H}^+]$$

$$0.1 \times 0.01 \ (1\%) \ = 0.001 \text{ g } \text{H}^+/\text{L}$$

SECTION 8.2 USE OF pH

Trying to express the acidity or alkalinity of an aqueous solution by its H^+ concentration is quite often cumbersome and inconvenient. Sørensen developed a scale to use in measuring this. He also created the symbol *pH* (which can be taken to mean *potence in hydrogen ion* or *potential of hydrogen ion*). He defined pH as follows:

pH is the logarithm of the reciprocal of the H^+ concentration. Stated another way, pH is the negative logarithm of the molar concentration of the hydrogen ions.

Sørensen's scale permits the representation of the enormous range of the possible hydrogen ion concentration from a 1N (or M) H^+ to a 0.00000000000001N (or M) H^+, with numbers extending from 0 to 14.

Consider the scale presented in Table 8-1 and shown graphically in Fig. 8-1.

Notice in the acid column that as the $[\text{H}^+]$ decreases, the pH increases. Also notice that each increase of one unit on the pH scale corresponds to a tenfold decrease in the $[\text{H}^+]$. Therefore a change of $\frac{1}{10}$ or 10 times in hydrogen ion concentration will make a change of

Table 8-1

[H^+]	pH	[OH^-]	pH
1.0 molar	0	0.00000000000001	0
0.1	1	0.0000000000001	1
0.01	2	0.000000000001	2
0.001	3	0.00000000001	3
0.0001	4	0.0000000001	4
0.00001	5	0.000000001	5
0.000001	6	0.00000001	6
0.0000001	7	0.0000001	7
0.00000001	8	0.000001	8
0.000000001	9	0.00001	9
0.0000000001	10	0.0001	10
0.00000000001	11	0.001	11
0.000000000001	12	0.01	12
0.0000000000001	13	0.1	13
0.00000000000001	14	1.0	14

[H⁺]

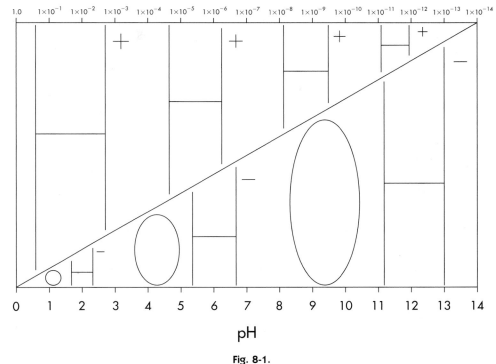

Fig. 8-1.

1 pH unit either up or down. The same holds true for bases. A change of either ¹⁄₁₀ or 10 times the base concentration will change the pH by 1 pH unit either up or down.

Recall that it was stated earlier that in all aqueous solutions the $[H^+] \times [OH^-] = 1 \times 10^{-14}$.

	[H⁺]	**[OH⁻]**		
For a pH of 4.0	0.0001	$\times$ 0.0000000001	$= 10^{-14}$	$= 1 \times 10^{-14}$
For a pH of 9.0	0.000000001	$\times$ 0.00001	$= 10^{-14}$	$= 1 \times 10^{-14}$

From the preceding definition of pH, two formulas for pH and, similarly, two formulas for pOH are derived.

pH

1. $pH = \log \dfrac{1}{[H^+]}$

$pH = \log 1 - \log [H^+]$

$pH = 0 - \log [H^+]$

2. $pH = -\log [H^+]$

pOH

1. $pOH = \log \dfrac{1}{[OH^-]}$

$pOH = \log 1 - \log [OH^-]$

$pOH = 0 - \log [OH^-]$

2. $pOH = -\log [OH^-]$

Table 8-2

[H^+]	pH	pOH	[OH^-]
1.0 molar	0	14	0.00000000000001 molar
0.1	1	13	0.0000000000001
0.01	2	12	0.000000000001
0.001	3	11	0.00000000001
0.0001	4	10	0.0000000001
0.00001	5	9	0.000000001
0.000001	6	8	0.00000001
0.0000001	7	7	0.0000001
0.00000001	8	6	0.000001
0.000000001	9	5	0.00001
0.0000000001	10	4	0.0001
0.00000000001	11	3	0.001
0.000000000001	12	2	0.01
0.0000000000001	13	1	0.1
0.00000000000001	14	0	1.0

In Table 8-2, notice again that the $[H^+] \times [OH^-] = 1 \times 10^{-14}$, but also notice the following:

$$pH + pOH = 14$$

This information may be used to solve certain types of problems. It is illustrated later in the chapter.

It can be shown that 10,000,000 liters of water will yield 1 gram of H^+ or that 1 liter of water contains 1/10,000,000 gram of H^+. Since numbers such as these are large and unwieldy, they are often expressed as powers of 10.

$$10,000,000 = 10^7$$

$$\frac{1}{10,000,000} = \frac{1}{10^7} = 0.0000001 = 10^{-7}$$

For pure water the $[H^+]$ is 10^{-7}. Using the two preceding formulas for pH, it can be seen that the pH for pure water is as follows:

1. $pH = \log \dfrac{1}{[H^+]}$

   $pH = \log \dfrac{1}{10^{-7}}$

   $pH = \log 1 - \log 0.0000001$

   $pH = 0 - \log 0.0000001$

   $pH = -\log 0.0000001$

   $pH = -(\bar{7}.0)$

   $pH = -(-7.0)$

   $pH = 7.0$

2. $pH = -\log [H^+]$

   $pH = -\log 10^{-7}$

   $pH = -\log 0.0000001$

   $pH = -(\bar{7}.0)$

   $pH = -(-7.0)$

   $pH = 7.0$

The relationship of pH to the hydrogen ion concentration can be expressed simply as long as the $[H^+]$ is equal to some negative power of 10. Such a value written in scientific notation would be 1×10^n, where n equals some whole number between 1 and 14. The pH value for such a $[H^+]$ will equal the value of n, which is a whole number. The same relationship applies between the concentration of hydroxyl ions and pOH values. Pure water has a $[H^+]$ of 10^{-7}. This is equal to 1×10^{-7} or pH 7. In an earlier example, 0.1N HCl had a $[H^+]$ of 0.1 gram per liter, or 10^{-1}, or pH 1. The 0.1N acetic acid had a $[H^+]$ of 0.001, 10^{-3}, 1×10^{-3}, or pH 3.

However, many solutions have a $[H^+]$ between exact negative powers of 10. The pH and pOH values of these must be calculated using logarithms. To calculate the pH or pOH value from the $[H^+]$ or $[OH^-]$, write the concentration using scientific notation. Then use the formula $a \times 10^{-b}$, where a equals the digits of the value and has a decimal point set between the first and second digit from the left and $-b$ equals the number of decimal places of the value. If this is not clear, review scientific notation in Chapter 1, p. 30.

EXAMPLE 8-1: Express a $[H^+]$ of 0.004 as $a \times 10^{-b}$.

$$[H^+] \text{ expressed as } a \times 10^{-b}$$
$$0.004 = 4.0 \times 10^{-3}$$

Substitute $a \times 10^{-b}$ in the formula for pH.

$$pH = -\log [H^+]$$
$$pH = -\log (a \times 10^{-b})$$
$$pH = -(\log a + \log 10^{-b})$$
$$pH = -(\log a + \bar{b})$$
$$pH = -(\log a + (-b))$$
$$pH = -(\log a - b)$$
$$pH = -\log a + b$$
$$pH = b - \log a$$

This is another formula for pH ($pH = b - \log a$) that is important for calculations.

EXAMPLE 8-2: $[H^+] = 0.004$ g/L; what is the pH of the solution?

$$[H^+] = a \times 10^{-b}$$
$$0.004 = 4 \times 10^{-3}$$

$$pH = -\log (a \times 10^{-b})$$
$$pH = -\log (4 \times 10^{-3})$$
$$pH = -(\log 4 + \log 10^{-3})$$
$$pH = -(\log 4 + \log 0.001)$$
$$pH = -(\log 4 + \bar{3}.0)$$
$$pH = -[\log 4 + (-3.0)]$$

$$pH = -(\log 4 - 3.0)$$
$$pH = -\log 4 + 3.0$$
$$pH = 3.0 - \log 4$$
$$(b - \log a)$$
$$pH = 3.0 - 0.6021$$
$$pH = 2.3979$$

IN REVIEW: At this point, review the formulas presented thus far for pH (and similarly for pOH). The formulas indicated by the asterisks are the most common.

$*pH = \log \dfrac{1}{[H^+]}$	$*pOH = \log \dfrac{1}{[OH^-]}$
$pH = \log 1 - \log [H^+]$	$pOH = \log 1 - \log [OH^-]$
$pH = 0 - \log [H^+]$	$pOH = 0 - \log [OH^-]$
$*pH = -\log [H^+]$	$*pOH = -\log [OH^-]$
$pH = -\log (a \times 10^{-b})$	$pOH = -\log (a \times 10^{-b})$
$pH = -(\log a + \log 10^{-b})$	$pOH = -(\log a + \log 10^{-b})$
$pH = -[\log a + (-b)]$	$pOH = -[\log a + (-b)]$
$pH = -(\log a - b)$	$pOH = -(\log a - b)$
$pH = -\log a + b$	$pOH = -\log a + b$
$*pH = b - \log a$	$*pOH = b - \log a$

Recall these known relationships for any ionic aqueous solution.
1. $[H^+] \times [OH^-] = 1 \times 10^{-14}$
2. $pH + pOH = 14$

EXAMPLE 8-3: A 0.1N acid solution is 70% ionized. Calculate the H^+ concentration.

$$N \times \% \text{ ionization} = [H^+]$$
$$0.1 \times \quad 0.7 \quad = 0.07 \text{ g } H^+/L$$

EXAMPLE 8-4: What would be the pH of the preceding solution?

$$[H^+] = 0.07 \text{ g/L}$$
$$0.07 = 7.0 \times 10^{-2}$$
$$pH = b - \log a$$
$$pH = 2 - \log 7.0$$
$$pH = 2 - 0.8451$$
$$pH = 1.1549$$

EXAMPLE 8-5: What would be the pOH of the solution in the two preceding examples?

$$pH + pOH = 14$$
$$1.1549 + pOH = 14$$
$$pOH = 14 - 1.1549$$
$$pOH = 12.8451$$

EXAMPLE 8-6: What would be the [OH⁻] in the preceding example?

$$[H^+] \times [OH^-] = 1 \times 10^{-14}$$

$$(7.0 \times 10^{-2}) \times [OH^-] = 1 \times 10^{-14}$$

$$[OH^-] = \frac{1 \times 10^{-14}}{7 \times 10^{-2}}$$

$$[OH^-] = \frac{1}{7} \times 10^{-12}$$

$$[OH^-] = 0.1428 \times 10^{-12}$$

EXAMPLE 8-7: An acid solution has 1/100,000 g of H⁺/L. Express this as pH.

$$\frac{1}{100,000} = 0.00001 = 10^{-5}$$

$$pH = -\log [H^+]$$

$$pH = -\log 10^{-5}$$

$$pH = -(\log 0.00001)$$

$$pH = -(\bar{5}.0)$$

$$pH = -(-5.0)$$

$$pH = 5.0$$

EXAMPLE 8-8: What is the [H⁺] of a solution having a pH of 8.95?

REMEMBER:

$$pH = \log \frac{1}{[H^+]} = b - \log a$$

In working problems of this type, the relationship between a and b is such that b may be any value and the [H⁺] will always be the same. The easiest way to work these problems is to assign b the value that is the smallest whole number that is equal to or greater than the pH or pOH value. In this problem, b would equal 9.

$$8.95 = 9 - \log a$$

$$\log a = 9 - 8.95$$

$$\log a = 0.05$$

$$a = 1.12$$

$$[H^+] = a \times 10^{-b}$$

$$[H^+] = 1.12 \times 10^{-9}$$

The hydrogen ion concentration that has a pH of 8.95 is 1.12×10^{-9} mol/L.

If another value were used for b in the example, the result would be the same, as demonstrated in the following calculation:

$$pH = b - \log a$$

$$8.95 = 10 - \log a$$

$$\log a = 10 - 8.95$$

$$\log a = 1.05$$

$$a = 11.2$$

$$[H^+] = a \times 10^{-b}$$

$$[H^+] = 11.2 \times 10^{-10} = 1.12 \times 10^{-9}$$

EXAMPLE 8-9: To prepare 400 ml of a solution of NaOH with a pH of 12, how much NaOH is needed?

NaOH is a strong base that dissociates completely.

$$NaOH \rightarrow Na^+ + OH^-$$

Since $[Na^+] = [OH^-] =$ the original $[NaOH]$, in terms of molarity the molar concentration of OH^- will equal the molar concentration of the NaOH.

$$pH + pOH = 14$$
$$12 + pOH = 14$$
$$pOH = 14 - 12$$
$$pOH = 2$$

$$pOH = -\log [OH^-]$$
$$2 = -\log [OH^-]$$
$$2 = -\log (a \times 10^{-b})$$
$$2 = b - \log a$$
$$2 = 2 - \log a$$
$$\log a = 2 - 2$$
$$\log a = 0$$
$$a = 1.0$$
$$a \times 10^{-b} = 1.0 \times 10^{-2} = 0.01 \text{ mol/L NaOH}$$

$$0.01 \text{ mol/L} = 0.01\text{M solution}$$

$$M = \frac{g/L}{mol\ wt}$$

$$0.01 = \frac{x}{40}$$
$$x = 40 \times 0.01$$
$$x = 0.4 \text{ g/L}$$

It would take 0.4 g to make 1 L of this solution. However, the problem called for 400 ml; therefore 0.4 g are to 1,000 ml as x g are to 400 ml.

$$0.4:1,000 = x:400$$

$$\frac{0.4}{1,000} = \frac{x}{400}$$

$$1,000x = 160.0$$

$$x = 0.16 \text{ g NaOH} \uparrow 400 \text{ ml} \rightarrow 400 \text{ ml of } 0.01\text{M NaOH}$$

EXAMPLE 8-10: Convert a $[H^+]$ of 0.45×10^{-9} to a pH value.

$$pH = b - \log a$$
$$pH = 9 - \log 0.45$$
$$pH = 9 - (\bar{1}.653)$$
$$pH = 9 - (-0.347)$$
$$pH = 9 + 0.347$$
$$pH = 9.347$$

In reality a logarithm consists of two numbers, the characteristic and the mantissa (see Chapter 7). Each of these numbers has its own sign; the characteristic can be either negative or positive, whereas the mantissa is always positive. In the preceding example, log *a* consists of a negative characteristic and a positive mantissa. The pH value is expressed as a single number. To get a pH value, it is necessary to combine the values of the characteristic and the mantissa. If these two numbers carry the same sign (in which case they will both be positive), they are added, and there is no change in the logarithm.

EXAMPLE 8-11: Log *a* = 1.216.

$$\text{Characteristic} = +1.0000$$
$$\text{Mantissa} = \underline{+ \ .2160}$$
$$\text{Added together} \ +1.2160$$

However, if the characteristic is negative, it is necessary to add the positive mantissa to the negative characteristic; this produces one number with a negative sign.

EXAMPLE 8-12: Log *a* = $\bar{1}$.653.

$$\text{Characteristic} = -1.0000$$
$$\text{Mantissa} = \underline{+ \ .653}$$
$$\text{Added together} - .347$$

The negative characteristic and the positive mantissa were combined by algebraic addition to form the single negative number. Remember that such a number does not exist in a table of logarithms.

Frequently in calculations using logarithms, a single negative number results as a logarithm. This is not a desirable form of a logarithm, and one cannot find the antilogarithm of such a number. Remember, the characteristic may be positive or negative, but *the mantissa of a logarithm is always positive*. To change a negative logarithm to the correct form, add the next highest whole number above the characteristic to the entire negative number. This will always result in a positive decimal fraction and will be the positive mantissa. Now use the negative form of the whole number, which was added, as the characteristic of the corrected logarithm. Indicate its sign with a bar over the number rather than the minus sign to show a negative characteristic and a positive mantissa.

EXAMPLE 8-13: Find the antilog of log *a* = −7.4.

Convert this log to a correct form having a negative characteristic and a positive mantissa. Add the next highest whole number above the characteristic to the negative logarithm.

$$\begin{array}{r} + \ 8.00 \\ \underline{- \ 7.40} \\ + \ 0.6 \end{array}$$

This is the mantissa of the corrected logarithm. Next use the negative form of the whole number added as the characteristic. Indicate its sign with a bar over the number.

$$\log a = \bar{8}.6$$

Find the antilog of mantissa 0.60, and set the decimal place according to the characteristic, $\bar{8}$.

$$\text{antilog of mantissa } 0.60 = 3981 = 4000 \text{ (rounded off)}$$
$$\text{antilog of } \overline{8}.6 = 4 \times 10^{-8} = 0.00000004$$

Hence,

$$\log a = -7.4$$
$$\log a = \overline{8}.6$$
$$a = 0.00000004 = 4 \times 10^{-8}$$

SECTION 8.3 ACID-BASE RELATIONSHIPS

The calculations involving the acid-base balance of the cells and fluids of the body involve some rather complex relationships that a book of this type should consider. The major buffer system of the body involves the following reactions:

$$CO_2 + H_2O \rightleftarrows H_2CO_3 \rightleftarrows H^+ + HCO_3^-$$

Carbon dioxide combines with water to form carbonic acid. Carbonic acid dissociates into hydrogen and bicarbonate ions. This system in relation with the reactions of hemoglobin maintains the pH of the body fluids at a remarkably constant value of 7.35 to 7.45.

All acids, bases, and salts ionize to a certain degree when dissolved in a solvent such as water. The proportion of the material that ionizes is called the **degree of dissociation.** When carbonic acid is dissolved in water, some of it ionizes into hydrogen and bicarbonate ions.

$$H_2CO_3 \rightleftarrows H^+ + HCO_3^-$$

The law of mass action states that at a constant temperature the product of the concentration of the active substances on one side of a chemical equation, when divided by the product of the concentration of the active substances on the other side of the chemical equation, is a constant, regardless of the amounts of each substance present at the beginning of the reaction. This means that the product of the hydrogen ion concentration times the bicarbonate ion concentration divided by the concentration of carbonic acid always produces the same answer, no matter how much carbonic acid is added to a solution. In other words, the degree of dissociation of a substance at a particular temperature will always be the same.

$$\frac{[H^+][HCO_3^-]}{[H_2CO_3]} = K'$$

It is extremely difficult to measure the concentration of carbonic acid directly. However, it has been found that in water solutions the molar concentration of dissolved carbon dioxide is 1,000 times the molar concentration of carbonic acid.

$$[CO_2] = 1{,}000\,[H_2CO_3]$$

$$\frac{[H^+][HCO_3^-]}{[CO_2]} = K = \frac{1}{1{,}000}K'$$

The CO_2 of this formula refers to the carbon dioxide dissolved in the blood plasma.

The hydrogen ion concentration can be calculated using a rearrangement of the preceding formula.

$$[H^+] = K \times \frac{[CO_2]}{[HCO_3{}^-]}$$

Because the hydrogen ion concentration is usually expressed as pH, it is usually more convenient to express all concentrations in this equation in the logarithmic form.

$$\log [H^+] = \log K + \log \frac{[CO_2]}{[HCO_3{}^-]}$$

Since pH $= -\log [H^+]$, change the signs of all logarithms.

$$-\log [H^+] = -\log K + \left(-\log \frac{[CO_2]}{[HCO_3{}^-]}\right)$$

Stated another way:

$$-\log [H^+] = -\log K + \log \frac{[HCO_3{}^-]}{[CO_2]}$$

Since $-\log [H^+]$ is called the pH, the $-\log K$ can be called the pK.

$$pH = pK + \log \frac{[HCO_3{}^-]}{[CO_2]}$$

This is one form of the Henderson-Hasselbalch equation. The Henderson-Hasselbalch equation is used to calculate the pH of a mixture of a weak acid and its salt. This mixture is called a *buffer system*. The equation can be defined as follows:

$$pH = pK_a + \log \frac{[A^-]}{[HA]}$$

where [HA] is the molar concentration of the free acid, [A$^-$] is the concentration of the anion from the acid, and pK is the logarithm of the reciprocal of the acid's dissociation constant (K_a). A pK value is constant only for a specific set of conditions. It varies inversely with the degree of dissociation, temperature, and pH. It also varies with different solutions of the body. For example, the pK for serum and plasma is 6.10 at 37°C, whereas it is 6.18 for erythrocytes at this temperature.

Study of the Henderson-Hasselbalch relationship will show that an increase in the concentration of the bicarbonate ions will cause an increase in the pH of the solution. Similarly, an increase in the concentration of dissolved CO_2 will cause a decrease in the pH of the solution.

When a gas is dissolved in a liquid, the concentration of the gas in that liquid is directly proportional to the partial pressure of the gas. Hence, the dissolved carbon dioxide is proportional to the partial pressure of gaseous carbon dioxide. The partial pressure of CO_2 in millimeters of mercury (mm Hg) is designated by P_{CO_2},

$$[CO_2] = a \times P_{CO_2}$$

where a is the proportionality constant. This constant equals 0.0301 when the total carbon dioxide concentration is expressed as millimoles per liter and 0.07 when the total carbon dioxide concentration is expressed as ml%. If this information is added to the Henderson-Hasselbalch equation, the following formula results.

$$pH = pK + \log \frac{[HCO_3^-]}{a \times P_{CO_2}}$$

The total carbon dioxide is the dissolved CO_2 plus the bicarbonate ion. The small amount of carbonic acid is usually disregarded in these calculations.

$$\text{Total } CO_2 = [CO_2] + [HCO_3^-]$$

Remember, dissolved $CO_2 = a \times P_{CO_2}$. Hence,

$$\text{Total } CO_2 = a \times P_{CO_2} + [HCO_3^-]$$

If this formula is expressed differently:

$$[HCO_3^-] = \text{total } CO_2 - a \times P_{CO_2}$$

Substitute this in the Henderson-Hasselbalch formula:

$$pH = pK + \log \frac{\text{total } CO_2 - a \times P_{CO_2}}{a \times P_{CO_2}}$$

This form of the Henderson-Hasselbalch formula allows the calculation of any one of three values: pH, P_{CO_2}, or total CO_2. Recognize that two of the values must be known to calculate the third.

With the substitution of accepted values for pK (6.1) and a (0.03 for CO_2 in millimoles per liter), the equation becomes

$$pH = 6.10 + \log \frac{\text{total } CO_2 - 0.03 \, P_{CO_2}}{0.03 \, P_{CO_2}}$$

When the total CO_2 is expressed in millimoles per liter and the P_{CO_2} in mm Hg, the equation for expressing P_{CO_2} becomes:

$$P_{CO_2} \text{ (in mm Hg)} = \frac{\text{total } CO_2 \text{ (in mmol/L)}}{0.03 \, [\text{antilog (pH} - 6.1) + 1]}$$

The equation for determining the total CO_2 is:

$$\text{Total } CO_2 \text{ (in mmol/L)} = 0.03 \, P_{CO_2} \, [\text{antilog (pH} - 6.1) + 1]$$

Using the preceding formulas and the following values, calculate each parameter asked for in Examples 8-14, 8-15, and 8-16.

$$pH = 7.44, \, P_{CO_2} = 37.7, \, CO_2 = 26$$

EXAMPLE 8-14: Determine the pH.

$$pH = 6.10 + \log \frac{\text{total } CO_2 - 0.03 \, P_{CO_2}}{0.03 \, P_{CO_2}}$$

$$pH = 6.10 + \log \frac{26 - (0.03 \times 37.7)}{0.03 \times 37.7}$$

$$pH = 6.10 + \log \frac{26 - 1.131}{1.131}$$

$$pH = 6.10 + \log \frac{24.87}{1.131}$$

$$pH = 6.10 + \log 21.99$$
$$pH = 6.10 + 1.3422$$
$$pH = 7.44$$

EXAMPLE 8-15: Determine the P_{CO_2}.

$$P_{CO_2} = \frac{total\ CO_2}{0.03\ [antilog\ (pH - 6.1) + 1]}$$

$$P_{CO_2} = \frac{26}{0.03\ [antilog\ (7.44 - 6.1) + 1]}$$

$$P_{CO_2} = \frac{26}{0.03\ (antilog\ 1.34 + 1)}$$

$$P_{CO_2} = \frac{26}{0.03\ (21.88 + 1)}$$

$$P_{CO_2} = \frac{26}{0.03 \times 22.88}$$

$$P_{CO_2} = \frac{26}{0.6864}$$

$$P_{CO_2} = 37.9$$

EXAMPLE 8-16: Determine the total CO_2.

$$Total\ CO_2 = 0.03\ P_{CO_2}\ [antilog\ (pH - 6.1) + 1]$$
$$Total\ CO_2 = 0.03 \times 37.7\ [antilog\ (7.44 - 6.1) + 1]$$
$$Total\ CO_2 = 0.03 \times 37.7\ (antilog\ 1.34 + 1)$$
$$Total\ CO_2 = 0.03 \times 37.7\ (21.88 + 1)$$
$$Total\ CO_2 = 0.03 \times 37.7 \times 22.88$$
$$Total\ CO_2 = 25.9$$

SECTION 8.4 USE OF cH

Another method for expressing the concentration of the hydrogen ion in a solution is referred to as *cH*. This method is being advocated by many teachers of chemistry as well as technicians. This is the expression of the hydrogen or hydronium ion concentration directly in terms of moles per liter, moles per milliliter, nanomoles per liter, etc. One of the major reasons for the acceptance of Sørensen's pH scale was that it was a way to avoid the very small numbers involved with the concentration of free protons in solutions. With the introduction of methods to handle very small numbers, such as electronic calculators, the major reason for the pH scale becomes less important. The use of direct values has been recommended as a way to reduce the confusion involved with the measurement of this part of solutions. For example, the concentration of the hydrogen ion in normal serum is about 4×10^{-8} moles per liter. This value can also be expressed as pH 7.4. This is the same as 4×10^{-5} moles per milliliter or 40 nanomoles per liter. Using this system, there is no need to consider logarithmic calculations, because this method does not use logarithms. In those cases in which it may be necessary to convert from pH notation to some direct form of expression of the hydrogen ion concentration, the explanation to do this is given on pp. 191-195.

The reciprocal antilogarithm of the pH is equal to the moles per liter of H^+.

EXAMPLE 8-17: Report a pH of 7.4 as cH in nanomoles per liter.

Recall:

$$[H^+] = a \times 10^{-b}$$
$$pH = b - \log a$$
$$7.4 = 8 - \log a$$
$$\log a = 8 - 7.4$$
$$\log a = 0.6$$
$$a = 3.98 = 4.0 \text{ (rounded off)}$$

Hence:

$$[H^+] = 4.0 \times 10^{-8}$$

This is the H^+ concentration in moles per liter. To convert to nanomoles per liter, multiply this number by 10^9.

$$4.0 \times 10^{-8} \times 10^9 = 4.0 \times 10^1 = 4.0 \times 10 = 40 \text{ nmol/L}$$

Therefore to convert pH to cH into nanomoles per liter, multiply the H^+ concentration in moles per liter by 10^9.

Using the reciprocal antilog, make the conversion as follows.

$$pH = 7.4$$
$$\text{Antilog of } 7.4 = 25,120,000$$
$$\text{Reciprocal antilog of } 7.4 = \frac{1}{25,120,000}$$
$$= 0.0000000391$$
$$= 0.00000004 \text{ (rounded off)}$$

Hence,

$$0.00000004 = 4.0 \times 10^{-8}$$
$$4.0 \times 10^{-8} \times 10^9 = 4.0 \times 10^1 = 4.0 \times 10 = 40 \text{ nmol/L}$$

See Appendix X.3 for a table and simplified conversion method.

SECTION 8.5 BUFFER SYSTEMS

The addition of a mixture of a weak acid and its salt will cause a solution to resist change in pH when other acids or bases are added. Such a mixture is a **buffer system.** Buffer systems are vital to biological processes and many laboratory procedures.

To understand why buffers stabilize the pH of ionic solutions, one must consider **the common ion effect.** This is the term given the fact that if two substances that ionize to form the same ion (the common ion) are mixed in a solution, the amount of dissociation is less than expected if each is added alone.

Since salts usually dissociate completely, or nearly so, and weak acids dissociate slightly, most of the common ion of the acid and salt comes from the salt. This means that more of the weak acid remains undissociated than if it were in a solution without its salt. For example, in the buffer system consisting of acetic acid and sodium acetate, the sodium acetate dissociates almost completely into sodium and acetate ions. The acetic acid normally dissociates only slightly into hydronium and acetate ions. Because the acetate ion is common to both, the acetic acid dissociates even less than if it were alone in the solution, as a result of the common ion effect. This results in a low concentration of hydronium ions when the solution reaches equilibrium. Now if a strong acid is added to this solution, the extra hydronium ions react with the excess acetate ions to form undissociated acetic acid. If a strong base is added, the hydroxide ions produced react with the scarce hydronium ions to form water. Some of the acetic acid will then ionize to replace the hydronium ions. In both cases the concentration of hydronium ions, and hence the pH, change very little. The Henderson-Hasselbalch equation is used in the making of laboratory buffer solutions. The basic equation for this use is as follows:

$$pH = pK + \log \frac{[salt]}{[acid]}$$

In this formula the concentrations of the salt and the weak acid are usually expressed in moles per liter, millimoles per liter, or milliequivalents per liter. The pK values can be found in Appendix AA.

EXAMPLE 8-18: Calculate the pH of an acetate buffer composed of 0.15M sodium acetate and 0.06M acetic acid. From a reference source the pK value for acetic acid is known to be 4.76.

$$pH = pK + \log \frac{[salt]}{[acid]}$$

$$pH = 4.76 + \log \frac{0.15}{0.06}$$

$$pH = 4.76 + \log 2.5$$

$$pH = 4.76 + 0.3979$$

$$pH = 5.1579$$

$$pH = 5.16$$

If the pK of the acid of a buffer pair and the total concentration of the buffer are known, the amount of salt and acid required to prepare a buffer can be calculated.

EXAMPLE 8-19: Prepare an acetate buffer with a concentration of 0.1M and buffers at a pH of 5.5.

The pK of acetic acid is 4.76, the molecular weight of acetic acid is 60, and the molecular weight of sodium acetate is 82.

$$pH = pK + \log \frac{[salt]}{[acid]}$$

$$5.5 = 4.76 + \log \frac{[salt]}{[acid]}$$

$$\log \frac{[salt]}{[acid]} = 5.5 - 4.76$$

$$\log \frac{[salt]}{[acid]} = 0.74$$

antilog of 0.74 = 5.5; therefore

$$\frac{mol/L \; salt}{mol/L \; acid} = 5.5$$

These calculations show that the ratio of the moles per liter of salt divided by the moles per liter of acid is 5.5. Any ratio that gives this value may be used. One simple combination would be 5.5M salt and 1M acid. Remember that the ratio is based on molar concentration. This combination could be used only for buffer solutions having a total of 6.5 moles of buffer per liter of solution. However, the example calls for 0.1M. To find the amounts of buffer materials needed in a 0.1M buffer solution, use the ratio-proportion procedure. The known ratio is 6.5 moles per liter of total buffer materials to 1 mole per liter of acetic acid. The desired system has 0.1 mole per liter; hence,

$$\frac{6.5 \; total \; mol/L}{1 \; mol/L \; acid} = \frac{0.1 \; total \; mol \; desired}{x \; acid}$$

$$6.5x = 0.1$$

$$x = 0.015 \; mol/L \; acid$$

Out of the total moles per liter needed, 0.015 mol/L will be acid.

$$mol/L \; acid + mol/L \; salt = total \; mol/L$$

$$mol/L \; salt = total \; mol/L - mol/L \; acid$$

$$mol/L \; salt = 0.1 - 0.015$$

$$mol/L \; salt = 0.085$$

$$mol/L \; acid = 0.015M$$

$$mol \; wt \times M = g/L$$

$$60 \times 0.015 = 0.9 \; g/L$$

$$mol/L \; salt = 0.085M$$

$$mol \; wt \times M = g/L$$

$$82 \times 0.085 = 6.97 \; g/L$$

Therefore 0.9 g acid + 6.97 g salt ↑ 1,000 ml yield 1 L of 0.1M acetate buffer, which buffers at pH 5.5.

APPENDIXES RELATED TO THIS CHAPTER

PRACTICE PROBLEMS

Calculate the answer for each problem. Understand each portion of the calculation and determine whether the answer is logical. *Just because an answer can be calculated does not mean that it is reasonable.*

Use of pH

1. A 0.03N acid solution is 70% ionized. Give the following:
   a. $[H^+]$ c. pH
   b. $[OH^-]$ d. pOH
2. A 0.9N acid solution is 90% ionized. Give the $[H^+]$ concentration.
3. If the hydrogen ion concentration is 10^{-3}, what is the pH value?
4. If the pH value is 7, what is the hydrogen ion concentration?
5. If the pH of a solution changes from pH 5 to pH 3, the hydrogen ion concentration changes:
   a. twofold   c. twentyfold
   b. tenfold   d. one hundred-fold
6. Which of the following equals 10^{-6}?
   a. 0.0000006
   b. 0.000001
   c. 0.000006
   d. 0.0000001
7. The greater the hydrogen ion concentration $[H^+]$ of a solution, the more _____ it is.
   a. acid
   b. basic
8. A solution contains 1/100,000 g H^+/L of solution. What is its pH?
9. The greater the hydroxyl ion concentration $[OH^-]$, the more _____ the solution.
   a. acid
   b. basic
10. Give the pH if the pOH is known to be 11.0.
11. True or false: The higher the pH, the greater the acidity.
12. A 0.02N acid solution is 95% ionized. Give each of the following:
    a. $[H^+]$ c. pH
    b. $[OH^-]$ d. pOH
13. A solution of pH 6 has _____ times as many hydrogen ions as a solution of pH 7. Therefore the lower the pH the greater the (acidity, alkalinity) of the solution.
14. Each pH unit represents a multiple of 10; therefore a solution of pH 10 has _____ as many hydrogen ions as does neutral water.
15. If the $[H^+]$ is 1×10^{-4}, what is the $[OH^-]$?
16. Convert to $[OH^-]$
    a. $[H^+] = 1.9 \times 10^{-6}$
    b. $[H^+] = 0.03 \times 10^{-11}$
    c. $[H^+] = 5.2 \times 10^{-4}$
17. Convert to $[H^+]$
    a. $[OH^-] = 1.01 \times 10^{-7}$
    b. $[OH^-] = 0.19 \times 10^{-2}$
    c. $[OH^-] = 6.43 \times 10^{-10}$
18. Express the concentrations in question 16 as pH and pOH.
19. Express the concentrations in question 17 as pH and pOH.

20. What is the pH of a solution with a $[H^+]$ of 1×10^{-9}?
21. If the $[H^+]$ is 1×10^{-8}, what is the $[OH^-]$?
22. The $[H^+]$ of a solution is 1×10^{-4}. What is the pH of the solution?
23. Express the following as pH: $[H^+] = 4.2 \times 10^{-4}$.
24. What is the pH of a solution with a $[H^+]$ of 4×10^{-7}?
25. Express the following as pH and pOH: $[H^+] = 0.93 \times 10^{-2}$.
26. Express as pH and pOH: $[H^+] = 3.1 \times 10^{-6}$.
27. Express a pH of 8 as 1 g of $H^+/\underline{\quad}$ L.
28. Express a pH of 4 as grams of H^+ per liter.
29. Express as pH and pOH: $[H^+] = 0.876 \times 10^{-3}$.
30. Express as pH and pOH: $[OH^-] = 3.1 \times 10^{-6}$.
31. Express as $[H^+]$: pH $= 7.8$
32. Express as $[H^+]$: pH $= 3.26$.
33. Express as $[OH^-]$: pH $= 4.93$.
34. Express as $[H^+]$: pH $= 11.51$.
35. Express as $[H^+]$: pOH $= 6.37$.
36. To prepare 400 ml of a solution of NaOH with a pH of 10, how many grams of NaOH would need to be weighed out?
37. How much HCl would be required to make 600 ml of a solution with a pH of 4.5?
38. What is the pH of a 0.01M HCl solution?
39. Express the following as $[H^+]$ and $[OH^-]$: pH $= 8.4$.
40. Express the following as $[H^+]$ and $[OH^-]$: pOH $= 8.4$.
41. What is the pH of a 0.04M HCl solution?
42. Express the following as $[H^+]$: pH $= 1.93$.
43. Give the following information about a 0.2M NaOH solution:
    a. pH   c. $[H^+]$
    b. pOH   d. $[OH^-]$
44. What is the pH of a NaOH solution having a $[OH^-]$ of 0.03M?
45. What is the pH of a 0.0001M NaOH solution?
46. A solution has a pH of 4.0; 10 ml are diluted to 1,000 ml. What is the pH of the final solution?
47. Convert to pH: $[H^+] = 0.003$ mol/L.
48. Convert to $[H^+]$: pOH $= 8.95$.

Acid-Base Relationships

49. Calculate the blood pH using the Henderson-Hasselbalch equation:

$$pH = pK + \log \frac{[salt]}{[acid]}$$

Use the following information if and as needed:

$$Total\ CO_2 = 50\ mEq/L$$

$$P_{CO_2} = 70\ mm\ Hg$$

$$pK_1\ H_2CO_3 = 6.1$$

$$pK_2\ H_2CO_3 = 10.25$$

$$Solubility\ coefficient\ for\ CO_2 = 0.03$$

50. Given a pH of 7.29 and a P_{CO_2} of 36.1, calculate the CO_2.
51. Given a P_{CO_2} of 43 and a CO_2 of 28, calculate the pH.
52. Given a CO_2 of 45 and a pH of 7.49, calculate the P_{CO_2}.

Use of cH

53. Report as cH:
    a. pH 6.9
    b. pH 7.7

Buffer systems

54. What is the pH of a buffer solution containing equal concentrations of salt and acid?
55. How would one prepare an acetate buffer, concentration 0.3M, that has a pH of 6.5? (pK of acetic acid = 4.76)
56. The buffer capacity of a buffer is greatest when the pH = _____.
57. For maximal buffer capacity, the [salt] should _____ the [acid], so that the pH = _____.
58. Calculate the pH of a bicarbonate buffer that is composed of a solution that is 0.5M sodium carbonate and 0.05M carbonic acid. The pK is 6.10.
59. How would one prepare an acetate buffer, concentration 0.6M, that has a pH of 7.0? (pK of acetic acid = 4.76)

9

Colorimetry

EDUCATIONAL OBJECTIVES

To have successfully learned the material in this chapter, the student should be able to do the following properly:

- ◆ State Beer's Law, and describe the relationships included in this principle.
- ◆ Determine the concentration of a substance in solution using inverse colorimetry.
- ◆ Determine the concentration of a substance in solution using direct colorimetry.
- ◆ Describe the relationship between absorbance and percent transmittance.
- ◆ Convert absorbance to percent transmittance.
- ◆ Calculate the concentration of a substance in solution using molar absorptivity coefficients.

SECTION 9.1 INTRODUCTION

Colorimetry is a much used tool in the clinical laboratory; however, most workers do not realize this. Many of the automated analytical machines in the laboratory use colorimetry to determine the values printed out on the forms or presented on the monitors. This technique can be used in making qualitative and quantitative determinations of many biological materials. It works by measuring the kind and amount of light absorbed or transmitted by a substance. The materials tested in a clinical laboratory are usually in solution.

The wavelength determines the color of light. The color of a substance is determined by the wavelengths of the light transmitted from it. A colorimeter has a light source of known quality. The light is passed through a prism or a grating to separate the different wavelengths of light, resulting in individual color bands. Light of one wavelength is directed toward a vessel holding a solution of the material being examined. The amount of light allowed to pass through the solution is measured by a photometer as either the absorbance or the percent transmittance (%T).

For a complete explanation of the mechanics and theory of operation of a colorimeter, consult one of the standard texts listed at the end of the book.

There are several calculations involved in the use of colorimetry in the laboratory, particularly involving the use of curves and standards. The law forming the mathematical basis for colorimetry is really a combination of several laws that are often collectively called **Beer's**

law. Stated simply, it says that the absorbance, A, of a colored solution is equal to the product of the concentration of the color-producing substance, C, times the depth of the solution through which the light must travel, L, times a constant, K. Written as an equation, this law becomes the following:

$$A = C \times L \times K$$

It is from this relationship that some of the formulas are derived. There are two main types of colorimetry: visual and photometric. Visual colorimetry is seldom used and is presented here only as a mathematical contrast to photometric colorimetry.

SECTION 9.2 VISUAL COLORIMETRY (INVERSE COLORIMETRY)

In visual colorimetry the colors of a standard solution and an unknown solution are set equal to each other by varying the depth of solution through which one looks. The color is an indication of the absorbance of the solutions. Referring to the mathematical equation of Beer's law, $A = C \times L \times K$, there is one formula that refers to the standard and one that refers to the unknown.

Standard	**Unknown**
$A_s = C_s \times L_s \times K$	$A_u = C_u \times L_u \times K$

Since A_s has been set to equal A_u, it can be said that $A_s = A_u$. If this is true, then by substituting for A_s and A_u, one would have the following:

$$A_s = A_u$$
$$C_s \times L_s \times K = C_u \times L_u \times K$$

Since K appears on both sides of the equation, it may be cancelled out.

$$C_s \times L_s = C_u \times L_u$$

The concentration of the unknown is to be determined; therefore the following should be set up:

$$C_u \times L_u = C_s \times L_s$$
$$C_u = \frac{C_s \times L_s}{L_u}$$
$$C_u = \frac{L_s}{L_u} \times C_s$$

Visual colorimetry is referred to as *inverse* colorimetry because as the reading of the unknown, L_u, increases, the concentration of the unknown, C_u, decreases.

SECTION 9.3 PHOTOMETRIC COLORIMETRY (DIRECT COLORIMETRY)

In photometric colorimetry, the depth of the solution is held constant (cuvette diameter determines the depth) and the absorbance changes (the reading taken from the instrument). Here again, there is one formula for the standard and one for the unknown.

Standard	**Unknown**
$A_s = C_s \times L_s \times K$	$A_u = C_u \times L_u \times K$

In photometric colorimetry the depth is held constant, and the absorbances vary and are read from a scale; therefore:

$$L_s = L_u$$

$$L_s = \frac{A_s}{C_s \times K} \qquad L_u = \frac{A_u}{C_u \times K}$$

Therefore:

$$\frac{A_s}{C_s \times K} = \frac{A_u}{C_u \times K}$$

Or since K appears on both sides:

$$\frac{A_s}{C_s} = \frac{A_u}{C_u}$$

$$\frac{C_u}{A_u} = \frac{C_s}{A_s}$$

$$C_u = \frac{C_s}{A_s} \times A_u$$

$$C_u = \frac{A_u}{A_s} \times C_s$$

Photometric colorimetry is called *direct* colorimetry because as the absorbance of the unknown, A_u, increases, the concentration of the unknown, C_u, also increases.

This formula applies *only* when Beer's law is followed. If it is followed, the absorbance and concentration are directly related; that is, if the absorbance doubles, the concentration doubles; if the absorbance triples, the concentration triples; and so on. Some solutions do not show this relationship. In such cases a standard curve must be used to determine the concentration of the unknown (see Chapter 10).

SECTION 9.4 RELATIONSHIP BETWEEN ABSORBANCE AND %T

Look at the relationship between A (or *OD*, optical density) and %T presented in Fig. 9-1.

In Fig. 9-1 the divisions on the absorbance scale are unequal and almost impossible to separate on the left side. **Absorbance, A,** is a measure of the amount of light stopped, or absorbed, by a solution, and the absorbance of light is a logarithmic function. Hence, the A scale is a logarithmic scale. On the other hand, **transmittance, T,** is a measure of the amount of light allowed to pass through a solution (Fig. 9-2).

Since **transmission** is a mathematical comparison of the amount of light emerging from a solution to the amount of light entering the solution, and since **transmittance** is the comparison of the transmission of the unknown solution to the transmission of the blank

Absorbance

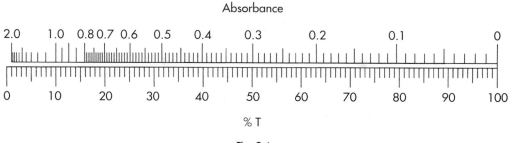

% T

Fig. 9-1.

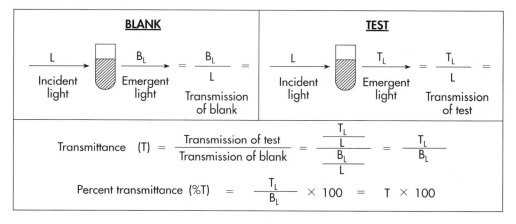

Fig. 9-2.

solution, the %*T* scale is a linear scale. The divisions on the %*T* scale are equally spaced and easy to read; thus these divisions are commonly seen on most instruments. Because the following relationship is true, *A* = light stopped and *T* = light passed through, *A* and *T* are inversely related. They are also logarithmically related, because the absorption of light is a logarithmic function. Therefore the following is the basic relationship between *A* and *T*:

$$A = \log \frac{1}{T}$$

This relationship may be rearranged to give a second relationship.

$$A = \log \frac{1}{T} \quad \text{(first relationship)}$$

$$A = \log 1 - \log T$$

$$A = 0 - \log T$$

$$A = -\log T \quad \text{(second relationship)}$$

From Fig. 9-2 it can be seen that:

$$\%T = T \times 100$$

Therefore:

$$T = \frac{\%T}{100}$$

With a little substitution in the formula $A = -\log T$, the most commonly seen relationship may be derived. If $\frac{\%T}{100}$ is substituted for T, the following becomes apparent:

$$A = -\log \frac{\%T}{100}$$
$$A = - (\log \%T - \log 100)$$
$$A = - (\log \%T - 2)$$
$$A = - \log \%T + 2$$
$$A = 2 - \log \%T \quad \text{(third relationship)}$$

Beginning with the first basic relationship, it is possible to derive the other two most commonly stated relationships (all denoted with an asterisk) as follows:

$$*A = \log \frac{1}{T}$$
$$A = \log 1 - \log T$$
$$A = 0 - \log T$$
$$*A = -\log T$$
$$A = -\log \frac{\%T}{100}$$
$$A = - (\log \%T - \log 100)$$
$$A = - (\log \%T - 2)$$
$$A = - \log \%T + 2$$
$$*A = 2 - \log \%T$$

Those relationships marked with an asterisk are the ones that laboratory workers see most often. Learn them. Understand them. They will be used in the next chapter.

SECTION 9.5 ABSORBANCE AND ITS RELATIONSHIP TO MOLAR ABSORPTIVITY

Colorimetry can be used to determine the actual concentration of materials in solution rather than simply a relative concentration. To do this the absorbance of a solution must be used in connection with a known coefficient for the particular compound being measured at a particular wavelength. This coefficient is known as the **molar absorptivity** (also known as ϵ, molar absorption coefficient, and molar extinction coefficient) and is usually the absorbance (at a given wavelength) of a 1M solution of the pure substance through a 1-centimeter light path. Stated another way, the absorbance is the product of absorptivity, the optical light path, and the substance concentration (usually in moles per liter). Molar absorbance coefficients for the substances being tested can usually be found from references. This coefficient can also be used to estimate the purity of the dissolved material.

To use the molar absorptivity for concentration determinations, one can include the results of a test in the following formula to calculate the concentration of the material in the sample:

$$A = \epsilon \times c \times d$$

where A is the absorbance of the sample at a given wavelength; ϵ is the molar absorptivity; c is the concentration in moles per liter; and d is the length of the light path in centimeters.

EXAMPLE 9-1: If ϵ is known, the concentration can be calculated from the absorbance.

$$c = \frac{A}{\epsilon \times d}$$

Since $d = 1.0$:

$$c = \frac{A}{\epsilon}$$

The ϵ of nicotinamide-adenine dinucleotide (NADH) for three different wavelengths is as follows: 340 nm $= 6.22 \times 10^3$, 366 nm $= 3.3 \times 10^3$, and 334 nm $= 6.0 \times 10^3$. The absorbance values at these wavelengths were found to be 340 nm $= 0.311$, 366 nm $= 0.165$, and 334 nm $= 0.300$. Insert these values to calculate the concentration of the solution.

$$(\text{at } 366 \text{ nm}) \ c = \frac{0.165}{3.3 \times 10^3} = 0.05 \times 10^{-3} \text{ mol/L}$$

$$(\text{at } 340 \text{ nm}) \ c = \frac{0.311}{6.22 \times 10^3} = 0.05 \times 10^{-3} \text{ mol/L}$$

$$(\text{at } 334 \text{ nm}) \ c = \frac{0.300}{6.0 \times 10^3} = 0.05 \times 10^{-3} \text{ mol/L}$$

One can determine the purity of a solution of known concentration by calculating the molar absorptivity if the concentration and absorbance values are known; this is then compared with the value for the pure substance. The following is a convenient formula for this determination:

$$\epsilon = \frac{A}{c \times d}$$

Since $d = 1.0$:

$$\epsilon = \frac{A}{c}$$

EXAMPLE 9-2: A solution of NADH has a concentration of 0.05×10^{-3} mol/L. What would the ϵ be at 340 nm, 366 nm, and 334 nm, using the absorbance values from the preceding example?

Using these values, one obtains the following information:

$$\epsilon_{366} = \frac{0.165}{0.05 \times 10^{-3}} = 3.3 \times 10^3$$

$$\epsilon_{340} = \frac{0.311}{0.05 \times 10^{-3}} = 6.22 \times 10^3$$

$$\epsilon_{334} = \frac{0.300}{0.05 \times 10^{-3}} = 6.0 \times 10^3$$

One can further derive that the amount of NADH reduced in a reaction can be computed from the measured change in absorbance, ΔA.

EXAMPLE 9-3: Using the preceding values, if a change in absorbance of 1.000 is obtained at the three wavelengths, one would find that the concentration of NADH is the following:

$$\Delta A_{340} = 1.000: \quad c = \frac{1.000}{6.22 \times 10^3} = 1.608 \times 10^{-4} \text{ mol/L}$$

$$\Delta A_{366} = 1.000: \quad c = \frac{1.000}{3.3 \times 10^3} = 3.030 \times 10^{-4} \text{ mol/L}$$

$$\Delta A_{344} = 1.000: \quad c = \frac{1.000}{6.0 \times 10^3} = 1.667 \times 10^{-4} \text{ mol/L}$$

Before these coefficients can be used with most analytical instruments, they must be adjusted to conform to the range of the instrument. This is done by diluting the sample and then making a mathematical correction of the results. For example, a 1M solution of bilirubin suitable for use as a standard should have an absorbance of 60,700 (mean) $\pm$ 800 at 453 nanometers in chloroform at 25°C, when measured in a cuvette with a 1-centimeter light path. Since the most accurate range in spectrophotometry is approximately 0.2 to 0.8A, the dilution should be made so that readings will fall within these limits. If a 1M solution had an absorbance of 60,700, a 1/60,700M (a 1/60,700 dilution of a 1M) would have an absorbance of 1.0. Hence, a 1/121,400M solution would have an absorbance of 0.5, which is within the desired range.

If the instrument being used has a light path of other than 1 centimeter, correction must be made for this difference.

EXAMPLE 9-4: What would be the molar absorptivity of a 1M solution of bilirubin diluted 1:121,400 and giving an absorbance of 0.73 on a machine using a light path of 1.5 cm?

$$\epsilon = \frac{A}{c \times d}$$

$$\epsilon = \frac{0.73}{\dfrac{1}{121,400} \times 15}$$

$\epsilon = 59,350$ (which would not be within the acceptable range)

APPENDIXES RELATED TO THIS CHAPTER

P Transmission—Optical Density Table
Q Formulas Presented In This Book

PRACTICE PROBLEMS

Calculate the answer for each problem. Understand each portion of the calculation and determine whether the answer is logical. *Just because an answer can be calculated does not mean that it is reasonable.*

Colorimetry

1. You are using a visual colorimeter and have the following data:

Reading of standard	25
Reading of unknown	18
Concentration of standard	200 mg/100 ml

   What is the concentration of the unknown?
2. Using a photoelectric colorimeter, the OD reading of the standard is 0.420, the reading of the unknown is 0.210, and the concentration of the standard represents 150 mg/dl. What is the concentration of the unknown?
3. What is the absorbance of a solution having an 85%T?
4. The absorbance of an unknown is 0.17; the absorbance of the standard is 0.13. The concentration of the standard = 100 μg/dl. What is the concentration of the unknown?
5. The percent transmittance of an unknown solution is 48%. What is the concentration of this solution if a standard solution of 100 mg/dl of this substance has a 75%T reading?
6. A solution of 150 μg/dl of ammonia nitrogen has an OD of 0.14. The OD of an unknown blood sample is 0.12. What is the concentration of the blood sample?
7. Convert to OD using the formula, not a table:
   a. 10%T c. 61%T
   b. 35%T d. 92%T
8. Convert to %T using the formula, not a table:
   a. 0.009 OD   c. 0.732 OD
   b. 0.206 OD   d. 0.913 OD

Molar absorptivity

9. The absorbency of a 2.0 g/100 ml standard is usually 0.300 when measured at a wavelength of 545 nm in a 19 × 105-mm cuvette. If one uses 10-mm cuvettes, the absorbency of the 2.0 g/100 ml standard would be approximately:
   a. 0.150   d. 0.600
   b. 0.300   e. not predictable
   c. 0.450
10. Calculate the concentration from the information given below:

	ϵ	A	Light path
a.	1.1 × 10^3	0.163	1.0 cm
b.	6.4 × 10^3	0.391	12 mm
c.	2.9 × 10^3	0.404	1.5 cm
d.	0.7 × 10^4	0.710	19 mm
e.	0.092 × 10^4	0.263	16 mm
f.	1.1 × 10^3	0.163	10 mm

11. Calculate the ϵ from the information given below:

	c	A	Light path
a.	0.03 × 10^{-3} mol/L	0.216	19 mm
b.	0.16 × 10^{-4} mol/L	0.099	1 cm
c.	0.09 × 10^{-3} mol/L	0.3000	10 mm

12. A 1M solution of a substance should have an absorbance of 50,000 ± 500 at 450 nm at room temperature. How would you dilute this solution so that it reads between 0.2 and 0.8 A? What absorbance would the diluted solution have?

13. A 1:125,000 dilution of a 1M substance has an OD of 0.46. The ϵ of the pure substance should be 60,000 ± 700. Would you say that this solution was suitable for use?

14. What would be the ϵ of a 1M bilirubin solution diluted 1:150,000 and giving an absorbance of 0.63 on an instrument with a 12-mm light path?

15. What should the absorbance be for a solution with an ϵ of 55,200 if it is diluted 1:150,000, read on an instrument with a 19-mm light path, and has an original concentration of 1.1×10^{-3}?

16. Given: A divalent substance with a molecular weight of 140 with an ϵ of 60,300. It is diluted 1:100,000 and read in an instrument with a 1.5-cm light path; it gives an absorbance of 0.561. Give the concentration of the diluted substance in:

   a. mol/L   e. mEq/L
   b. M   f. ppm
   c. N   g. $\%^{w/v}$
   d. mg/dl

10

Graphs and Standard Curves

EDUCATIONAL OBJECTIVES

To have successfully learned the material in this chapter, the student should be able to do the following properly:

- ◆ Describe the current use of graphs and standard curves in the clinical laboratory.
- ◆ Describe the organization of linear, semilog, and log-log graphs.
- ◆ Establish a standard curve using a set of data.
- ◆ Calculate the concentration of a substance in solution using a standard curve.

SECTION 10.1 INTRODUCTION

The use of graphs and standard curves has declined greatly in the clinical laboratory. Most of the tests formally using these techniques now use computers or some other manner of automation. This chapter is presented so students can gain an understanding of the concepts and vocabulary of graphs and standard curves.

SECTION 10.2 GRAPHS

Graphs are grids of lines used to show a relationship between properties. Most graphs use some form of the Cartesian coordinate system, in which paired values of two related properties are used to determine the placement of a point on an array of lines. Several such pairs produce a pattern of points that demonstrates the relationship between the properties. The values are the **variables** of the coordinate pairs. A line through a series of points is called a **curve.** The curve is the demonstration of the relationship.

The foundation for a graph consists of two straight lines set at right angles to one another. These are the major axes of the graph. The horizontal line is the ***x* axis,** and the vertical line is the ***y* axis.** The intersection of the two axes is the **origin** of the graph. Other lines parallel to these two axes complete the graph array (Fig. 10-1).

The origin of the graph is usually taken as the zero point for both axes. Positive and negative values are assigned from this point along both major axes. On the x axis, negative values are assigned progressively to the left of the origin and positive values are arranged to the right. On the y axis, negative values are below the origin and positive values are distributed above the origin. Hence, a complete graph is divided into four quadrants by the axes (Fig. 10-1). Points are plotted in each of these quadrants according to the signs of the variables in the coordinate pairs. If both variables of a pair are positive, the point is plotted in the

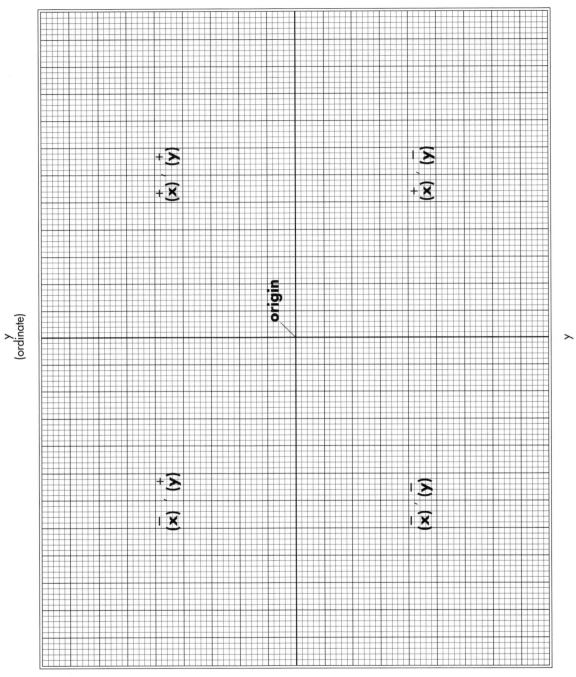

Fig. 10-1.

upper right quadrant. If both variables are negative, the point is in the lower left quadrant. If the x variable is positive and the y variable is negative, the point is placed in the lower right quadrant. The upper left quadrant contains points from coordinate pairs with negative x variables and positive y variables. Most graphs occur only in the upper right hand quadrant, since this is where positive values are plotted.

The data used to create a graph are several related measurements of two properties. Measurements of one property are coordinated with measurements of the other to produce the coordinate pairs of variables. In most cases only one variable of a pair changes as a result of a change in the other. This is the **dependent variable.** The other variable is the **independent variable,** and changes in it are not a result of any change in the dependent variable. For example, consider a chemical reaction in which the concentration of a product is directly proportional to the length of time the reaction is allowed to proceed. Since the concentration of the product changes with a change in the length of time, the concentration is the dependent variable. Changes in the length of time are not due to a change in concentration; hence, length of time is the independent variable. The x axis is usually used to plot the independent variable, whereas the y axis is used for the dependent variable.

To prepare a graph array for the plotting of variables, appropriate values must be assigned to the x and y axes. These values must be compatible with the data to be plotted. The range of values assigned to an axis has to be greater than the range of the variables plotted along it. Additionally, the values must be uniformly distributed along the axis. Any equal portion of the length of an axis must include an equal portion of the range of values along the axis. However, the values along one axis are not necessarily the same as the values on the other axis.

When the values have been properly assigned to the axes, the graph is ready for the plotting of the variables. To plot a point determined by a coordinate pair of variables, first move along the x axis to the value equal to the independent variable of the pair. Now move vertically from this value to a point opposite the value on the y axis equal to the dependent variable. Mark this point. The distance of this point to the y axis is the **abscissa** of the point, and the distance to the x axis is the **ordinate** of the point. Stated another way, the x value is called the abscissa of the point and the y value is called the ordinate of the point. Repeat this procedure for each coordinate pair. All of these points are used to place the **curve** on the graph. The most common way to place the curve is to simply connect the points with a line. The shape and direction of this curve indicate the relationship of the two properties. The curve may actually be a curved line, although it can also be a straight line.

Kinds of Graphs

The **linear graph** is a common type of graph used for laboratory work. The rulings of this type of graph are equally spaced along both axes. Any range of values can be used along an axis of this kind of graph, as long as the values are distributed uniformly (Fig. 10-2).

The **semilog graph** is another common kind of graph used in laboratories. One axis of a semilog graph is linear, and the other has logarithmic rulings. This results in a straight line curve if the properties are related logarithmically (Fig. 10-3).

Log-log graphs have both axes with logarithmic rulings. This is used when the independent variable is a logarithmic function and the dependent variable varies logarithmically with the independent variable (Fig. 10-4).

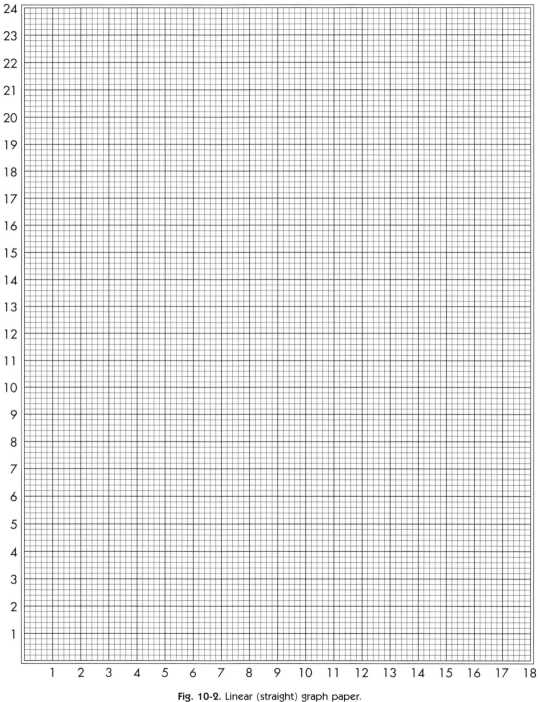

Fig. 10-2. Linear (straight) graph paper.

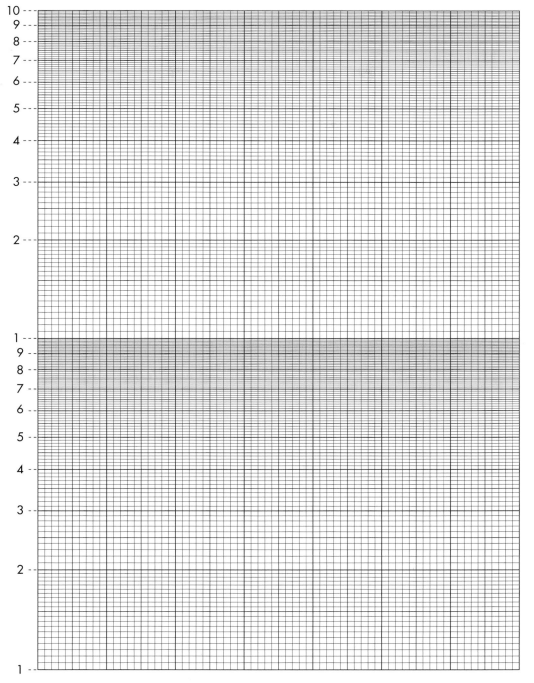

Fig. 10-3. 2-cycle semilog-graph paper.

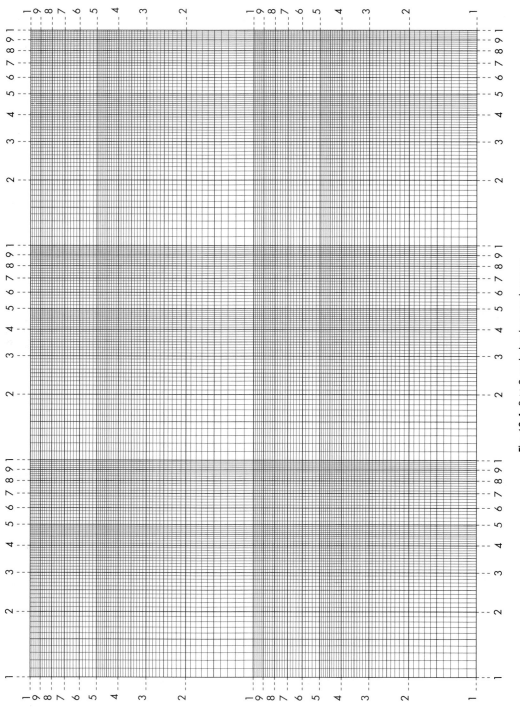

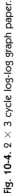

Fig. 10-4. 2 × 3 cycle log-log graph paper.

With the semilog and log-log graphs, a complete order of magnitude must be used for a complete cycle of a logarithmic axis. Ranges of values such as 1 to 10, 10 to 100, 100 to 1,000, etc. must be used for one cycle of this kind of axis. This is necessary because the distances between the lines of one cycle vary according to the mantissa of the logarithm of the portion of the order of magnitude used for the particular space. Hence, the distribution of values along this kind of axis must match the variation of the distance between any two lines.

When there is more than one logarithmic cycle on a graph, each cycle is 10 times the value of the preceding one. For example, if the first cycle is labelled from 1 to 10, the second cycle must be labelled from 10 to 100. However, if the first cycle is labelled 10 to 100, the second cycle should be labeled 100 to 1,000 (Figs. 10-5 to 10-7).

Slope

Another property of a graph is called **slope.** This refers to the direction of the curve of the graph. It is calculated as the ratio of the portion of the y axis included in a convenient length of the curve to the portion of the x axis included by the same part of the curve. If this is placed in a formula, then:

$$\text{Slope} = \frac{\Delta y}{\Delta x}$$

The slope of a curve is usually calculated using the relative lengths of the two axes and not necessarily the values assigned to the particular axis. Consider the example in Fig. 10-8.

A study of curve 1 shows that when the concentration changes from 30 millimoles per liter to 80 millimoles per liter, the time varies from 3 seconds to 8 seconds. Notice that the range of 30 to 80 millimoles per liter takes 5 centimeters on the y axis and the range 3 to 8 seconds takes 5 centimeters on the x axis. The length of the portions of the two axes is the same, although the actual values are different. Hence, the slope of this curve is 1.0

$$\text{Slope} = \frac{\Delta y}{\Delta x} = \frac{5}{5} = 1.0$$

Now consider curve 2. A change in the concentration from 30 to 80 millimoles per liter results in a change in time from 1.9 to 5 seconds. The length of the y axis is 5 centimeters, whereas the length of the x axis is 3.1 centimeters within these ranges. The slope of this curve is 1.6.

$$\text{Slope} = \frac{\Delta y}{\Delta x} = \frac{5}{3.1} = 1.6$$

The portion of a curve considered for the calculation of the slope is arbitrary within the limits of reason and convenience. The slope is the same at every portion of a straight line curve. One may choose any point along the curve from which to obtain the data needed to calculate the slope. If done correctly, the answers will be the same (Fig. 10-9).

Caution must be used when comparing the slopes of graph curves. The graph array must be the same for such comparisons to be valid.

Text continued on p. 229.

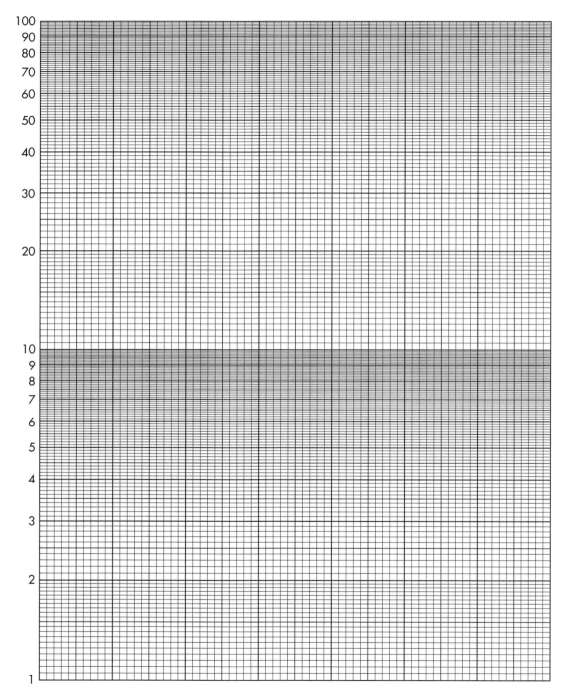

Fig. 10-5.

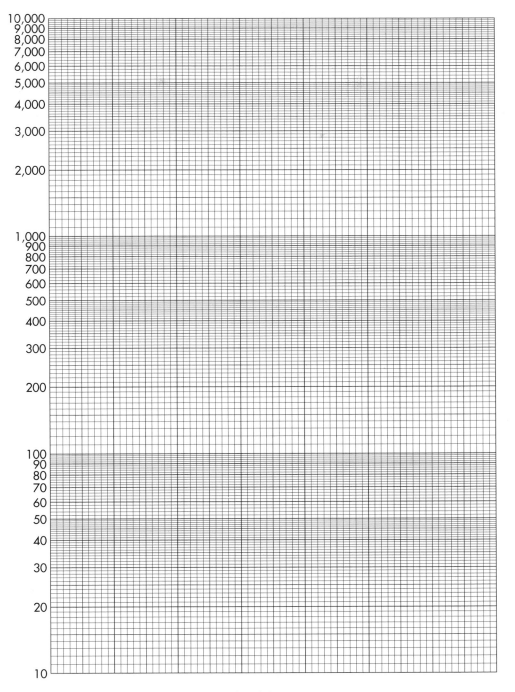

Fig. 10-6.

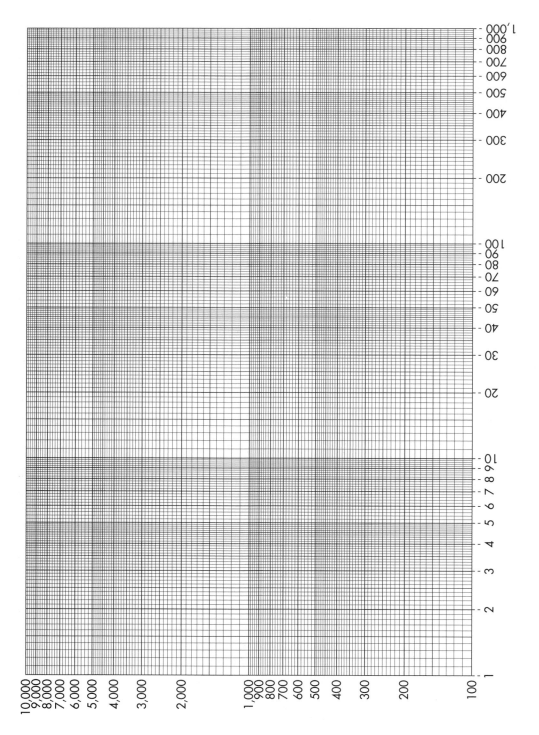

Fig. 10-7.

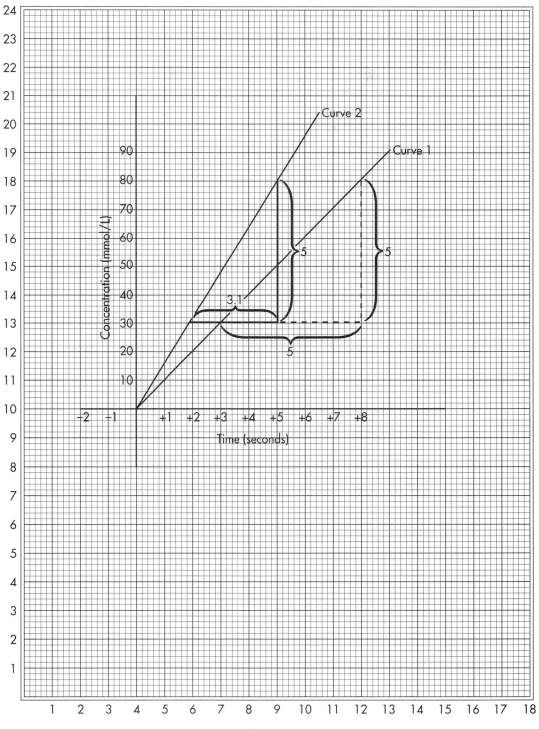

Fig. 10-8.

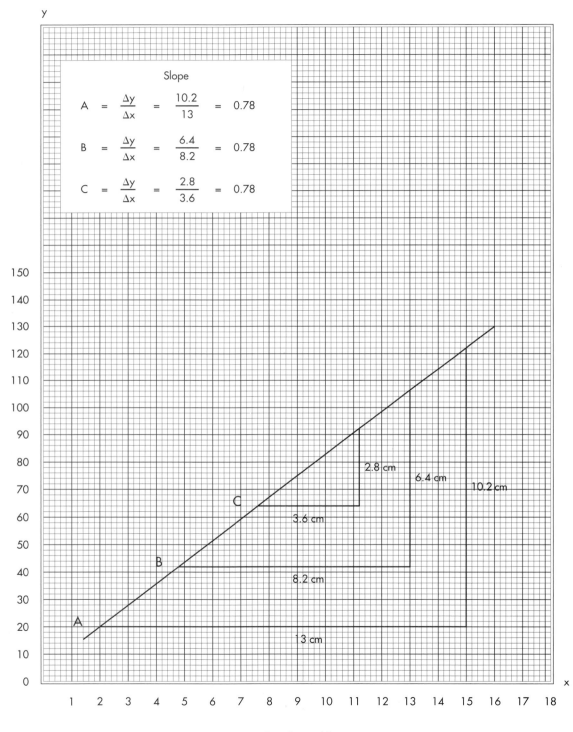

Fig. 10-9.

Intercept

Another property of curves is the point at which the curve intercepts (or meets) the x or y axis of the graph. On the examples in Fig. 10-8, the intercept of both curves is the origin of the graph. In other words, the curves meet the x and y axes at the zero point. The intercept of most curves is at this point. However, in those curves involving negative values, the intercept can be anywhere along the two axes.

"Slope and Calibrate" and Related Terms

The terms **slope and calibrate** and the **calibration of the slope and intercept** refer to the procedures used to determine the proper adjustment of laboratory instruments to account for changes in such factors as new reagent lots, temperature, or pressure. In such cases the instrument values are usually plotted against standardized values. The instrument is adjusted, or calibrated, so that the slope and intercept of the resulting curve conforms to the proper operation of the instrument. When carrying out such procedures, it is important that the instructions for the procedures for each particular instrument be followed carefully.

Extrapolation

The extension of a curve beyond the limits imposed by the highest and lowest points placed from observed coordinate pairs is called **extrapolation.** If information is taken from an extrapolated portion of a curve, extreme caution should be observed with regard to its accuracy. Usually before such information is accepted, it is supported in some other manner.

SECTION 10.3 STANDARD CURVES

Many procedures conducted in clinical and biological laboratories involve the use of standard curves. A **standard curve** as used in this context is a line plotted on graph paper that reflects the pattern of values from a test procedure or instrument in response to variations in the concentration of the material being tested. This curve is usually established by using several known values of the test material. Once this curve is established, it is used in several ways.

1. It may be used to determine an unknown value. This is probably the most common use of standard curves in most laboratories; that is, it is used in the determination of concentration by colorimetric procedures. The general principle governing the pattern of variation of most procedures is Beer's law. Remember, Beer's law may be expressed as $A = C \times L \times K$. In other words, absorbance is directly proportional to concentration. If the cause of the variation of the absorbance values *does not* conform to Beer's law, the following formula:

$$C_u = \frac{A_u}{A_s} \times C_s$$

for the determination of the concentration of the unknown value *may not* be used and a standard curve must be made.
2. If many test determinations are performed at one time, it is an arduous task to calculate each one using the formula; hence, a standard curve may be used to expedite the completion of a large number of similar tests.

3. Still another common use of standard curves is to determine whether a series of values conforms to some general principle. In this respect, a standard curve may be used to determine whether a new or unknown procedure conforms to Beer's law.

The details of the formulation of a standard curve vary with each procedure. However, there are some general guidelines to follow.

1. The range of values on the curve should correspond to the most efficient range of the test system or instrument.
2. The curve should be based on at least three known values. This is a minimum. More should be used where possible. For most procedures, a good curve can be produced from five to seven well-distributed points.
3. If possible, the values of each end of the curve should be beyond the values of any unknown used with the curve.
4. As with most endeavors of life, common sense and sound logic must be used in the development and use of a standard curve.

Because the most common use of standard curves is to convert colorimeter readings to concentrations of materials in solution, the rest of the chapter deals principally with the procedures relating to this use.

Colorimetric values reflect the color intensity of a solution placed in the light path of the machine. The color intensity is related to the amount of the color-producing substance in the light path. If the distance of the path of light through the solution is constant, the *concentration* of the test solution is the property that determines the amount of material in the light path. It is important to remember that in general, the same concentration of a given material produces the same response by the machine. The *meaning* of any concentration measurement is determined by the procedures used to obtain the concentration.

The points on which a standard curve is drawn are based on the response of the colorimeter to the known concentrations of a series of standard solutions. To greatly increase the convenience of a curve, it is necessary that the concentration notation on the graph be in terms of the equivalent concentration of the material on which the tests are to be made. For example, if a standard curve is made for the determination of milligrams of glucose per deciliter of blood, then the concentration notation on the graph should be in terms of milligrams of glucose per deciliter of blood and not in the concentration of the standard solutions used to establish the curve.

Aqueous Standards

The methods used to adjust the standard concentrations to concentrations of the test material depend on the procedures used in the preparation of the solution for use in the colorimeter. One of the most complex of such adjustments is that needed when a simple aqueous solution is used as the standard solution for the establishment of a standard curve to be used for serum concentration determinations. The following formula for this adjustment is given in some textbooks:

$$C_u = \frac{A_u}{A_s} \times \left[W_s \times \frac{V_u}{V_s} \times D \times \frac{V_c}{V_t} \right] \qquad \textbf{Formula 1}$$

where C_u is the concentration of the test (unknown) solution; A_u is the absorbance of the test solution; A_s is the absorbance of the standard solution; W_s is the total weight (mass) of the standard substance used; V_u is the final volume of the test solution; V_s is the final volume of the standard solution; D is a factor to correct for any dilution made in the test sample, that is, serum, blood, or urine; V_c is the volume base of the reported values; and V_t is the volume of test solution taken for analysis.

On first examination, this could be accurately termed an unholy mess. However, if careful study is made of each part of this formula, some sense can be made of it. Formula 1 is an expanded form of formula 2, which is the formula used for the practical expression and use of Beer's law.

$$C_u = \frac{A_u}{A_s} \times C_s \qquad\qquad \textbf{Formula 2}$$

Note that the last portion of formula 1 (the part within brackets) is simply an expression of the calculation of the concentration of the standard solution (C_s) in formula 2, in terms compatible with a particular test procedure.

The separate parts of the long formula are explained in the following list.

1. W_s: The W_s equals the total weight or the mass of the standard substance taken for color development. The mass of the standard substance used can be calculated by multiplying the number of milliliters of the working standard used by the amount of the substance per milliliter in the standard solution (see Example 10-1).

    EXAMPLE 10-1: A working standard has a concentration of 10 mg/50 ml, and 2 ml of this working standard are used. What would the W_s be for this problem?

    Concentration of working standard = 10 mg/50 ml = 1 mg/5 ml = 0.2 mg/ml. If 2 ml of this standard are used, there would be a total of:

    $$2 \times 0.2 \text{ mg} = 0.4 \text{ mg}$$
    $$W_s = 0.4 \text{ mg}$$

2. V_u, V_s: The final volumes of the test and standard solutions (V_u and V_s, respectively) are the total volumes of the solutions at the end of the test procedure. Both of these volumes are usually the same. If this is the case, the result of this fraction (V_u/V_s) is 1. This would have no effect on the final answer and can be deleted from the formula, which would leave $W_s \times D \times V_c/V_t$. If these two volumes are not equal, the result of the expression is something other than 1 and must be included in the calculation.

3. D: The part of the formula designated D is the dilution factor, which corrects the calculation for any dilutions made of the test sample. See Chapter 5, p. 113, for a discussion of dilution factors and, if necessary, for a review of how to calculate a dilution factor.

4. V_c: The factor V_c is equal to the volume on which the report of the test results is based. The concentration of substances in the body fluids is most often reported as parts per deciliter (100 milliters) or liter (1,000 milliliters) of fluid. For example, blood sugar concentrations are reported as milligrams of glucose per deciliter of blood or serum. In this kind of test V_c would be equal to 100 (1 deciliter equals 100 milliters).

5. V_t: The part of the formula designated V_t is equal to the amount of the test sample used in the analysis. If a dilution has been made of the test sample, V_t refers to the volume of diluted sample used for color development, and D is included in the formula to correct for the dilution that was made. If there has been no dilution of the test sample, V_t refers

to the actual amount of test sample (such as blood, serum, or urine) used and D would not be needed.

The last three values (D, V_c, and V_t) correct the formula for differences in the reporting base (such as milligrams per deciliter) and the volume of sample tested. If a test result for blood sugar is reported as 25 milligrams per deciliter, this means that there are 25 milligrams of glucose per 100 milliliters blood. However, 100 milliliters of blood would not normally be taken for analysis. Usually, much less blood or sample is used. Hence, a correction is made for this difference by the inclusion in the formula of the following expression:

$$D \times \frac{V_c}{V_t}$$

A rearrangement of the last portion of formula 1 ($W_s \times D \times V_c/V_t$) yields a simpler formula for everyday use in producing a standard of some desired concentration:

$$\text{ml std} \times \frac{100}{\text{quantity of test sample}} \times \text{conc. of WS/ml} = C_s \qquad \textbf{Formula 3}$$

where *ml std* is the number of milliliters of the working standard used in the test procedure; *100* is used to produce results reported in percent concentration, such as milligrams per deciliter (if the results are to be reported in parts per liter, this factor is changed to 1,000); *quantity of test sample* is the actual quantity (usually in milliliters) of the sample being tested before any alteration in volume (if procedures calling for filtrates or dilution are used, this is the actual amount of the test sample present in the final solution taken for analysis); *conc. of WS/ml* is the concentration in parts per milliliter of the working standard; and C_s is the *equivalent* concentration of the standard with which one is working for *this* procedure.

◆ ◆ ◆

NOTE: There is an important difference in the meaning of the terms **working standard** and **stock standard.** The stock standard, *SS,* refers to the solution that is normally stored, whereas the working standard, *WS,* is the solution used in the test procedure. These terms may refer to the same solution. However, on occasion low concentrations of some materials are not stable; therefore higher concentrations are used for storage. In these cases a dilution of the stock standard is made to produce a working standard with the desired concentration.

EXAMPLE 10-2: Make a working standard from a stock standard. The concentration of a stock standard is 1,000 mg/dl; a working standard with a concentration of 0.2 mg/ml is desired.

$$SS = 1{,}000 \text{ mg/dl}$$

$$SS = 1{,}000 \text{ mg/100 ml}$$

$$SS = 10 \text{ mg/ml}$$

A dilution procedure may be used to figure out how to make the needed concentration. Set up the dilution problem by putting down the original concentration (what is on hand) and the final concentration (what is desired), and make the denominator of the first dilution the volume that is desired. If 100 ml of the preceding working standard is desired, the problem is filled in as follows:

Available stock		Dilution needed		Desired concentration
$\dfrac{10 \text{ mg}}{1 \text{ ml}}$	$\times$	$\dfrac{x}{100}$	$=$	$\dfrac{0.2 \text{ mg}}{1 \text{ ml}}$

$$\frac{10}{1} \times \frac{x}{100} = \frac{0.2}{1}$$

$$10x = 0.2 \times 100$$

$$10x = 20$$

$$x = 2$$

A $^2/_{100}$ dilution of the stock standard is needed; that is, 2 ml stock standard ↑ 100 ml would give 100 ml of a working standard with a concentration of 0.2 mg/ml. Another way to think about this type of problem would be:

$$SS = 1,000 \text{ mg/dl}$$

$$SS = 1,000 \text{ mg/100 ml}$$

$$SS = 10 \text{ mg/ml}$$

In every milliliter of stock standard there are 10 mg glucose. Set up a ratio and proportion as follows: 0.2 mg in 1 ml would be the same as 10 mg in x ml.

$$\frac{0.2 \text{ mg}}{1 \text{ ml}} = \frac{10 \text{ mg}}{x \text{ ml}}$$

$$0.2x = 10$$

$$x = 50$$

If there were 10 mg in 50 ml, the desired concentration would be attained. To get 10 mg in 50 ml, take 1 ml stock standard (which contains 10 mg) and dilute this up to 50 ml. This would then be a concentration of 10 mg/50 ml, or 0.2 mg/ml. Likewise, 2 ml stock standard diluted up to 100 ml = 20 mg/100 ml or 0.2 mg/ml. Use whichever method makes most sense to you!

◆ ◆ ◆

Compare the two formulas:

$$W_s \times D \times \frac{V_c}{V_t} = C_s$$

$$\text{ml std} \times \frac{100}{\text{quantity of test sample}} \times \text{conc } WS/ml = C_s$$

The W_s of the long formula is represented by the *ml std* and the *conc of WS/ml* because the product of the concentration per milliliter times the number of milliliters used is the total weight of standard used in the procedure.

$$D \times \frac{V_c}{V_t}$$

is represented by:

$$\frac{100}{\text{Quantity of test sample}}$$

EXAMPLE 10-3: A 1:10 filtrate (which is a dilution) is made in a serum sample, and 5 ml of filtrate is used in a test reported in mg/dl.

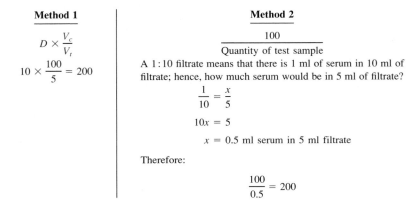

Method 1	Method 2

Method 1

$$D \times \frac{V_c}{V_t}$$

$$10 \times \frac{100}{5} = 200$$

Method 2

$$\frac{100}{\text{Quantity of test sample}}$$

A $1:10$ filtrate means that there is 1 ml of serum in 10 ml of filtrate; hence, how much serum would be in 5 ml of filtrate?

$$\frac{1}{10} = \frac{x}{5}$$

$$10x = 5$$

$$x = 0.5 \text{ ml serum in 5 ml filtrate}$$

Therefore:

$$\frac{100}{0.5} = 200$$

The same value, 200, is obtained from both procedures.

The last part of formula 1 (the part within brackets), which represents C_s:

$$C_s = \frac{A_u}{A_s} \times C_s$$

$$C_u = \frac{A_u}{A_s} \times \left[W_s \times D \times \frac{V_c}{V_t} \right]$$

has been made into a workable formula:

$$\text{ml std} \times \frac{100}{\text{quantity of test sample}} \times \text{conc. } WS/ml$$

Be sure the following relationships are understood before continuing:

$$C_u = \frac{A_u}{A_s} \times C_s$$

$$\times W_s \times D \times \frac{V_c}{V_t}$$

$$\times \text{ml std} \times \frac{100}{\text{quantity of test sample}} \times \text{conc. } WS/ml$$

A colorimetric standard is functionally a solution of known concentration of any substance that produces a given color of a given intensity under the particular conditions of the test procedure. One may then compare the color produced by a certain quantity of substance, for example, serum, blood, or urine, to that amount of the standard giving the same intensity of color.

EXAMPLE 10-4: A sugar procedure uses 1 ml of a glucose standard with a concentration of 0.1 mg/ml. The total weight of standard would be 0.1 mg (1×0.1) glucose. The color produced read $50\%T$ (obtained from the instrument reading). If the test sample, 0.5 ml serum, gave the same color for that particular test procedure, the following is known:
1. 0.1 mg glucose gave a reading of $50\%T$.

2. 0.5 ml serum under the same conditions also gave a reading of 50%*T*.
3. Therefore there must be 0.1 mg glucose in that 0.5 ml serum.
4. However, the test is not to be reported as glucose per 0.5 ml serum. It is to be reported as glucose per 100 ml serum; hence, use ratio and proportion.

$$\frac{0.1 \text{ mg}}{0.5 \text{ ml}} = \frac{x \text{ mg}}{100 \text{ ml}}$$

$$0.5x = 10$$

$$x = 20 \text{ mg/dl (per 100 ml)}$$

In *this* test procedure, using *this* amount of serum, the color produced by 0.1 mg glucose is equivalent to a blood glucose of 20 mg/dl; hence, this standard, *in this case,* is equivalent to 20 mg/dl. This is the same information that is obtained from the following formula:

$$\left(\text{ml std} \times \frac{100}{\text{quantity of blood used}} \right) \text{conc. of std/ml} = C_s$$

$$\left(1 \times \frac{100}{0.5} \right) 0.1 = C_s$$

$$200 \times 0.1 = C_s$$

$$C_s = 20 \text{ mg/dl}$$

Compare the preceding information with the formula until the relationship between the two is fully understood.

Bear in the mind that a given amount of an *aqueous* standard *will not* always have the same value in different procedures. *The value an aqueous standard has in any procedure depends on the amount of sample giving the same intensity of color.*

EXAMPLE 10-5: 1 ml of an aqueous glucose standard (conc = 0.1 mg/ml) is used in each of two procedures. One procedure calls for 0.2 ml serum, and the other uses 0.5 ml serum.

0.2 ml serum	**0.5 ml serum**
If 0.2 ml serum gives the same intensity of color as the standard, then 0.2 ml serum must contain 0.1 mg glucose.	If 0.5 ml serum gives the same intensity of color as the standard, then 0.5 ml serum must contain 0.1 mg glucose.
$$\frac{0.1 \text{ mg}}{0.2 \text{ ml}} = \frac{x \text{ mg}}{100 \text{ ml}}$$	$$\frac{0.1 \text{ mg}}{0.5 \text{ ml}} = \frac{x \text{ mg}}{100 \text{ ml}}$$
$$0.2x = 10$$	$$0.5x = 10$$
$$x = 50$$	$$x = 20$$
1 ml of this standard, *in this procedure,* equals 50 mg/dl glucose.	1 ml of this standard, *in this procedure,* equals 20 mg/dl glucose.

EXAMPLE 10-6: Work Example 10-5 using the formula.

0.2 ml serum	**0.5 ml serum**
$$1 \times \frac{100}{0.2} \times 0.1 = C_s$$	$$1 \times \frac{100}{0.5} \times 0.1 = C_s$$
$$C_s = 50 \text{ mg/dl glucose}$$	$$C_s = 20 \text{ mg/dl glucose}$$

The value for any standard in any given procedure is determined by the quantity of serum that produces the same intensity of color *under those particular test conditions.*

SECTION 10.4 PROCEDURE FOR ESTABLISHING A STANDARD CURVE

There is a general rule that should (in most cases) be followed. When setting up a standard curve, never use more standard, that is, a greater number of milliliters, than the amount of sample (or filtrate) called for in the test procedure. If the test procedure uses 0.5 milliliter of whole blood or serum, the most standard that should be used is 0.5 milliliter; if the test procedure uses 3 milliliters of filtrate, 3 milliliters of standard is the most that should be used. The reason for this is to keep the total volume of the test and standard the same.

One exception to the general rule on the volume of standard should be considered. Whenever a very small quantity (such as 0.1 or 0.05 milliliter) of sample—and hence, standard— is used and the total volume in the test procedure is relatively large (that is, 10 milliliters or so), the addition of another 0.1 milliliter or so in volume would not really alter the total volume enough to affect it appreciably, and a little extra quantity of standard would be acceptable. Use common sense and logic to decide if more standard is acceptable.

EXAMPLE 10-7: Set up a blood urea nitrogen (BUN) procedure to read from 0 mg/dl to 60 mg/dl. The procedure uses 0.02 ml serum and the only standard available has a concentration of 0.2 mg/ml.

First, calculate the concentration of this standard for this procedure in milligrams per deciliter.

$$0.02 \times \frac{100}{0.02} \times 0.2 = 20 \text{ mg/dl}$$

The highest point (when one is obeying the general rule) for this standard and in this procedure would be 20 mg/dl.

In this test procedure the following is done: to 0.02 ml serum (Fig. 10-10A):
1. Add 1 ml reagent A.
2. Add 1 ml reagent B.
3. Add 8 ml H$_2$O.

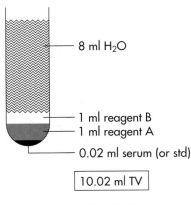

8 ml H$_2$O

1 ml reagent B
1 ml reagent A
0.02 ml serum (or std)

10.02 ml TV

Fig. 10-10A.

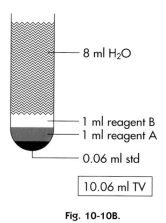

8 ml H₂O

1 ml reagent B
1 ml reagent A

0.06 ml std

10.06 ml TV

Fig. 10-10B.

20 mg/dl is not enough; 60 mg/dl is needed.

If 0.06 ml standard were used in the standard tube instead of the 0.02 ml as before (Fig. 10-10*B*):

$$0.06 \times \frac{100}{0.02} \times 0.2 = 60 \text{ mg/dl}$$

The total volume has been changed from 10.02 to 10.06 ml, a change of 0.04 ml, hardly enough to make any difference in the calculations (remember V_u/V_s is omitted when the total volumes are the same). Use common sense when deciding whether or not to follow the general rule.

Consider the following situation: There is on hand a glucose standard for which the concentration on the bottle is stated as 1,000 mg/dl. It is to be used in a glucose procedure that uses 5 milliliters of a 1:20 filtrate solution.

There are several ways to approach the establishment of a standard curve for this procedure. Probably the easiest way would be to decide first (using past experience as a guide) on the highest point needed for the standard. Experience shows that a standard as high as 400 milligrams per deciliter could be read on the available instrument when one is using this procedure. Go to the formula and begin to fill it in.

$$\text{ml std} \times \frac{100}{\text{quantity of sample used}} \times \text{conc. of } WS/\text{ml} = C_s$$

Fill in the formula one section at a time.
1. C_s: It was decided that the highest point on the curve should be 400 milligrams per deciliter. Therefore put 400 in place of C_s.
2. ml std: The largest quantity of standard to give this value is required. Since the procedure uses 5 milliliters of filtrate, 5 milliliters is the largest quantity of standard that one may use following the general rule. Hence, put 5 in place of the *ml std*.
3. Quantity of sample used: Referring to the procedure, notice that 5 milliliters of a 1:20 filtrate is used. Since this figure (quantity of sample used) is the *actual amount of blood or serum* (*not* the amount of filtrate), it must be determined how much serum is in the 5

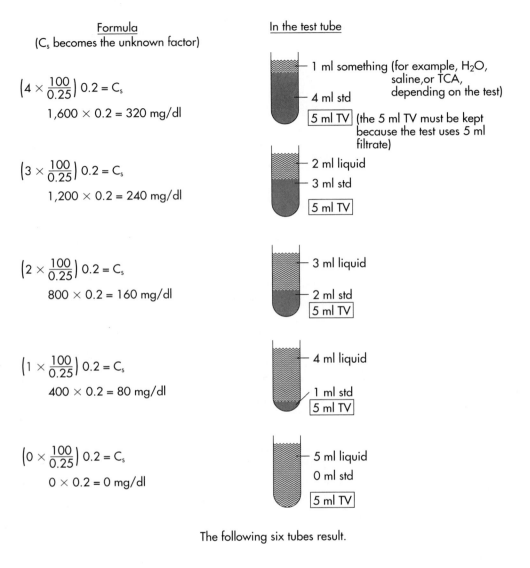

Formula
(C_s becomes the unknown factor)

In the test tube

$\left(4 \times \dfrac{100}{0.25}\right) 0.2 = C_s$

$1{,}600 \times 0.2 = 320 \text{ mg/dl}$

— 1 ml something (for example, H_2O, saline, or TCA, depending on the test)
— 4 ml std
5 ml TV (the 5 ml TV must be kept because the test uses 5 ml filtrate)

$\left(3 \times \dfrac{100}{0.25}\right) 0.2 = C_s$

$1{,}200 \times 0.2 = 240 \text{ mg/dl}$

— 2 ml liquid
— 3 ml std
5 ml TV

$\left(2 \times \dfrac{100}{0.25}\right) 0.2 = C_s$

$800 \times 0.2 = 160 \text{ mg/dl}$

— 3 ml liquid
— 2 ml std
5 ml TV

$\left(1 \times \dfrac{100}{0.25}\right) 0.2 = C_s$

$400 \times 0.2 = 80 \text{ mg/dl}$

— 4 ml liquid
— 1 ml std
5 ml TV

$\left(0 \times \dfrac{100}{0.25}\right) 0.2 = C_s$

$0 \times 0.2 = 0 \text{ mg/dl}$

— 5 ml liquid
0 ml std
5 ml TV

The following six tubes result.

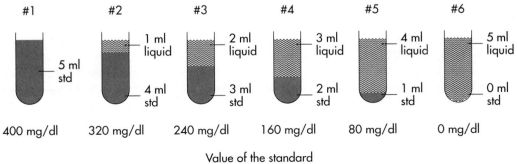

#1	#2	#3	#4	#5	#6
5 ml std	1 ml liquid / 4 ml std	2 ml liquid / 3 ml std	3 ml liquid / 2 ml std	4 ml liquid / 1 ml std	5 ml liquid / 0 ml std
400 mg/dl	320 mg/dl	240 mg/dl	160 mg/dl	80 mg/dl	0 mg/dl

Value of the standard

Fig. 10-11.

milliliters of filtrate. A 1:20 filtrate means that there is 1 milliliter of serum for every 20 milliliters of filtrate; therefore:

$$\frac{1}{20} = \frac{x}{5}$$

$$20x = 5$$

$$x = 0.25 \text{ ml serum in 5 ml filtrate}$$

Put 0.25 in place of *quantity of sample used*. The problem now stands as follows:

$$\left(5 \times \frac{100}{0.25}\right)x = 400$$

The only information not known is what concentration of standard per milliliter will yield the value 400 milligrams per deciliter (in this procedure); hence, *conc. of std/ml* is the unknown, or *x*.

$$\left(5 \times \frac{100}{0.25}\right)x = 400$$

$$2,000x = 400$$

$$x = 0.2$$

The concentration of the working standard must be 0.2 mg/ml.

To establish a curve, at least three points are needed, preferably more. The different points may be determined several ways; one is presented here.

Recall that the total volume of the standard and the unknown (used in the test procedure) should be the same; keep this in mind.

It is known that 5 milliliters of this particular standard, in this procedure, is equivalent to 400 milligrams per deciliter. If less standard is used, it would be equivalent to fewer milligrams per deciliter. Therefore fill in the formula using fewer milliliters of standard. Study Fig. 10-11. Take each tube, run each one through the procedure, and read it in the instrument as would be done with the test. The reading taken from the instrument and the corresponding concentrations will now be used to plot the curve.

SECTION 10.15 PLOTTING THE STANDARD CURVE

There are two main types of graph paper generally used in the laboratory: semilog and linear (equal or straight).

Semilog (half-log) graph paper is exactly what the name implies. The scale for the *%T* instrument reading is a log scale, and the scale for the concentration values is a straight (linear) scale (Fig. 10-12). **Linear** graph paper has both scales set off in equal units (Fig. 10-13).

These two kinds of graph paper are used because there are two units of measure on the instruments commonly employed in the laboratory: percent transmittance (*%T*), and absorbance or optical density (*A* or OD). Recall that the absorption of light is a logarithmic function and that the absorbance scale is a logarithmic scale that compensates for this. Therefore

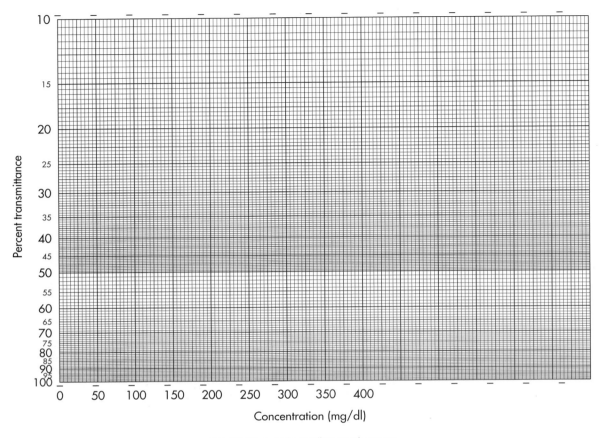

Fig. 10-12. 1-cycle semilog graph paper.

absorbance values or readings are usually plotted on straight graph paper because the logarithmic absorbance of light has already been taken care of by the *A* scale. However, the percent transmittance scale is a linear (straight) scale, and when test values are read in *%T*, there has been no compensation for the logarithmic absorption of light. Hence, *%T* readings are usually plotted on semilog paper because this corrects for the logarithmic function.

Either type reading may be plotted on either type graph paper; however, consider the following: To see if a straight line is formed, that is, to see whether Beer's law is followed, absorbance must be plotted on straight paper and *%T* must be plotted on semilog paper. If there is no desire to know whether Beer's law is followed and the proper paper is not available, use the other type. It is easier and a little more accurate to read values from a straight curve rather than one that is not straight, but it is by no means mandatory. Do not decide against using a curve just because the correct paper is not available. Simply be sure the limitations are clearly understood!

CAUTION: Never draw the lines of the curve past the last point on the curve! What happens to the relationship between the readings and the concentration is not known beyond the

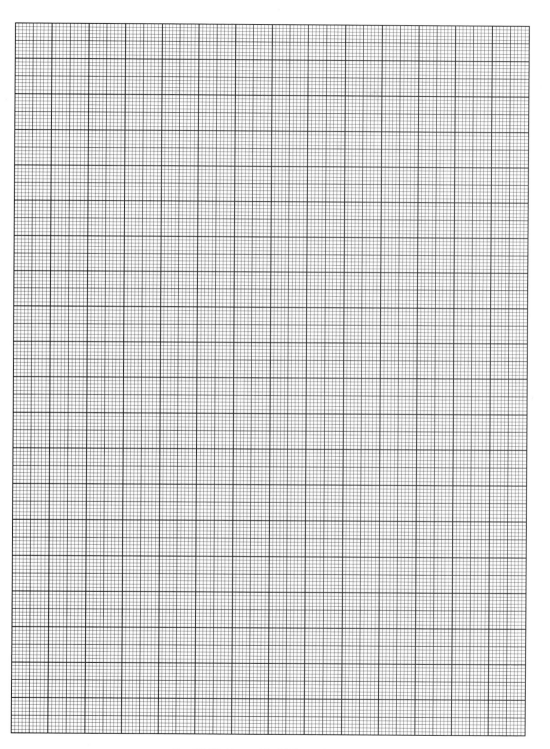

Fig. 10-13. Linear (straight) graph paper.

extremes of the curve. Additionally, values as low as 10 (in %T readings) should not be used in actual practice. They are used here for convenience and simplicity.

Using the values from the glucose problem earlier and the %T and A values given below, plot a curve each of the four possible ways (Figs. 10-14, 10-15, 10-16, and 10-17).

Standard value	%T readings	A readings
400 mg/dl	10	1.0
320 mg/dl	16	0.8
240 mg/dl	25	0.6
160 mg/dl	39.5	0.4
80 mg/dl	63	0.2
0 mg/dl (reagent blank)	100	0.0

Notice here the percent transmittance (%T) readings and the absorbance (A) readings in relation to the concentration of the standard. Recall that when Beer's law is followed, absorbance is directly related to the concentration. Notice that the absorbance reading that corresponds to 80 mg/dl is 0.2. As the concentration doubles (to 160 mg/dl) the absorbance doubles (to 0.4A). When the concentration is 4 times greater (80 × 4 = 320 mg/dL), the absorbance is four times greater (4 × 0.2 = 0.8). However, no such relationship exists between the %T readings and the concentration, for there has been no adjustment for the logarithmic relationship of the absorption of light by the substance.

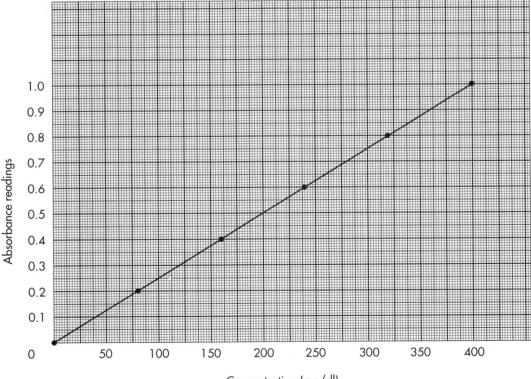

Fig. 10-14. Absorbance plotted on straight paper.

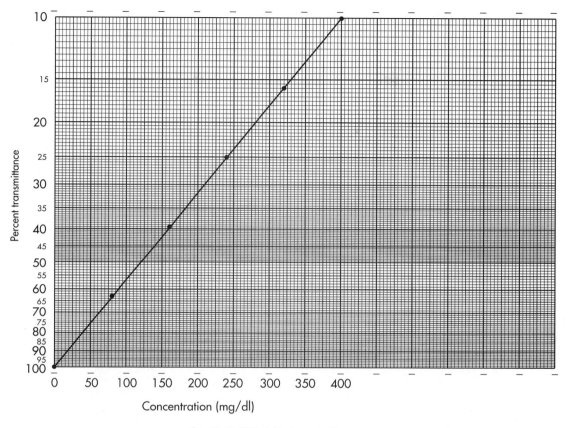

Fig. 10-15. %*T* plotted on semilog paper.

The four types of plots to make are shown in Figs. 10-14 to 10-17 (first on the correct paper, then on the opposite paper). Consider the following:

Fig. 10-14: With absorbance readings plotted on straight paper, it is evident that Beer's law is followed.

Fig. 10-15: With %*T* readings plotted on semilog paper, it is evident that Beer's law is followed.

Fig. 10-16: With absorbance readings plotted on semilog paper, it is not known whether the curve develops because of the semilog paper or because the procedure does not follow Beer's law.

Fig. 10-17: With %*T* readings plotted on straight paper, it is not known if the curve develops because of the straight paper or because the procedure does not follow Beer's law.

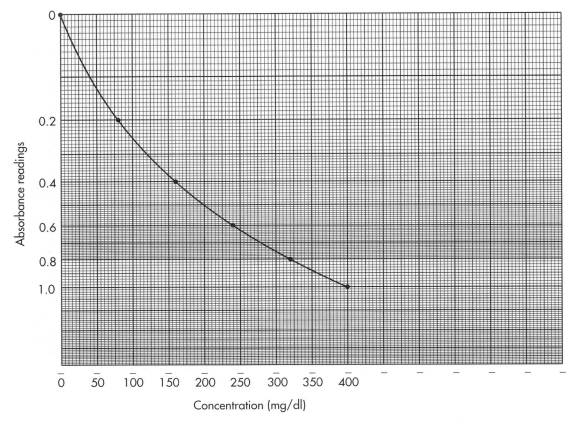

Fig. 10-16. Absorbance plotted on semilog paper

If readings are taken from each curve, the following values result (Figs. 10-14 through 10-17):

Sample Number	Instrument Reading		Value from curve used			
	%T	A	%T (semilog) Fig. 10-15	%T (straight) Fig. 10-17	A (semilog) Fig. 10-16	A (straight) Fig. 10-14
1	50	0.3	120 mg/dl	120 mg/dl	120 mg/dl	120 mg/dl
2	80	0.097	38 mg/dl	39 mg/dl	40 mg/dl	38 mg/dl
3	30	0.52	208 mg/dl	208 mg/dl	208 mg/dl	208 mg/dl

Essentially, the same answer is obtained from each curve. Those plotted on the correct paper are just a little easier to read and also give some information about Beer's law.

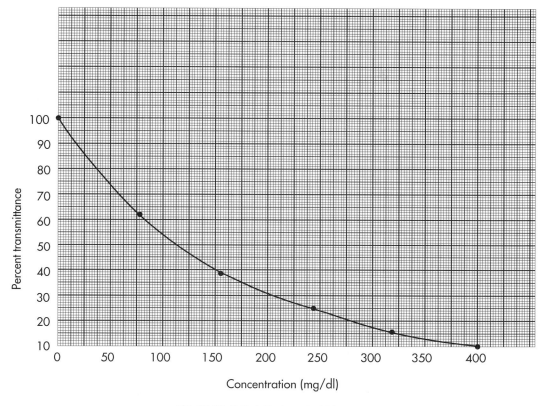

Fig. 10-17. %*T* plotted on straight paper.

SECTION 10.6 USE OF REFERENCE (BLANK) SOLUTIONS

Most colorimetric procedures use some kind of reference solution to set the colorimeter for the particular test solution used. These reference solutions are usually referred to as blank solutions. The most convenient, common type of blank solution is the reagent blank. This solution contains the same concentration of all the reagents used in the preparation of the standard and test solutions. However, it does not contain any of the substance for which the test is being made.

When a reagent blank is put into a colorimeter, any response is due to factors other than the test substance. The machine is then set on 100%*T* or 0 *A*. These values are used to represent zero concentration, and any response of the machine would be due to the substance for which the test is being made.

In some test procedures a specialized reference solution may be used to modify the colorimeter readings. In many of these procedures the instrument is set at 0 *A* or 100%*T* using only distilled water as a blank. In such cases the reading of the test solution must be adjusted using the reading of the specialized blank solution.

In these procedures there is one common pitfall in the adjustment of the readings. One must not use the percent transmittance scale without the proper consideration of the logarithmic absorption of light by substances. This mistake is commonly made.

There are several ways the colorimetric readings may be corrected using the specialized blank solution. Three are considered here.

One method commonly used is to mentally move the reading of the specialized blank down the scale to 0 *A* or 100%*T*. The readings of the standard or test solutions are moved a corresponding number of units down the scale. *This procedure will produce accurate results with the absorbance scale. It will **not** make a proper adjustment of the percent transmittance readings.*

> EXAMPLE 10-8: A test was made using a procedure directing that the colorimeter be adjusted to 0 *A* or 100%*T* using distilled water for the blank solution. A specialized blank was used to compare with the test solution. The absorbance of the specialized blank was 0.1, and the absorbance of the test was 0.5. The test reading can be adjusted by mentally moving the reading down the scale 0.1 *A* units, so the absorbance reading of the specialized blank can be thought of as 0 *A*. The test reading is then mentally moved the same number of units down the scale and will now be 0.4 *A* (Fig. 10-18).

If this same general procedure were done using the percent transmittance scale, the test reading would be incorrect (Fig. 10-19). The corresponding percent transmittance of the specialized blank is 79.5, and the percent transmittance of the test is 31.5. If the readings are moved down the scale 20.5 units so the specialized blank is at 100%*T*, the test reading would be at 52. This is *not* equal to 0.4 *A*.

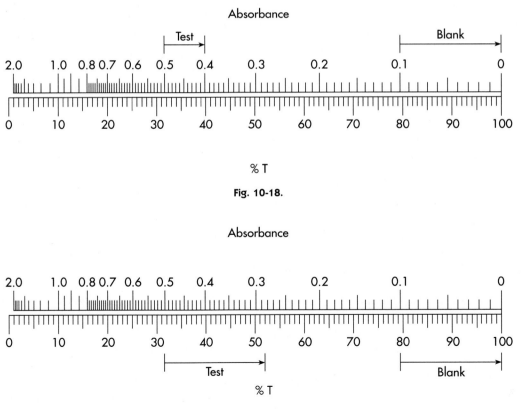

Fig. 10-18.

Fig. 10-19.

Table 10-1

Procedure	Value from the appropriate curve	
	%*T* curve (Fig. 10-15)	*A* curve (Fig. 10-14)
1. Move down the scale and read. $0.5 \to 0.1 = 0.4; A = 0.4$ $31.5 \to 20.5 = 52; \%T = 52$	113 mg/dl	160 mg/dl
2. Subtract readings. $A = 0.5 - 0.1 = 0.4$ $\%T = 79.5 - 31.5 = 48$	126 mg/dl	160 mg/dl
3. Read values from curve; subtract values. $A = 0.5; 0.1$ $\%T = 31.5; 79.5$	$31.5 = 200$ $79.5 = \underline{40}$ 160 mg/dl	$0.5 = 200$ $0.1 = \underline{40}$ 160 mg/dl

Another method of adjusting a test reading with a specialized blank is to subtract the smaller reading from the larger. Again, *this will work for the absorbance scale, but it will* ***not*** *work for percent transmittance.* Consider the values from the preceding example.

Absorbance	Percent transmittance
0.5	79.5
$- \underline{0.1}$	$- \underline{31.5}$
0.4	48.0

A third method would be to take the concentration value of the specialized blank and the test solution from the standard curve. The value for the specialized blank is then subtracted from the value for the test. *This method will work for readings taken as absorbance or percent transmittance* (Table 10-1).

Note the final concentration values when absorbance and percent transmittance are used in these three ways. The same answer is obtained for the test values using absorbance (*A* or OD) readings all three ways. This is true for two main reasons: (1) absorbance is *directly* related to concentration, and (2) the logarithmic absorption of light is taken care of at the time of reading. However, notice that the only way to obtain the correct answer (160 milligrams per deciliter) using percent transmittance readings is to get the values from the percent transmittance curve and then to subtract the blank value from the test value; the reason for this is that until the readings have been taken from the curve there has been no correction for the logarithmic absorption of light, and percent transmittance readings are *not* directly related to concentration.

Study the preceding relationships until they are thoroughly understood.

SECTION 10.7 SERUM CONTROLS

The aqueous standards discussed previously are not always treated exactly as the sample all the way through the procedure. For this reason the value (concentration) given on the aqueous standard bottle may or may not be the equivalent concentration for the standard in that particular procedure. The same standard may be equivalent to more than one sample concentration, depending on the procedure used.

Serum controls, on the other hand, are usually treated exactly as the test sample all the way through the procedure. For this reason the concentration on the bottle usually *is* the equivalent concentration for that procedure, and the concentration for a serum control is usually the same no matter what procedure it is used in.

EXAMPLE 10-9: Consider a serum control for glucose. A concentration of 100 mg/dl is stated on the bottle; therefore the value expected for this control when it is used in a procedure is 100 mg/dl. Use this same control in two different glucose procedures.

1. This procedure used 5 ml of a 1:10 filtrate.	2. This procedure used 3 ml of a 1:20 filtrate.
Control = 100 mg/dl Control = 100 mg/100 ml Control = 1 mg/ml	Control = 100 mg/dl Control = 100 mg/100 ml Control = 1 mg/dl
A 1:10 filtrate = 1 ml serum/10 filtrate.	A 1:20 filtrate = 1 ml serum/20 ml filtrate.
$$\frac{1}{10} = \frac{x}{5}$$ $$10x = 5$$ $$x = 0.5 \text{ ml serum/5 ml filtrate}$$	$$\frac{1}{20} = \frac{x}{3}$$ $$20x = 3$$ $$x = 0.15 \text{ ml serum/3 ml filtrate}$$
Fill in the formula:	Fill in the formula:
$$\text{ml std} \times \frac{100}{0.5} \times 1 = C_s$$	$$\text{ml std} \times \frac{100}{0.15} \times 1 = C_s$$

The information missing in the last expression of each preceding method is the number of milliliters of control used. This makes serum controls different in calculations from aqueous standards. Since serum controls are treated *exactly* as the unknowns, a filtrate is made of them also. And since the *ml std* means the number of milliliters of *actual control* (not filtrate), one must calculate the amount of control present in the quantity of filtrate used.

EXAMPLE 10-10: Consider the control for the two procedures in Example 10-9.

1. 1:10 filtrate = 1 ml control/10 ml filtrate.	2. 1:20 filtrate = 1 ml control/20 ml filtrate.
$$\frac{1}{10} = \frac{x}{5}$$ $$10x = 5$$ $$x = 0.5 \text{ ml control/5 ml filtrate}$$	$$\frac{1}{20} = \frac{x}{3}$$ $$20x = 3$$ $$x = 0.15 \text{ ml control/3 ml filtrate}$$
Therefore:	Therefore:
$$0.5 \times \frac{100}{0.5} \times 1 = C_s$$ $$C_s = 100 \text{ mg/dl}$$	$$0.15 \times \frac{100}{0.15} \times 1 = C_s$$ $$C_s = 100 \text{ mg/dl}$$

Think carefully about these examples and be sure the principles are understood before continuing.

In some instances a substance needed for a standard is not available, for one reason or another, in pure form. In this case a compound is used that contains this specific substance but that also contains other substances. For example, if a nitrogen standard is needed, $(NH_4)_2SO_4$ may be used. Figure out how much of the compound used would contain the quantity of nitrogen desired.

EXAMPLE 10-11: Make a 4 mg/dl nitrogen standard using $(NH_4)_2SO_4$.

The molecular weight of $(NH_4)_2SO_4$ is 132; the molecular weight of nitrogen is 14; there are two atoms of nitrogen in the compound; hence, there would be 28 mg of nitrogen in every 132 mg $(NH_4)_2SO_4$. If 100 ml of this standard is to be made, 4 mg of nitrogen are needed.

$$\frac{28 \text{ mg N}}{132} = \frac{4 \text{ mg N}}{x}$$

$$28x = 528$$

$$x = 18.86 \text{ mg } (NH_4)_2SO_4 \text{ (contains 4 mg nitrogen)}$$

Therefore dilute 18.86 mg $(NH_4)_2SO_4$ up to 100 ml to yield a nitrogen standard with a concentration of 4 mg N/dl.

APPENDIXES RELATED TO THIS CHAPTER

Q Formulas Presented in this Book
Z Atomic Weights

PRACTICE PROBLEMS

Calculate the answer for each problem. Understand each portion of the calculation and determine whether the answer is logical. *Just because an answer can be calculated does not mean that it is reasonable.*

In all the following problems assume Beer's law to be followed unless stated otherwise.

Standard Curves

1. A stock standard is available; stated on the label is a concentration of 250 mg/dl. How would 50 ml of a 0.03 mg/dl working standard be prepared?
2. A glucose standard contains 50 mg/ml. A 1/5 dilution of this standard would contain how much glucose per 100 ml?
3. You have a stock standard, and stated on the label is a concentration of 1,000 mg/dl. How would you prepare 50 ml of a 0.5 mg/dl working standard?
4. A stock standard solution of glucose contains 1 g of glucose/5,000 ml. The working standard is prepared by diluting 5 ml of the stock solution to 100 ml. What is the concentration of glucose in the working standard in milligrams per deciliter?
5. The concentration of the glucose standard reads 41%*T* on the spectrophotometer. The label on the container says *250 mg/100 ml.* The reading of the unknown sample is 53%T. What is the concentration of glucose in the unknown sample?
6. A bilirubin standard of 10 ml/dl is read on the spectrophotometer and has an OD of 0.30. The unknown has an OD of 0.15. What answer would you report? (Give answer in milligrams per deciliter and SI units.)

7. The following optical density values were obtained and recorded for a glucose procedure.

Reagent blank	0.1
Unknown sample	0.2
Standard	0.3

The known value for the standard solution is 250 mg/dl. What glucose value should be reported for this sample?

8. Given the following information, calculate the value for the unknown glucose level:

OD reading of standard	0.382
OD reading of unknown	0.501
Concentration of standard	200 mg/dl

Establishing a Standard Curve

9. A certain procedure uses 5 ml of a $1:20$ filtrate. What concentration of working standard would be needed to set up a curve on which the highest point was 500 mg/dl? How would the working standard be made from a stock standard with a concentration of 1,000 mg/dl?

10. In a procedure that uses 0.05 ml serum in the test and reports in milligrams per deciliter, what would be the value of 1.0 ml of a standard whose concentration was 15 mg/dl? What would be the standard's value in a test reported in micrograms per milliliter?

11. The following represents a scheme for the colorimetric determination of magnesium in serum. (Concentration of the working standard = $25/\mu g$ magnesium/10 ml).

Reagents	Reagent blank (ml)	Working standard (ml)	Serum (ml)
Serum			1
H_2O	5		5
$CaCl_2$	1		
Working standard		5	
Sodium tungstate	2		2
H_2SO_4	2		2
Mix and filter: use filtrate			
Filtrate	5		5
H_2O	1		1
$CaCl_2$		1	
Polyvinyl alcohol	1	1	1
Titan yellow	1	1	1
NaOH	2	2	2

The serum and working standard were compared photometrically at 540 nm against the reagent blank. The following absorbances were recorded:

Absorbance of standard	0.440
Absorbance of unknown	0.390

What is the serum magnesium concentration in micrograms per milliliter?

12. A new glucose curve is needed. The usual readable range is 0 to 400 mg/dl. The procedure uses 0.5 ml of a $1:10$ filtrate. The concentration of the stock standard is 100 mg/dl.
   a. What is the highest point you would make for the curve?
   b. How much standard (*WS*) will be used to give this point?

c. What concentration of *WS* will be needed?

d. How will this working standard be made from the stock standard?

e. What other points will there be on the curve, and how will they be determined? (Show formulas and work.)

13. Stock standard = 1,500 mg/dl; dilute 15 ml of stock standard to 150 ml for working standard. Use 2 ml of working standard in a procedure that uses 2 ml of a 1:20 filtrate. What blood concentration in milligrams per deciliter would this standard equal?

14. A certain procedure says to use 5 ml of a 1:20 filtrate. What concentration of working standard would be needed to set up a curve on which the highest point was 400 mg/dl?

15. A new glucose curve is needed. The usual readable range is 0 to 350 mg/dl. The procedure uses 0.3 ml of a 1:10 filtrate. The concentration of the stock standard is 50 mg/10 ml.

a. What is the highest point you would make for this curve?

b. How much standard (working standard) will you use to give this point?

c. What concentration of working standard will you need?

d. How will you make this concentration from the stock standard?

e. What other points will there be on the curve, and how will you arrive at them? (Show formulas and work.)

16. A procedure requires 5 ml of a 5:25 filtrate. As you prepared to run the test, you spilled the filtrate and only had 4 ml left to run the test. The standard and test gave the same reading. The value for the standard is 200 mg/dl. What is the true value for your patient?

17. Given: A stock standard of 100 mg/dl to use in a procedure that requires 5 ml of a 1:20 filtrate. Give the dilution and the concentration of working standard you need to use 5 ml and have it equal 300 mg/dl.

18. If you are working with a procedure that uses 0.02 ml of serum in the test, reported in micrograms per milliliter, what would be the value of 0.05 ml of a standard with a concentration of 40 mg/dl?

19. A new glucose curve is needed. The usual readable range is 0 to 600 mg/dl. The procedure uses 1 ml of a 1:10 filtrate. The concentration of the stock standard is 250 mg/dl.

a. What is the highest point you would make for the curve?

b. How much standard (*WS*) will you use to give this point?

c. What concentration of *WS* will you need?

d. How will you make it from the stock standard?

e. What other points will there be on the curve, and how will you arrive at them? (Show formulas and work.)

Plotting the Standard Curve

20. If Beer's law is followed, a straight line results if one plots the points of the graph using:

a. Concentration vs. wavelength on semilog graph paper

b. Concentration vs. absorbance on straight graph paper

c. Concentration vs. log %T on straight graph paper

d. Concentration vs. %T on semilog graph paper

e. Absorbance vs. wavelength on straight graph paper

Serum Controls

21. How much $(NH_4)_2SO_4$ would be needed to make a nitrogen standard with a concentration of 6 mg of N/dl?

22. A technologist prepared a stock standard for a lead determination by weighing 0.1500 mg $Pb(NO_3)_2$, dissolving it in HNO_3, and diluting to 1 L. He prepared a working standard by taking

40 ml of the stock solution and adding 150 ml of diluent. What is the concentration of the working standard in micrograms of lead per milliliter?

23. A mixed sodium and potassium standard was prepared by weighing 0.52 g KCl and 6.49 g NaCl, quantitatively transferring to a 1,000 ml volumetric flask, and diluting to the mark with distilled water. What is the concentration of the standard in mEq/L Na^+ and mEq/L K^+?

24. How many milligrams of $(NH_4)_2SO_4$ are needed to make 1 L of a 3 mg/dl nitrogen standard?

25. How many milligrams of urea, $CO(NH_2)_2$, are needed to make 600 ml of solution containing 5 mg of nitrogen/100 ml?

26. How much $(NH_4)_2SO_4$ would need to be weighed out to make a nitrogen standard of 4 mg/dl if you wanted to make 500 ml of the standard?

27. What would be the value for a phosphorus standard if it contained 0.035% KH_2PO_4 and if 0.2 ml of the standard was used in a procedure that required 0.2 ml of serum? Report in millimoles per liter.

28. How much $(NH_4)_2SO_4$ would be needed to make a nitrogen standard with a concentration of 10 mg of N/dl?

11

Hematology Math

EDUCATIONAL OBJECTIVES

To have successfully learned the material in this chapter, the student should be able do the following properly:

- ◆ Calculate the dilution factor for an amount of blood diluted with white blood cell (WBC) and red blood cell (RBC) pipettes.
- ◆ Calculate the final factor used to convert a blood count from a Neubauer hemocytometer to the number of cells per microliter of blood.
- ◆ Correct a white count for nucleated red blood cells (NRBCs).
- ◆ Calculate the final factors used to convert blood counts from the Fuchs-Rosenthal and Speirs-Levy hemocytometers to the number of cells per microliter of blood.
- ◆ Calculate the mean corpuscular volume, mean corpuscular hemoglobin, and mean corpuscular hemoglobin concentration from the hemoglobin, hematocrit, and RBC count.
- ◆ Establish a hemoglobin curve using the aqueous standard, or cyanmethemoglobin, method.

There are three main areas in hematology that have some mathematics connected with them: (1) the dilution of blood in the RBC and WBC pipettes and the counting chamber; (2) the indices; and (3) the establishment of a hemoglobin curve.

It is true that today the majority of laboratories make cell counts on particle counters. Even so, there are times when the laboratory worker needs to be able to use, and compute the results using, a counting chamber and the pipettes.

SECTION 11.1 PIPETTES

The pipettes used in hematology are composed of two main parts. The first part is a stem, subdivided into two (or sometimes 10) equal parts, and the second is a bulb containing a bead, which serves three purposes: (1) to identify (white or clear bead for a WBC pipette and a red bead for an RBC pipette), (2) to aid in mixing when the pipette is full or partially full, and (3) to indicate dryness when the pipette is empty and clean.

The dilutions used in these calculations are based on the fact that the volume of the bulb is 10 times the volume of the stem in the WBC pipette and 100 times the volume of the stem in the RBC pipette. Since the blood in the stem is drawn up into the bulb for dilution and since the total capacity of the bulb is 10 volumes for the WBC pipettes and 100 volumes for the RBC pipettes, the denominators for the WBC and the RBC dilutions are always 10 and 100, respectively (Fig. 11-1).

Notice the WBC pipette in Fig. 11-1. There are 11 total parts (or volumes) from the tip of the stem to the 11 mark. There is 1 volume from the tip to the 1 mark, and there are 10 volumes from the 1 mark to the 11 mark. Since the diluting fluid remaining in the stem (1 part) does not take part in the dilution, the total volume for the dilution process is 10 parts (11 total parts minus 1 part in the stem). If the blood had been drawn up to the 0.5 mark in a WBC pipette and diluted up to the 11 mark with diluting fluid, there would be 0.5 parts of blood in a total volume of 10 parts: a 0.5/10 dilution.

Remember, for ease of understanding and to have a factor that is easy to work with, one usually expresses a dilution as a 1-to-something dilution; therefore:

$$\frac{0.5}{10} = \frac{1}{x}$$

$$0.5x = 10$$

$$x = 20$$

1/20 dilution

Recall that to correct for a dilution, one must multiply by the reciprocal. Hence, the dilution factor for blood drawn to the 0.5 mark in a WBC pipette is 20 (the reciprocal of $\frac{1}{20}$).

WBC pipette

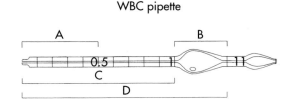

A. 0.5 parts blood
C. 1 part diluting fluid remains in stem

B. 10 parts total volume in bulb
D. 11 parts total volume in pipette

RBC pipette

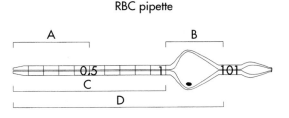

A. 0.5 parts blood
C. 1 part diluting fluid remains in stem

B. 100 parts total volume in bulb
D. 101 parts total volume in pipette

Fig. 11-1. Explanation of dilution of blood in red and white cell counting pipettes. (Modified from Bauer JD: *Clinical laboratory methods,* ed. 9, St. Louis, 1982, Mosby.)

Now look at the RBC pipette in Fig. 11-1. The stem has a smaller bore, and the bulb is larger. The total number of parts from the tip of the stem to the 101 mark is 101 total parts, but again, because the 1 part of fluid remaining in the stem does not enter into the dilution, the total parts for diluting purposes are 100 (101 total parts minus 1 part in the stem equals 100 parts). If the blood were drawn to the 0.5 mark in an RBC pipette and diluted up to the 101 mark, the dilution would be:

$$\frac{0.5}{100} = \frac{1}{x}$$

$$0.5x = 100$$

$$x = 200$$

1/200 dilution

Dilution factor = 200

EXAMPLE 11-1: What would be the dilution and the dilution factor in the following instances?
1. In a WBC pipette the blood is drawn to the 0.4 mark.

$$\frac{0.4}{10} = \frac{1}{x}$$

$$0.4x = 10$$

$$x = 25$$

1/25 dilution

Dilution factor = 25

2. In an RBC pipette the blood is drawn to the 0.2 mark.

$$\frac{0.2}{100} = \frac{1}{x}$$

$$0.2x = 100$$

$$x = 500$$

1/500 dilution

Dilution factor = 500

SECTION 11.2 HEMOCYTOMETERS

There are three main types of hemocytometers: the Neubauer, the Fuchs-Rosenthal, and the Speirs-Levy. The Neubauer hemocytometer is used for most types of blood counts, whereas the other two are used for such tests as eosinophil counts, which need a larger volume of blood for an acceptable level of precision.

Neubauer Hemocytometer

The Neubauer hemocytometer is the most common type in use. For this reason the principles of the calculations related to these instruments are explained using this type of ruling.

There are three dimensions of the counting chamber with which one should be thoroughly familiar:
1. Length (L) = one dimension = millimeters (in this case) = mm
2. Area = two dimensions = length × width (W) = square millimeters = mm^2
3. Volume = three dimensions = length × width × height (H) (depth) = cubic millimeters = mm^3

It has been recommended that red and white cell counts be reported as the number of cells per microliter (μl). Since the dimensions of the counting chambers of hemocytometers are measured in millimeters, it is much easier to calculate the volume of the blood in the chamber in terms of cubic millimeters. This requires the conversion of cubic millimeters to microliters. One cubic millimeter is equal to 1 microliter. Hence, to convert a value in terms of cubic millimeters to microliters, simply change the unit term. The numbers are not changed. For example, a white cell count of 7,500/mm^3 is equal to 7,500/μl.

The counting chamber is mainly used for performing red and white blood counts and platelet counts. The ruled area (Fig. 11-2A) is presented enlarged in Fig. 11-2B. Examine it closely.

Notice that the entire length (or width) of the ruled area is 3 mm (Fig. 11-3A, [1]). That means that the *entire* area of one ruled area (on one side on the counting chamber) is 9 mm^2 (area = $L \times W$; $3 \times 3 = 9$ mm^2). The entire ruled area is composed of nine squares, each 1 mm^2. The length of the sides of these largest squares is 1 mm; $1 \times 1 = 1$ mm^2 (Fig. 11-3A, [2]). These squares (1 mm^2) are referred to as *white squares,* because the four corner squares (Fig. 11-3A) are usually used for the white blood count.

These white squares are further divided into 16 smaller squares (Fig. 11-3A, [3]), which have sides that are 0.25 mm in length (1 mm $\div$ 4 = 0.25; there are four divisions on that 1 mm).

The central square millimeter (Fig. 11-3B) is subdivided into 25 squares, sometimes referred to as *red squares,* because the four corner squares and the central square are usually used to perform the manual red blood count. Each of these 25 squares is subdivided into 16 smaller squares. The length of one of the 25 squares is 0.2 mm (1 $\div$ 5 = 0.2; Fig. 11-3B, [5]). The length of one of the 16 subdivisions is 0.05 mm (0.2 $\div$ 4 = 0.05; Fig. 11-3B [6]). The entire length (or width) of this central area is 1 mm (Fig. 11-3B, [4]).

It seems confusing at first, but try to remember two main things: (1) the length of each of the nine large squares is 1 millimeter; and (2) the squares are subdivided—16, 25, and 16 (the white squares into 16, the middle square into 25, and each of the 25 into 16). Remembering this, the length of any line and the area of any square can always be figured out (not memorized).

Examine Fig. 11-4. Neubauer hemocytometers are made so that the center platform, *A,* which bears the ruled areas, is exactly 0.1 millimeter lower than the raised side ridges, *B,* which support the cover slip, *C.* It is into this space between the coverslip and this center platform, *D,* that the diluted blood, which is to be counted, flows. Therefore the depth of the fluid being counted is 0.1 millimeter.

Factors

There are three factors to be considered when calculating the results obtained from the use of the pipettes and counting chamber; the first factor pertains to the pipettes, and the next two pertain to the counting chamber.

1. Whole blood was not used; therefore a *dilution factor* is needed.
2. Depth counted: the counts are reported in the number of cells per cubic millimeter (microliter). If one could count a space 1 mm $\times$ 1 mm $\times$ 1 mm, one would have 1 mm^3.

Ruled area

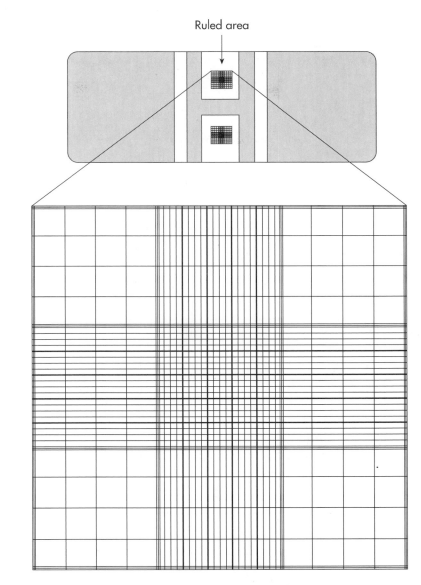

A

B

Fig. 11-2. Area for counting cells, Neubauer hemocytometer.

$$\underbrace{1 \text{ mm} \times 1 \text{ mm}}_{\text{area}} \times \underbrace{1 \text{ mm} = 1 \text{ mm}^3}_{\text{depth}}$$

But the depth is 0.1 millimeter, not 1 millimeter ($\frac{1}{10}$ what it should be); therefore a *depth factor* (10) is needed to correct for this. Unless stated otherwise, the depth factor for problems presented here will always be 10.

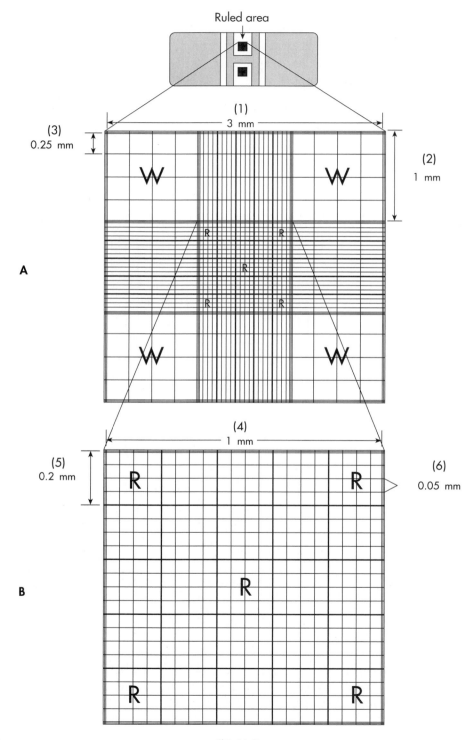

Ruled area

(1)
3 mm

(3)
0.25 mm

(2)
1 mm

A

(4)
1 mm

(5)
0.2 mm

(6)
0.05 mm

B

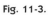

Fig. 11-3.

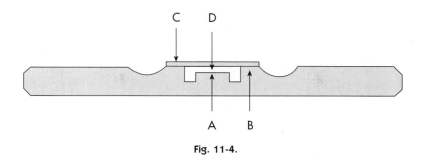

Fig. 11-4.

3. Area counted: if 1 mm² were counted, an *area factor* would not be needed. If more or less than 1 mm² is counted, this should be corrected for. Use

$$\frac{1}{\text{Area counted (in mm}^2)}$$

for determining the area factor (recall: divide by what was used and multiply by what should have been used). Notice that the area counted in square millimeters and the area factor *are not* the same thing.

Using these three factors, one obtains the following basic formula:

$$\text{Depth factor} \times \text{area factor} \times \text{dilution factor} = \text{final factor}$$

$$\text{Final factor} \times \text{cells counted (in the area used for the area factor)} = \text{cells/mm}^3 \ (\mu l)$$

If the area factor is expanded, the following formula develops:

$$\text{Depth factor} \times \frac{1}{\text{area counted (in mm}^2)} \times \text{dilution factor} = \text{final factor}$$

When it is combined, the formula becomes:

$$\frac{\text{Depth factor} \times \text{dilution factor}}{\text{area counted (in mm}^2) \text{ (not area factor)}} = \text{final factor}$$

There is one other factor that may, at times, be seen. Some authors refer to a *volume correction factor* (or volume factor). The volume factor is one factor that is a combination of the depth factor and the area factor. Since volume is $L \times W \times H$, the factor may be arrived at in the following two ways:

1. The volume that should be counted is 1 mm³. Using the rule, divide by what was used and multiply by what should have been used, one may find the volume factor by

$$\frac{1}{\text{Volume counted (in mm}^3)}$$

Divide by the volume actually counted (length of area counted × width of area counted × depth = volume in mm³; or since length × width = area, area × depth = volume in mm³) and multiply by 1 (the 1 mm³ that should have been counted). Again, notice that the volume counted and the volume factor are not the same thing.

2. One may multiply the *area factor,* not area counted, times the *depth factor* to obtain the volume factor.

The formula presented earlier for calculating the final factor may be expressed in several ways. Four other expressions of this formula are presented below. Understand the relationships and the fact that they are all different expressions of the same thing before continuing!

$$\text{Dilution factor} \times \text{depth factor} \times \frac{1}{\text{area counted (in mm}^2)} = \text{final factor}$$

$$\text{Dilution factor} \times \text{depth factor} \times \text{area factor} = \text{final factor}$$

$$\text{Dilution factor} \times \frac{1}{\text{volume counted (in mm}^3)} = \text{final factor}$$

$$\text{Dilution factor} \times \text{volume factor} = \text{final factor}$$

In everyday practice, use the one that seems easiest for you. Study the following examples, and give the following information for each:

A. Dilution of blood
B. Dilution factor
C. Depth factor
D. Area factor (expressed two ways)
E. Volume factor (determined two ways)
F. Final factor
G. Cells/mm^3 (μl)

EXAMPLE 11-2: In a WBC pipette the blood is drawn to the 0.8 mark. Six *white* squares are counted. One hundred cells are counted.
  A. Dilution:

$$\frac{0.8}{10} = \frac{1}{x}$$

$$0.8x = 10$$

$$x = 12.5$$

1/12.5 dilution

B. Dilution factor: reciprocal of 1/12.5 = 12.5.
C. Depth factor: since no information was given concerning the counting chamber depth, assume a standard counting chamber with a depth of 0.1 mm. This is ⅒ of 1 mm, so the depth factor is 10.
D. Area factor:

$$\frac{1}{\text{Area counted (in mm}^2)}$$

One has been asked to count six *white* squares. A white square is one of the nine larger squares, each 1 mm^2. Therefore if six of them are counted, 6 mm^2 have been counted. Hence, the area factor may be either of the following:

1.

$$\frac{1}{\text{Area counted (in mm}^2)}$$

$\frac{1}{6}$ (left as a fraction)

2.

$$\frac{1}{\text{Area counted (in mm}^2)}$$

$\frac{1}{6} = 0.167$

E. Volume factor: determined two ways.

1. Volume factor =

$$\frac{1}{\text{volume counted (in mm}^3)}$$

$L \times W \times H = \text{volume in mm}^3$

2. Area factor $\times$ depth factor $=$ volume factor

$0.167 \times 10 = 1.67$

The squares counted would not be lined up as below on the counting chamber; they are presented this way so the length and width can be easily figured. If 6 mm^2 were counted, the L and W would be:

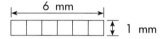

$L = 6 \text{ mm}, W = 1 \text{ mm}, H = 0.1$
$6 \times 1 \times 0.1 = 0.6 \text{ mm}^3 \text{ counted}$
$1/0.6 \text{ or } 1.67 = \text{volume factor}$

F. Final factor:

1.

$$\frac{\text{Depth factor} \times \text{dilution factor}}{\text{area counted (in mm}^2)} = \text{final factor}$$

$$\frac{10 \times 12.5}{6} = 20.8$$

2.

Depth factor $\times$ area factor $\times$ dilution factor $=$ final factor

$10 \quad \times \quad 0.167 \quad \times \quad 12.5 \quad = \quad 20.8$

G. Cells/mm^3

Cells counted $\times$ final factor $=$ cells/mm^3 (μl)

$100 \quad \times \quad 20.8 \quad = 2{,}080 \text{ cells/mm}^3$

EXAMPLE 11-3: In a RBC pipette the blood is diluted to the 0.2 mark. Five red squares are counted. A counting chamber with a depth of 0.2 mm was used. 150 cells were counted.

A. Dilution:

$$\frac{0.2}{100} = \frac{1}{x}$$

$$0.2x = 100$$

$$x = 500$$

1/500 dilution

B. Dilution factor: Reciprocal of ⅟₅₀₀ is 500.

C. Depth factor: 0.2 mm is ⅕ the depth that should have been counted. Therefore the depth factor is 5.

$$\frac{1}{0.2} \text{ or } 5$$

D. Area factor: The central square used for red counts is 1 mm^2, subdivided into 25 smaller squares, each of which is $\frac{1}{25}$ mm^2. If five of these smaller squares were counted, $\frac{5}{25} = \frac{1}{5} = 0.2$ mm^2 would have been counted (area counted in mm^2).

1/0.2 or 5

area factor = 5

E. Volume factor:

1.

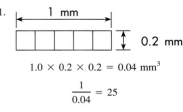

$$1.0 \times 0.2 \times 0.2 = 0.04 \text{ mm}^3$$

$$\frac{1}{0.04} = 25$$

Volume factor = 25

2. Depth factor $\times$ area factor = volume factor

5   $\times$ 5   =   25

Volume factor = 25

F. Final factor:

$$\frac{5 \times 500}{0.2} = 12{,}500$$

G. Cells/mm^3: $150 \times 12{,}500 = 1{,}875{,}000$ cells/mm^3 (μl).

Correction for Nucleated Red Blood Cells

Sometimes it is necessary to correct a white count if there are many nucleated red blood cells (NRBCs) present. This is because the white cell diluting fluids and the substances used in electronic counting procedures lyse the red cells as usual, but the nuclei (which are not usually present) remain and are counted as white cells.

There are several ways to correct for this extra counting. The method presented below does not rely on memorization. It is a ratio-proportion setup.

	Differential		Counting chamber
Actual count (WBC only)	100	=	x
Combined count (WBC + NRBC)	100 + NRBC/100 WBC		WBC counted

Look at the preceding formula. There are two ratios. The one on the left pertains to the differential; the one on the right pertains to the counting chamber. The top figure in each ratio is the number of *actual* white cells (100 is the actual number of white cells counted on the differential, and x is the true white count, which is the figure desired). The bottom numbers in each ratio are the combined counts, white cells plus nucleated red blood cells (100 + NRBC is the number of white cells counted on the differential, 100, plus the number of NRBC present along with those 100 white cells). The *WBC counted* is the number of white blood cells counted by whatever method was used. This count includes both white cells and the nuclei of the NRBC.

EXAMPLE 11-4: A white count of 25,000 is obtained. When the differential is performed, 100 white cells were counted, and along with these 100 white cells, 50 NRBC were seen. That means there were 150 cells counted, 100 of which were white cells. Using this information, fill in the ratio and proportion. If there are 100 WBC in every 150 cells, then there will be x WBC in 25,000 cells.

$$\frac{100}{150} = \frac{x}{25,000}$$

$$150x = 2,500,000$$

$$x = 16,667$$

The actual (corrected) white count is 16,667/mm^3.

Fuchs-Rosenthal Hemocytometer

The Fuchs-Rosenthal hemocytometer is a counting chamber with two platforms or counting areas. The chamber is 0.2 millimeter deep. Each ruled counting area consists of one large, 4 mm $\times$ 4 mm square. Since the depth of the chamber is 0.2 millimeter, the volume under each square is 4 mm $\times$ 4 mm $\times$ 0.2 mm, or 3.2 mm^3. Each large square is divided into 16 smaller squares, each of which is 1 millimeter long and 1 millimeter wide. These 1-millimeter squares are in turn divided into 16 even smaller squares (Fig. 11-5).

The calculations involved with this instrument are the same as those of the Neubauer hemocytometer, except for the depth factor. Because the depth of the counting chamber is 0.2 millimeter, a factor of 5 is used to correct for the 1 millimeter that should be counted.

$$\frac{1}{0.2} = 5$$

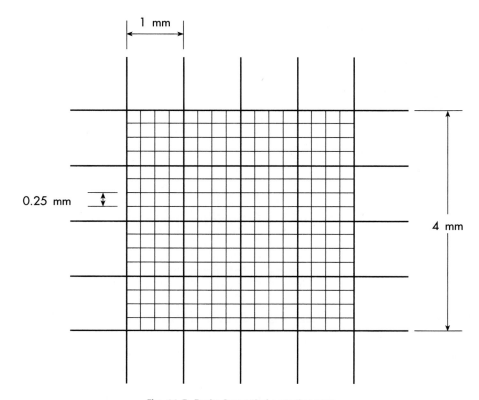

Fig. 11-5. Fuchs-Rosenthal counting area.

EXAMPLE 11-5: Using a WBC pipette, blood was drawn to the 0.5 mark and diluting fluid was drawn to the 11 mark. This gives a 1:20 dilution of the blood with the diluting fluid. The cells in all 32 squares of both sides of the counting chamber were counted; 53 cells were seen. The total area counted was 32 mm². The depth of the counting chamber is 0.2 mm. Using the formula, find the factor necessary to calculate the number of cells per microliter.

$$\frac{\text{Depth factor} \times \text{dilution factor}}{\text{area counted (in mm}^2)} = \text{final factor}$$

$$\frac{5 \times 20}{32} = 3.1$$

Multiply the number of cells counted by this factor.

$$53 \times 3.1 = 164.3$$

Hence, the sample would be reported as having 164 cell/μl.

Speirs-Levy Hemocytometer

The Speirs-Levy hemocytometer has a counting chamber that is 0.2 millimeter deep with four platforms or counting areas (Fig. 11-6). Each counting area consists of 10 squares that are each 1 millimeter long and 1 millimeter wide. These are arranged in two horizontal rows of five squares each. Each square is divided into 16 smaller squares. The volume of one counting area is 2.0 cubic millimeters (2 mm $\times$ 5 mm $\times$ 0.2 mm).

The depth factor for this instrument is the same as with the Fuchs-Rosenthal counter, that is, 5.

$$\frac{1}{0.2} = 5$$

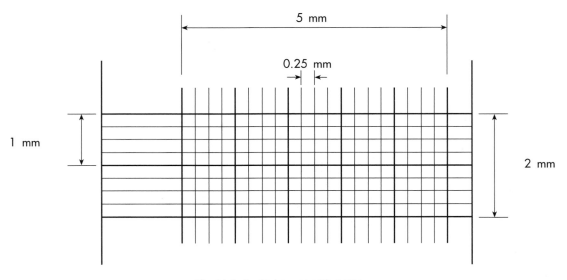

Fig. 11-6. Speirs-Levy counting area.

EXAMPLE 11-6: A 1:20 dilution of blood was made using a WBC pipette. This solution was placed in the Speirs-Levy counting chamber. The cells in all 40 1-mm² squares of the counting areas were counted; 45 cells were seen. Use the formula to find the number of cells per microliter.

$$\frac{\text{Depth factor} \times \text{dilution factor}}{\text{area counted (in mm}^2\text{)}} = \text{final factor}$$

$$\frac{5 \times 20}{40} = 2.5$$

Multiply the number of cells counted by the final factor.

$$2.5 \times 45 = 112.5$$

Report the number of cells as 112 cells/μl.

SECTION 11.3 INDICES

There are three mean corpuscular values (indices) that are commonly calculated. They are as follows:
1. Mean corpuscular volume (MCV)
2. Mean corpuscular hemoglobin (MCH)
3. Mean corpuscular hemoglobin concentration (MCHC)

These values are concerned with the volume of the average erythrocyte and the amount of hemoglobin in the average erythrocyte.

For all of the examples presented here, the following values will be used: hemoglobin (Hb), 15 g%; hematocrit (Hct), 50%; RBC count, 5,000,000.

Mean Corpuscular Volume

The mean corpuscular volume is the *volume* of the average erythrocyte. Normal values lie between 80 to 90 cubic micrometers (cubic because it concerns volume).

The following formula is used to calculate the mean corpuscular volume:

$$\text{MCV} = \frac{\text{Hct} \times 10}{\text{RBC (in millions)}} \qquad \textbf{Formula 1}$$

Since the mean corpuscular volume is the volume (in cubic micrometers) of the average erythrocyte, if the number of cubic micrometers of cells in 1 cubic millimeter is known and that number is divided by the number of cells per cubic millimeter, the volume (in cubic micrometers) of one erythrocyte would be known. Therefore:

$$\text{MCV} = \frac{\text{cubic micrometers of cells in 1 mm}^3 \text{ of blood}}{\text{cells/mm}^3 \text{ of blood}} \qquad \textbf{Formula 2}$$

To find the number of cubic micrometers of cells per cubic millimeter of blood, which is the numerator in formula 2, one needs to know the following:
1. How many cubic micrometers = 1 mm³ (See Appendix V)

$$1 \text{ mm} = 1{,}000 \ \mu\text{m}$$

$$1 \text{ mm} \times 1 \text{ mm} \quad \times 1 \text{ mm} \quad = 1 \text{ mm}^3$$
$$1{,}000 \ \mu\text{m} \times 1{,}000 \ \mu\text{m} \times 1{,}000 \ \mu\text{m} = 1{,}000{,}000{,}000 \ \mu\text{m}^3$$

$$1 \text{ mm}^3 = 10^9 \ \mu\text{m}^3$$

Hence, 1 mm³ of blood equals $10^9 \ \mu\text{m}^3$ of blood.

2. How much of the 10^9 μm^3 of blood is cells? The hematocrit determines what percentage of blood is erythrocytes; therefore multiply 10^9 μm^3 by the hematocrit to find out how much of the blood is erythrocytes.

$$10^9 \times 0.50$$

The cells/mm^3 of blood, which is the denominator in formula 2, has been given as 5,000,000 (5×10^6) cells/mm^3. Hence:

$$\text{MCV} = \frac{10^9 \times 0.50}{5 \times 10^6} \qquad \textbf{(Step 1)}$$

$$\text{MCV} = \frac{0.05 \times 10^9}{5 \times 10^6} \qquad \textbf{(Step 2)}$$

$$\text{MCV} = \frac{0.50 \times 10^{9-6}}{5} \qquad \textbf{(Step 3)}$$

$$\text{MCV} = \frac{0.50 \times 10^3}{5} \qquad \textbf{(Step 4)}$$

$$\text{MCV} = \frac{0.50 \times 1{,}000}{5} \qquad \textbf{(Step 5)}$$

$$\text{MCV} = \frac{500}{5} \qquad \textbf{(Step 6)}$$

$$\text{MCV} = 100 \ \mu m^3 \qquad \textbf{(Step 7)}$$

Look at step 6:

$$\text{MCV} = \frac{500}{5} = \frac{50 \ (\text{Hct}) \times 10}{5 \ (\text{RBC in millions})} = \frac{500}{5} = 100 \ \mu m^3$$

Steps 1 through 7 (and formula 2) are what the calculations for the mean corpuscular volume are actually based on, but since the numbers representing the hematocrit and RBC (in millions) give the same answer and are much easier to work with in daily calculations, formula 1 is the one usually given. However, one should know what it represents.

Mean Corpuscular Hemoglobin

The mean corpuscular hemoglobin is the *weight* of hemoglobin in the average erythrocyte. Normal values lie between 27 and 32 micromicrograms (written $\mu\mu g$ or pg [picograms]; *grams* because of *weight*). The following formula is used to calculate the mean corpuscular hemoglobin:

$$\text{MCH} = \frac{\text{Hb (in grams)} \times 10}{\text{RBC (in millions)}} \qquad \textbf{Formula 3}$$

Mean corpuscular hemoglobin is the weight of hemoglobin in the average red blood cell. If the number of picograms in 1 cubic millimeter of blood is known and that number is divided by the number of red cells in 1 cubic millimeter of blood, the number of picograms of hemoglobin per erythrocyte will be known.

$$\text{MCH} = \frac{\text{pg hemoglobin/mm}^3 \text{ of blood}}{\text{cells/mm}^3} \qquad \textbf{Formula 4}$$

To find pg hemoglobin/mm^3 of blood, which is the numerator in formula 4, convert the patient's hemoglobin value per 100 milliliter of blood (in grams%) to picograms of hemoglobin per cubic millimeter of blood.

$$1 \text{ g} = 10^{12} \text{ pg}$$
$$1 \text{ ml} = 1 \text{ cm}^3$$
$$1 \text{ cm} \times 1 \text{ cm} \times 1 \text{ cm} = 1 \text{ cm}^3$$
$$10 \text{ mm} \times 10 \text{ mm} \times 10 \text{ mm} = 1{,}000 \text{ mm}^3$$

Hence, 1 ml = 1,000 mm^3.

For example, 15 g/100 ml converted to picograms per cubic millimeter would be:

$$\frac{\text{g} \times 10^{12}}{\text{ml} \times 10^3} = \frac{15 \times 10^{12}}{100 \times 10^3} = 15 \times 10^7 \text{ pg Hb/mm}^3 \text{ of blood (the numerator)}$$

The cells/mm^3 of blood, the denominator in formula 4, has been given as 5,000,000 (5×10^6) cells/mm^3; hence:

$$\text{MCH} = \frac{15 \times 10^7}{5 \times 10^6} \qquad \textbf{(Step 1)}$$

$$\text{MCH} = \frac{15 \times 10^{7-6}}{5} \qquad \textbf{(Step 2)}$$

$$\text{MCH} = \frac{15 \times 10}{5} \qquad \textbf{(Step 3)}$$

$$\text{MCH} = \frac{150}{5} \qquad \textbf{(Step 4)}$$

$$\text{MCH} = 30 \text{ pg Hb/erythrocyte} \qquad \textbf{(Step 5)}$$

Notice step 3:

$$\text{MCH} = \frac{15 \times 10}{5} = \frac{15 \text{ (Hb in grams)} \times 10}{5 \text{ (RBC in millions)}} = \frac{15 \times 10}{5} = 30 \text{ pg Hb/erythrocyte}$$

Again, formula 3 is usually given because it is simple and because the numbers give the correct answer.

Mean Corpuscular Hemoglobin Concentration

The mean[*] corpuscular hemoglobin concentration is the *percentage* of hemoglobin in the patient's packed cell volume. Normal values range from 33% to 38%. The following is the

---

[*]Using the term *mean* in the name is not mathematically correct. Whenever the word *average* or *mean* is used in connection with a mathematical formula, it indicates that the number of particles used to arrive at the average must be included in the denominator. In the formula for the MCHC this does not occur. The formula, in reality, finds the number of grams of hemoglobin per milliliter of packed cells and then multiplies this by 100 to arrive at a *percent.*

formula for the mean corpuscular hemoglobin concentration:

$$\text{MCHC} = \frac{\text{Hb (in grams)} \times 100}{\text{Hct}} \qquad \textbf{Formula 5}$$

The mean corpuscular hemoglobin concentration is the *percentage* of hemoglobin in the packed cell volume. If the number of grams of hemoglobin in 100 milliliters of blood is divided by the number of milliliters of packed cells in 100 milliliters of blood and then this number multiplied by 100, the result would be the percentage of hemoglobin in the packed cell volume.

$$\text{MCHC} = \frac{\text{grams of Hb in 100 ml blood}}{\text{milliliters of packed cells in 100 ml blood}} \times 100 \qquad \textbf{Formula 6}$$

The numerator in formula 6 is the number of grams of hemoglobin per 100 milliliters of blood (g%).

To find the milliliters of packed cells in 100 milliliters of blood, the denominator in formula 6, take the amount of blood (100 ml) and multiply it by the percentage of packed cells (in this case 50%).

$$100 \times 0.50 = 50 \text{ ml packed cells}$$

To work the formula, fill in the preceding information.

$$\text{MCHC} = \frac{15 \times 100}{50} \qquad \textbf{(Step 1)}$$

$$\text{MCHC} = \frac{1,500}{50} \qquad \textbf{(Step 2)}$$

$$\text{MCHC} = 30\% \qquad \textbf{(Step 3)}$$

Look at step 1:

$$\text{MCHC} = \frac{15 \times 100}{50} = \frac{15 \text{ (Hb in grams)} \times 100}{50 \text{ (Hct)}} = \frac{15 \times 100}{50} = 30\%$$

Examine the short formulas 1, 3, and 5, and be sure it is understood why they may be used and exactly what they represent.

Calculating Indices Using Ratios

Since the mean corpuscular hemoglobin concentration (MCHC) is the ratio of the mass of the mean corpuscular hemoglobin (MCH) to the mean corpuscular volume (MCV) expressed as a percentage, any one of these values can be calculated from the other two. The following are the formulas for these calculations:

$$\text{MCHC} = \frac{\text{MCH}}{\text{MCV}} \times 100$$

$$\text{MCH} = 0.01 \text{ MCHC} \times \text{MCV}$$

$$\text{MCV} = \frac{\text{MCH}}{0.01 \text{ MCHC}}$$

SECTION 11.4 HEMOGLOBIN CURVE USING THE CYANMETHEMOGLOBIN METHOD (Aqueous Standard)

The following is a basic formula that may be used to establish a hemoglobin curve:

$$\frac{\text{Concentration of standard} \times \text{dilution factor}}{1,000} = \text{g\%}$$

The concentration of the standard is the assay on the bottle. For example, it may state 80 mg/dl on the label; this is the assay or concentration in the bottle.

The dilution factor is for the blood dilution made in that particular procedure. For example, if 0.02 milliliter blood is added to 5.0 milliliter diluent, the blood dilution is 0.02/5.02, or

$$\frac{0.02}{5.02} = \frac{1}{x}$$

$$0.02x = 5.02$$

$$x = 251$$

1/251 dilution

Dilution factor = 251

As was true in Chapter 10, the concentration of the standard for any procedure depends on the amount of blood giving the same intensity of color. The assay on the bottle (in this case 80 mg/dl) means that that intensity of color was produced by 80 milligrams per deciliter of hemoglobin; that is, there are 80 milligrams of hemoglobin in 100 milliliters of solution. If the test sample gives the same intensity of color, then in that test sample there are 80 milligrams per deciliter of hemoglobin. But if the sample had been diluted 1/251, then whole blood would contain 251 times as much hemoglobin. Therefore multiply the assay times the blood dilution to get the amount of hemoglobin in whole (undiluted) blood.

$$80 \times 251 = 20{,}080 \text{ mg/dl}$$

However, hemoglobin values are reported in g% *(not mg/dl)*. Mg/dl may be converted to g% by dividing by 1,000.

$$\frac{80 \times 251}{1,000} = 20.08 \text{ g\%}$$

The value for this standard in *this* procedure is 20.08 g%. This is the highest value for the standard. To set up a curve, make dilutions of the standard and calculate the corresponding values. Study the following examples.

	Amount* of diluent (ml)	Amount of standard (ml)	Value of standard (g%)
Example 1			
Pure standard	0	5	20
First dilution	1	4	16
Second dilution	2	3	12
Third dilution	3	2	8
Fourth dilution	4	1	4
Pure diluent	5	0	0
Example 2			
Pure standard	0	8	20
First dilution	2	6	15
Second dilution	4	4	10
Third dilution	6	2	5
Pure diluent	8	0	0

*The actual amount is not important as long as the minimum quantity demanded by the instrument is available. It is the way the standard is diluted that is important. The correct value must be calculated.

The values for the diluted standards may be calculated two ways: (1) as a dilution problem, and (2) as a ratio-proportion problem. Look at the first dilution in example 1 and consider the following two solutions:

1. As a dilution problem:

$$20 \text{ g\%} \times \frac{4}{5} \text{ (4 ml std + 1 ml diluent = 5 ml total volume)} = 16 \text{ g\%}$$

2. As a ratio-proportion problem: if there are 20 g% in 5 ml, there will be x g% in 4 ml.

$$\frac{20}{5} = \frac{x}{4}$$

$$5x = 80$$

$$x = 16 \text{ g\%}$$

Try to determine the concentration for the first dilution in example 2.

These samples are read in the instrument, and the readings and corresponding values are plotted on the appropriate graph paper.

APPENDIXES RELATED TO THIS CHAPTER

Q Formulas Presented in this Book
T Conversions Among Metric Prefixes
U Conversions Among Square Metric Units
V Conversions Among Cubic Metric Units
X Conversions Between Liter Units and Cubic Metric Units

PRACTICE PROBLEMS

Calculate the answer for each problem. Understand each portion of the calculation and determine whether the answer is logical. *Just because an answer can be calculated does not mean that it is reasonable.*

Pipette dilutions

1. In a WBC pipette, blood is drawn to the 0.5 mark and diluted to the 11 mark. What is the dilution?
2. In a WBC pipette, blood is drawn to the 0.6 mark and diluted to the 11 mark. What is the dilution?
3. In an RBC pipette, blood is drawn to the 0.8 mark and diluted to the 101 mark. What is the dilution?
4. If blood is drawn to the 0.3 mark in a WBC pipette and diluted to the 11 mark, what is the dilution?
5. If blood is drawn to the 1 mark in an RBC pipette and diluted to the 101 mark, what is the dilution?
6. In an RBC pipette, blood is drawn to the 0.7 mark and diluted to the 101 mark. What is the dilution?
7. The amount of blood used for a routine manual blood count is:
   - a. 0.5 vol
   - b. 0.5 mm^3
   - c. 0.5 vol%
   - d. 0.5 cm^3
8. If blood is drawn to the 0.9 mark in an RBC pipette and diluted to the 101 mark, what is the dilution?

Counting chamber

(assume a standard Neubauer Counting Chamber unless stated otherwise)

9. The usual volume for a manual white cell count is:
   - a. 1.6 mm^3
   - b. 4 mm^3
   - c. 0.5 mm^3
   - d. 0.4 mm^3
10. Blood is drawn to the 1.0 mark in an RBC pipette and diluted to the 101 mark with 2% acetic acid, and the total number of cells is counted in the four large corner squares of the hemocytometer. The total is 200 cells counted. What is the total count per cubic millimeter?
    - a. 2,200 white cells
    - b. 22,500 white cells
    - c. 50,000 white cells
    - c. 5.5 million red cells
    - e. 2.2 million red cells
11. Situation: A spinal fluid is drawn up in a WBC pipette to the 1.0 mark and diluted to the 11 mark. The total number of red cells counted in the four large corner squares is 472. The red cell count should be reported as:
    - a. 10,620/mm^3
    - b. 11,800/mm^3
    - c. 15,410/mm^3
    - d. 4,720/mm^3
12. In a WBC pipette, blood is drawn to the 0.2 mark and diluted to the 11 mark. Ten red squares are counted, and 50 cells are seen. Give the number of cells per cubic millimeter.
13. Give the report for a spinal fluid count in which 11 cells are counted on both sides of the counting chamber (assume 9 mm^2 per side) when the spinal fluid is drawn to the 1 mark in a WBC pipette and counted in a chamber with a depth of 0.2 mm.
14. One square millimeter of the counting chamber with Neubauer ruling represents a volume of:
    - a. 1 mm^3
    - b. 0.1 mm^3
    - c. 0.1 mm^3

15. A convenient procedure in performing an erythrocyte count with a dilution of $1:200$ is to count 80 of the smallest red squares (on a counting chamber with Neubauer ruling), which is a volume of _____.

16. The RBC pipette is filled to the 0.6 mark with blood, and in 10 regular red squares 205 cells are counted. What is the count?

17. The WBC pipette is filled to the 0.5 mark with blood, and in seven white squares 106 cells are counted. What is the count?

18. The routine depth of the counting chamber is:
   a. 1 mm^3
   b. 0.1 mm
   c. 1 mm
   d. 0.1 mm^3

19. Look at the counting chamber below and give the following:
   a. Length of: b. Area of:
       A   F
       B   G
       C   H
       D   I
       E

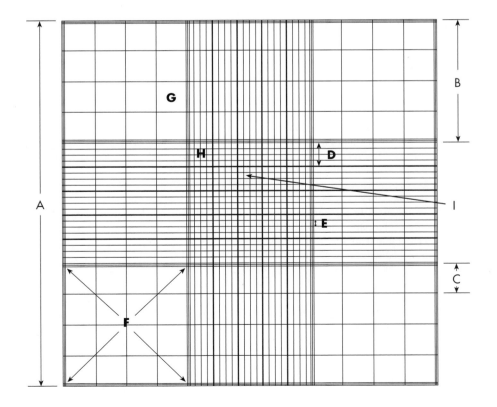

Factors

20. If blood is drawn to the 0.2 mark in a WBC pipette and diluted to the 11 mark, what is the dilution? What is the dilution factor?

21. Blood is drawn to the 0.4 mark in a WBC pipette. Ten white squares are counted. Give the following:
    - a. Dilution factor
    - b. Depth factor
    - c. Area factor
    - d. Volume correction factor
    - e. Final factor

22. Blood is drawn to the 0.3 mark in a WBC pipette. Six white squares are counted. One hundred cells are counted. Give the following:
    - a. Dilution
    - b. Dilution factor
    - c. Depth factor
    - d. Area factor
    - e. Area counted
    - f. Volume counted
    - g. Volume factor
    - h. Final factor
    - i. Number of cells/mm^3

23. In a certain platelet count procedure you draw up the blood to the 0.5 mark in an RBC pipette and count all nine squares on both sides of the counting chamber. Give the following:
    - a. Dilution factor
    - b. Area factor
    - c. Final factor
    - d. If 102 platelets were counted on both sides of the chamber, what would be the platelet count?

24. In a certain platelet count procedure you draw up the blood to the 1 mark in an RBC pipette and count all nine squares on both sides of the counting chamber. Give the following:
    - a. Dilution factor
    - b. Area factor
    - c. Final factor
    - d. If 50 platelets were counted on both sides on the chamber in the above, what would be the platelet count per cubic millimeter?

25. You have obtained a WBC count of 40,000. On doing the differential you find 125 NRBC/100 WBC. Give the following:
    - a. Corrected WBC count
    - b. Number of NRBC/mm^3

26. Blood is drawn to the 0.8 mark in an RBC pipette. Nine white squares are counted on each side of the counting chamber. One hundred cells are seen. Give the following:
    - a. Final factor
    - b. Number of cells/mm^3

27. A total WBC count of 30,000 was obtained. If 20 NRBC/100 WBC were found on the differential, what would you report as the actual WBC count?

28. Blood is drawn to the 0.3 mark in a WBC pipette. Ten white squares are counted. Give the following:
    - a. Dilution factor
    - b. Depth factor
    - c. Area factor
    - d. Volume correction factor
    - e. Final factor

29. You have obtained a WBC count of 95,000. On doing the differential you find 135 NRBC/100 WBC. Give the following:
    - a. Corrected WBC count
    - b. Number of NRBC/mm^3

30. In an RBC pipette, blood is drawn up to the 0.4 mark, 10 red squares are counted, the chamber depth is 0.2 mm, and 100 cells are found (assume Neubauer ruling with a depth of 0.2 mm). Give the following:
    a. Depth factor
    b. Area factor
    c. Volume factor
    d. Factor for multiplying number of cells counted to obtain number of cells/mm^3
    e. Cells/mm^3
    f. Cells/ml

31. White count = 65,000; differential = 57 NRBC/100 WBC; give the corrected WBC count.

32. If blood is drawn to the 0.4 mark in a WBC pipette, what is the dilution? What is the dilution factor?

33. If blood is drawn to the 0.3 mark in an RBC pipette, what is the dilution? What is the dilution factor?

34. Blood is drawn to the 0.2 mark in an RBC pipette. Four white squares are counted. Three hundred cells are found. Give the following:
    a. Depth factor
    b. Dilution factor
    c. Area factor (express two ways)
    d. Volume factor (express two ways)

35. Blood is drawn to the 0.8 mark in a WBC pipette. Five red squares are counted. The depth of the counting chamber is 0.2 mm (assume Neubauer ruling with a depth of 0.2 mm). One hundred cells are found. Give the following:
    a. Depth factor
    b. Dilution
    c. Dilution factor
    d. Area factor (express two ways)
    e. Volume factor (express two ways)
    f. Final factor
    g. Number of cells/mm^3

36. In a certain platelet count procedure you draw the blood up to the 0.5 mark in an RBC pipette, count all nine squares on both sides of the counting chamber, and get the average number of cells for one side (total cells on both sides = 450). Give the following:
    a. Dilution factor
    b. Area factor
    c. Final factor
    d. Volume factor
    e. Number of cells/mm^3

37. Blood is drawn to the 0.6 mark in an RBC pipette. Two white squares are counted. One hundred cells are found. Give the following:
    a. Depth factor
    b. Dilution
    c. Dilution factor
    d. Area factor (express two ways)
    e. Volume factor (express two ways)
    f. Final factor
    g. Number of cells/mm^3

38. Blood is drawn to the 0.8 mark in a WBC pipette. Fifteen red squares are counted. The depth of the counting chamber is 0.2 mm. Fifty cells are found. Give the following:
    a. Depth factor
    b. Dilution
    c. Dilution factor
    d. Area factor (express two ways)
    e. Volume factor (express two ways)
    f. Final factor
    g. Number of cells/m^3

39. Blood is drawn to the 0.3 mark in a WBC pipette. Eighteen WBC squares are counted. Fifty cells are found. Give the following:
    a. Dilution
    b. Dilution factor
    c. Depth factor
    d. Area counted
    e. Area factor
    f. Volume counted
    g. Volume factor
    h. Final factor
    i. Number of cells/mm^3
    j. Express i in SI units

40. In a certain platelet count procedure you draw the blood to the 1 mark in an RBC pipette, count 5 white squares on both sides of the chamber, and get the average. Give the following:
    a. Dilution factor
    b. Area factor
    c. Final factor
    d. If 68 platelets were counted on both sides of the chamber in the above procedure, what would be the reported platelet count?

41. You have obtained a WBC count of 10,000. On doing the differential you find 3 NRBC/100 WBC. Give the following:
    a. Corrected WBC count
    b. Number of NRBC/mm^3

42. A total leukocyte count is 35,000/mm^3, and the differential count on this same patient shows 110 nucleated erythrocytes/100 leukocytes. Give the following:
    a. Corrected WBC count
    b. Number of NRBC/mm^3

43. For each of the following give: (1) dilution, (2) dilution factor, (3) depth factor, (4) area counted, (5) area factor, (6) volume counted, (7) volume factor, (8) final factor, and (9) number of cells/μl.
    a. WBC pipette, chamber depth 0.1 mm.
       1. Blood to 0.2; six red squares counted; 130 cells found
       2. Blood to 0.5; eight red squares counted; 162 cells found
       3. Blood to 0.6; 18 white squares counted; 820 cells found
       4. Blood to 0.7; 10 white squares counted; 264 cells found
       5. Blood to 0.8; 10 red squares counted; 373 cells found
    b. RBC pipette, chamber depth 0.1 mm.
       1. Blood to 0.3; four white squares counted; 206 cells found
       2. Blood to 0.4; 20 red squares counted; 179 cells found
       3. Blood to 0.6; 10 red squares counted; 410 cells found
       4. Blood to 0.7; three red squares counted; 371 cells found
       5. Blood to 1.0; two white squares counted; 50 cells found
    c. Repeat *a* using chamber depth of 0.2 mm. (assume Neubauer ruling)
    d. Repeat *b* using chamber depth of 0.2 mm. (assume Neubauer ruling)

44. A patient has a WBC count of 7,500/μl, and the differential shows 20% small lymphocytes. The absolute lymphocyte count is:
    a. 7,500/μl   c. 1,500/μl
    b. 20%   d. 1,500%

45. In performing a white blood count, blood is brought up to the 0.2 mark, and diluting fluid is brought up to the 11 mark in a WBC pipette. The usual squares are counted and the total number of white blood cells counted is 250. What is the count per cubic millimeter?
    a. 6,000   c. 27,500
    b. 15,000   d. 31,250

46. In examining a stained blood smear, 15 NRBC are counted as the technician counts the 100 white cells for the differential. The total white count for the patient is 24,000/μl. What is the corrected WBC?

47. If a patient has a white cell count of 10,000 and a differential showing 30% monocytes and 70% lymphocytes, his absolute monocyte count would be:
    a. 7,000/μl   d. 3.5
    b. 10,000/μl   e. Could not calculate from above data
    c. 3,000/μl

Indices

48. Given: RBC = 4,500,000; Hb = 14 g; Hct = 41%. Calculate the following:
    a. MCV
    b. MCH
    c. MCHC
49. Given: RBC = 4,900,000; Hb = 15.0 g; Hct = 47%. Give the following:
    a. MCV
    b. MCH
    c. MCHC
50. Given: RBC = 5,100,000; Hb = 15.5 g; Hct = 45%. Give the following:
    a. MCV
    b. MCH
    c. MCHC
51. Calculate the indices for the following (RBC is in millions, for example, 4.9 *million*).
    a. RBC = 4.9   d. RBC = 5.3
       Hb   = 11.2 g   Hb   = 13.5 g
       Hct = 37%   Hct = 44%
    b. RBC = 3.6   e. RBC = 1.2
       Hb   = 12.5 g   Hb   = 3 g
       Hct = 36%   Hct = 9%
    c. RBC = 5.7   f. RBC = 3.10
       Hb   = 16.7 g   Hg   = 13.1 g
       Hct = 46%   Hct = 31%
52. Calculate the indices for the following (RBC in millions, for example, 5.2 *million*).
    a. RBC = 5.2   d. RBC = 4.5
       Hb   = 15.1 g   Hb   = 10.4 g
       Hct = 45%   Hct = 31%
    b. RBC = 2.7   e. RBC = 2.4
       Hb   = 4.3 g   Hb   = 8.1 g
       Hct = 28%   Hct = 26%
    c. RBC = 4.3   f. RBC = 2.1
       Hb   = 11.6 g   Hb   = 4.8 g
       Hct = 41%   Hct = 24%
53. Calculate problem 52 using ratios.

Hemoglobin curve

54. In a given hemoglobin procedure 0.05 ml blood is diluted with 6 ml diluent. The standard used for the curve is assayed at 85 mg/dl.
    a. What would be the highest value for this standard in this procedure?
    b. Set up a curve using at least four points.
55. In a given hemoglobin procedure 0.05 ml blood is diluted with 5 ml diluent. The standard used for the curve is assayed at 85 mg/dl.
    a. What would be the highest value for this standard in this procedure?
    b. Explain exactly how a curve would be set up for this procedure using this standard. Show all work.
56. In a given hemoglobin procedure 0.05 ml blood is diluted with 6 ml diluent. The standard used for the curve is assayed at 80 mg/dl.
    a. What would be the highest value for this standard in this procedure?
    b. Explain exactly how you would set up a curve for this procedure using this standard.

57. In a given hemoglobin procedure 0.05 ml blood is diluted with 9.5 ml diluent. The standard used for the curve is assayed at 85 mg/dl.
    a. What would be the highest value for this standard in this procedure?
    b. Set up a curve using at least four points.
    c. If a hemoglobin test sample read $40\%T$ from your curve and the $10.8g\%$ standard read $29\%T$, what would be the value reported (assume Beer's law is followed)?

12

Enzyme Calculations

◼ EDUCATIONAL OBJECTIVES

To have successfully learned the material in this chapter, the student should be able to do the following properly:

- ◆ Describe the relationship between enzyme activity and the change in the absorbance of a reacting solution.
- ◆ Calculate the international units (*IU*) of an enzyme from a change in absorbance of a substrate during an enzyme reaction.
- ◆ Convert King-Armstrong acid phosphatase units to international units per liter.
- ◆ Calculate enzyme units using the molar extinction coefficient of a reaction product.

SECTION 12.1 INTRODUCTION

This chapter is concerned mainly with the mathematical calculations necessary to determine enzyme activity in international units and the conversion of conventional units to the newer, more consistent international units.

An enzyme reaction is a complex biochemical process in which an enzyme present in the biological sample combines with a substrate to form an enzyme-substrate complex. The complex then separates into a reaction product, or products, releasing the enzyme. The released enzyme molecule can usually repeat the reaction. Because an enzyme can enter into a reaction and remain unchanged, it is referred to as a catalyst:

$$S + E \rightleftarrows ES \rightleftarrows P + E$$

where *S* is the substrate; *E* is the enzyme; *P* is the product; and *ES* is the enzyme-substrate complex.

Enzyme activity is usually determined either by the kinetic method or the endpoint method. In the **kinetic method** the rate of the enzyme-catalyzed reaction is measured while the reaction is in progress. In the **endpoint method** a product or residual reactant is color complexed with a suitable reagent after the completion of the enzyme-catalyzed reaction. The absorbance of the complex is then measured.

SECTION 12.2 KINETIC METHOD

The reaction rate is proportional to time and enzyme concentration. The concentration of the substrate must be relatively large in comparison to the quantity of enzyme present, so the reaction time will be independent of substrate concentration. The enzyme concentration and the time interval of the reaction determine the quantity of substrate consumed or the amount of product formed:

$$Q = E \times t$$

where Q is the quantity of product formed; E is the enzyme concentration; and t is the time interval of the reaction.

If the quantity of enzyme is doubled, the rate of the reaction will be doubled. The quantity of product formed in a fixed interval of time will then be doubled.

$$Q = (t) \times E$$
$$Q = 2 \times 4$$
$$Q = 8$$

If E is doubled:

$$Q = 2 \times 8$$
$$Q = 16$$

Likewise, if the concentration of enzyme is kept constant and the reaction period is doubled, the amount of product formed will be doubled.

$$Q = (E) \times t$$
$$Q = 4 \times 2$$
$$Q = 8$$

If t is doubled:

$$Q = 4 \times 4$$
$$Q = 16$$

As can be seen from the preceding equations, the quantity of product formed or substrate consumed is a straight line function of either enzyme concentration or time, providing the other is kept constant. If $Q = E \times t$, then $Q/t = E$, where Q/t is the rate of product formed.

Hence, the *rate* of product formation or substrate utilization may be used as a means of determining the enzyme concentration. This can be done conveniently and efficiently by spectrophotometry if one of the reactants or products is a chromogen, that is, a light-absorbing substance. The change in absorbance of the reacting solution over a period of time can be measured ($\Delta A/\Delta t$). With proper concentration of initial substrate, the absorbance change (increase in product or decrease in substrate) is *directly proportional* to the activity of the enzyme. If the activity of the enzyme is doubled, the rate will also be doubled. Therefore the following is true:

$$\text{Enzyme activity} = K \frac{\Delta A}{\Delta t}$$

The constant, K, is a function of temperature, pH, sample volume, and substrate concentration.

SECTION 12.3 INTERNATIONAL UNIT

As the field of enzymology progressed and new enzymes were discovered and analyzed, their activity was expressed in various units. In some cases, different units were used to express the activity of the same enzyme. In 1961 the International Union of Biochemistry, through its Commission on Enzymes, recommended a standard unit known as the **international unit,** which was defined as follows: One unit (U) of any enzyme is that which will catalyze the transformation of 1 micromole of the substrate per minute under standard conditions. Concentration is to be expressed in terms of units per milliliter (U/ml) of serum, or milliunits per milliliter (mU/ml, which is the same as units per liter [U/L]), whichever gives the more convenient numerical value.

$$\text{International units} = \mu\text{mol/min/ml of serum}$$

Whereas the 1961 report of the International Union of Biochemistry recommended 25°C for the temperature of the determination, the 1964 commission suggested a change to 30°C.

A widely used method for kinetic enzyme determinations is the *optical test* method introduced by Otto Warburg in 1936. This method is based on the fact that reduced nicotinamide-adenine dinucleotide (NADH) absorbs light with an absorption maximum at 340 nanometers, whereas the oxidized form (NAD) shows no absorption between 300 and 400 nanometers. Reactions based on these compounds can involve either oxidation of NADH to NAD or the reduction of NAD to NADH. In the first case the absorbance at 340 nanometers decreases during the reaction; in the second case, it increases.

The following explanation of the derivation or source of the basic formula for calculating international units may seem confusing at first. Read through all the explanation before giving up. Do *not* try to understand each sentence by itself.

The molar absorptivity of NADH at 340 nm is 6.22×10^3. This means that a solution containing 1 mol NADH/L has an absorbance of 6.22×10^3 A in a cell of 1-cm path length. Therefore a change in concentration of 1 mol/L/min would produce a change in absorbance of 6.22×10^3 A/min. Translation of this relationship to conditions encountered experimentally is summarized as follows:

Absorbance change per minute	Change in concentration per minute
6.22×10^3	1 mol/L
6.22×10^{-3}	1 μmol/L
6.22	1 μmol/ml
$6.22/V_t$	1 μmol in V_t ml

where V_t is the total volume of substrate and sample. Therefore if:

$$\frac{6.22}{V_t} \Delta A = 1 \ \mu\text{mol/min change in substrate}$$

Then:

$$1 \ \Delta A = \frac{V_t}{6.22} \ \mu\text{mol/min change in substrate}$$

If a change of ΔA/min is observed with a sample of serum volume, V_s, then:

$$\Delta A/\text{min}/V_s \text{ ml} = \Delta A/\text{min} \times \frac{V_t}{6.22} \, \mu\text{mol/min}/V_s \text{ of serum}$$

$$= \Delta A/\text{min} \times \frac{V_t}{6.22 \times V_s} \, \mu\text{mol/min/ml of serum}$$

To convert to 1 L:

$$\Delta A/\text{min}/V_s \text{ ml} = \Delta A/\text{min} \times \frac{V_t \times 1{,}000}{6.22 \times V_s} \, \mu\text{mol/min/L of serum} = \text{IU/L}$$

This is the basic equation for the conversion of absorbance data to international units (IU) in procedures using NADH or NAD. This equation must be further modified to include additional factors if the following are true:

1. The activity is determined at one temperature but reported at another.
2. The molar absorptivity is affected by instrument characteristics. It might be helpful to think about the preceding equation in another way.

$$6.22 \, A = 1 \, \mu\text{mol/min/ml of substrate}$$

If the volume of the substrate, sample, and reagents (the total volume) is more or less than 1 milliliter, then it becomes necessary to divide by that amount to give the absorbance change per milliliter. Therefore:

$$\frac{6.22}{V_t} A = 1 \, \mu\text{mol/min/ml}$$

Where V_t is total volume. Then:

$$1 \, \Delta A = \frac{V_t}{6.22} \, \mu\text{mol/min/ml}$$

or:

$$\Delta A \times \frac{V_t}{6.22} = \mu\text{mol/min/ml}$$

If the change in absorbance is brought about by 1 milliliter of serum, 1 milliliter of serum contains that number of μmol/min/ml of serum. If other than 1 milliliter of serum is used in the test, it must be taken into consideration by inserting the correction factor $1/V_s$; where V_s is the volume of sample used.

$$\Delta A/\text{min} \times \frac{V_t}{6.22} \times \frac{1}{V_s} = \mu\text{mol/min/ml of serum}$$

Therefore:

$$\frac{\Delta A \times V_t}{6.22 \times V_s} = \mu\text{mol/min/ml serum} = \text{IU/ml}$$

To convert this to micromoles per minute per liter of serum, it is necessary to multiply by 1,000. Finally,

$$\frac{\Delta A \times V_t \times 1{,}000}{6.22 \times V_s} = \mu\text{mol/min/L} = \text{IU/L}$$

The preceding formula assumes a reaction time of 1 minute. If the reaction time is other than 1 minute, the factor, $1/T$, must be added to the formula.

$$\frac{\Delta A/\text{min} \times V_t}{6.22 \times V_s} \times 1{,}000 \times \frac{1}{T} = \text{IU/L}$$

Although a wavelength setting of 340 nanometers is generally used to measure enzyme activity when NADH or NAD is used as substrate, 334 nanometers or 366 nanometers can be used if appropriate correction factors are applied. For example, 366 nanometers is recommended when a turbid serum sample or control used with a high-absorbance substrate causes the initial absorbance at 340 nanometers to exceed the absorbance specification of the spectrophotometer. The analyst must recognize the following differences in molar absorptivity at various wavelengths.

Wavelength	Molar absorptivity
334 nm	6.0×10^3
340 nm	6.22×10^3
366 nm	3.3×10^3

The basic formula for calculation of international units is based on a molar absorptivity for NADH of 6.22×10^3 at 340 nanometers. If a wavelength setting of 334 nanometers is used, the equation must be modified by replacing 6.22 with 6.0; if 366 nanometers is used, 6.22 is replaced by 3.3.

SECTION 12.4 CONVERSION OF CONVENTIONAL UNITS TO INTERNATIONAL UNITS
Non-NADH Methods

To convert conventional units from tests using other than NADH methods to international units, factors for each of the parts involved in the calculations must be used. These parts of the calculations are the mass of the substrate or product, the time over which the reaction is based, and the volume of the sample solution. Normally corrections for temperature and pH are unnecessary.

Remember that 1 international unit is defined as that amount of enzyme necessary to bring about the reaction of 1 micromole of substrate in 1 minute. These units are reported as international units per milliliter or units per liter, whichever results in the most convenient number. Other systems often use different quantities of mass, time, and volume as a base for their units. Hence, in the conversion of conventional units to international units, the mass of the substrate must be converted to micromoles, the reaction time must be converted to 1 minute, and the amount of the sample solution must be converted to either milliliters or liters.

EXAMPLE 12-1: How would King-Armstrong (KA) acid phosphatase units be converted to international units per liter?

One KA unit is the amount of phosphatase enzyme per 100 ml of serum that will split 1 mg of phenol from phenolphosphate in 60 minutes.

1 KA unit = 1 mg phenol/60 min/100 ml serum

1 IU/L = 1 μmol/min/L serum

To convert King-Armstrong units to international units, make the following calculations:
1. Convert milligrams to micrograms by multiplying by 1,000.
2. Convert micrograms to micromoles by dividing by the molecular weight of phenol (94).
3. Convert 60 minutes to 1 minute by dividing by 60.
4. Convert 100 milliliters of serum to 1 liter by multiplying by 10.

This results in the following equation:

$$1 \text{ KA unit} = \left(\frac{1,000}{94} \times \frac{1}{60} \times 10 \right) \text{ IU/L}$$

$$1 \text{ KA unit} = 1.77 \text{ IU/L}$$

NADH Methods

To convert units from a test using the NADH method, but reporting in other than international units, the same basic information is sought.

EXAMPLE 12-2: Convert Karmen transaminase units to international units per liter.

One Karmen transaminase unit is the amount of enzyme that will produce $\Delta 0.001$ *A* of NADH/min/ml of serum (in a total volume of 3 ml).

$$1 \text{ Karmen unit} = \Delta 0.001 \text{ } A/\text{min/ml serum}$$

$$\text{Wanted: } \mu\text{mol/min/L}$$

$$1 \text{ Karmen unit} = \frac{0.001 \times 3}{6.22} \times 1,000$$

$$1 \text{ Karmen unit} = 0.482 \text{ } \mu\text{mol/min/L} = 0.482 \text{ IU}$$

Notice that in either case the information desired is micromoles per minute per liter (or milliliter).

SECTION 12.5 COMPUTATION OF ENZYME UNITS

One of the basic formulas for calculating international units has been presented along with a method of converting some conventional units to international units.

The following presentation is a slightly rearranged, yet really more basic, computation of enzyme units (IU). Recall the information presented in Chapter 9 on molar absorptivity and the information presented in this chapter about international units. The following computations utilize the same information in a *slightly* different form. Why do the two different presentations give the same answer? Where do the differences lie?

Units of enzyme activity are computed with reference to a reaction product. The computation can be based on a *standard* by preparing a solution with an exactly known concentration of the reaction product. An aliquot of the standard solution is treated and measured together with the sample.

A standard is not required if the molar absorption coefficient, ϵ, of a reaction product is known at a given wavelength, for example, for NADH (and NADPH).

Calculation Based on a Standard

$$\frac{A \text{ of sample}}{A \text{ of standard}} \times 10^6 \times \text{standard} \times \frac{1}{T} \times \frac{V_t}{V_s} = \text{IU/L}$$

where *Standard* is the concentration of the standard (in moles per liter) in the assay volume; T is the reaction time in minutes; V_t is the total assay volume; V_s is the volume of sample; IU/L is μmoles per minute per liter; and 10^6 is the factor to convert moles per liter or millimoles per milliliter into micromoles per liter.

EXAMPLE 12-3: Calculate the value for alkaline phosphatase from the information given below.

$$p\text{-nitrophenylphosphate} \rightleftarrows p\text{-nitrophenol} + \text{phosphate}$$

The standard is *p*-nitrophenol; stock solution, 1×10^{-3} mol/L; concentration in the assay mixture, 9×10^{-6} mol/L; V_t, 555 μl; V_s, 5 μl (for example, serum); T, 30 min; A of sample, 0.080; and A of standard, 0.169.

$$\frac{0.080}{0.169} \times 10^6 \times (9 \times 10^{-6}) \times \frac{1}{30} \times \frac{555}{5} = 15.7 \text{ IU/L}$$

Calculation Based on the Molar Extinction Coefficient of a Reaction Product with the Absorbance

$$\frac{A \text{ of sample}}{\epsilon \times d} \times 10^6 \times \frac{1}{T} \times \frac{V_t}{V_s} = \text{IU/L}$$

where ϵ is the molar extinction coefficient and d is the diameter of the cuvette (light path) in centimeters. Using the preceding sample, $\epsilon_{400 \text{ nm}}$, *p*-nitrophenol $= 18.8 \times 10^3$, and $d = 1$.

$$\frac{0.080}{18.8 \times 10^3} \times 10^6 \times \frac{1}{30} \times \frac{555}{5} = 15.7 \text{ IU/L}$$

APPENDIXES RELATED TO THIS CHAPTER

M Conversion Factors for Converting Conventional Enzyme Units to International Units per Liter

Q Formulas Presented in this Book

PRACTICE PROBLEMS

Calcuate the answer for each problem. Understand each portion of the calculation and determine whether the answer is logical. *Just because an answer can be calculated does not mean that it is reasonable.*

Convert the following to international units per liter:

1. One King-Armstrong (KA) alkaline phosphatase unit is the amount of enzyme that will split 1 milligram of phenol from phenylphosphate in 30 minutes at 37°C and at a pH of 9.6. It is reported per 100 milliliters of serum. One KA unit/100 ml serum = 1 mg phenol/30 min/100 ml serum. One KA unit equals how many international units per liter?

2. One Shinowara-Jones-Reinhart (SJR) alkaline phosphatase unit is the amount of enzyme that will split 1 milligram phosphorus from β-glycerophosphate in 60 minutes at 37°C and at a pH of 9.8. It is reported per 100 milliliters of serum. One SJR unit/100 ml = 1 mg phosphorus/60 min/100 ml serum. One SJR unit/100 ml equals how many international units per liter?

3. A de la Huerga unit for serum cholinesterase is defined as the quantity of enzyme present in 1 milliliter of serum that will hydrolyze 1.0 micromole of acetylcholine in 60 minutes, under the

conditions of the assay. One de la Huerga unit $= 1$ μmol/60 min/ml. One de la Huerga unit equals how many international units per liter?

4. In a lactic dehydrogenase procedure, 1 spectrophotometric unit is defined as the amount of enzyme that will give a $\Delta 0.001$ A change/min/ml of serum (in a total volume of 3 ml). One spectrophotometric unit $= \Delta A$ of 0.001/min/ml (in a total volume of 3 ml). One spectrophotometric unit equals how many international units per liter?

13

Gastric Acidity

EDUCATIONAL OBJECTIVES

To have successfully learned the material in this chapter, the student should be able to do the following properly:

- Differentiate among combined acid, free acid, total acid, and titratable acidity.
- Calculate the degrees of acidity per 100 milliliters, milliequivalents per liter, and millimoles per liter from the titration of a small sample of gastric material.
- Explain the variation among the procedures used to calculate basal acid output (BAO), maximum acid output (MAO), and peak acid output (PAO).
- Calculate BAO, MAO, PAO, and BAO/MAO ratio from gastric samples.

Gastric acidity is the term used to refer to the acid content of the stomach. Most of this acidity is due to the presence of hydrochloric acid (HCl) secreted by the gastric mucosa. This HCl is necessary for the proper digestion of food. The clinical laboratory commonly makes two general kinds of determinations involving gastric acidity. These are the determination of the concentration of acid in the stomach contents and the rate of acid output by the mucosa.

SECTION 13.1 DETERMINATION OF ACID CONCENTRATION

The methods used to determine the concentration of acid in gastric material indicate two different concepts concerning the form of the acid in the stomach contents. The traditional concept of gastric acidity considers the acid to exist in two distinct components. One of these is called the **combined acid.** This is also called the nonionized acid. If the pH of the gastric material is greater than 3.5, the acid is considered to be present almost exclusively as a mixture of organic salts formed by the combination of the HCl with the proteins and peptones of the gastric material. The amount of this nonionized acid is thought to reflect the buffering capacity of the gastric proteins.

When enough acid is present to exceed the buffering capacity of the stomach, some HCl exists in the form of dissociated ions. This excess acid is called the **free acid.** Free acid is considered to be present in material having a pH of 3.0 or less.

Total acid is the term used to describe the amount of combined acid plus the free acid.

The tests for gastric acidity in this concept involve the use of two different pH indicators to differentiate the combined acid from the free acid. The free acid is determined by titration of a sample of gastric material with 0.1N NaOH to an endpoint of Töpfer's reagent. This indicates a pH of 2.8 to 3.5. Total acidity is determined with phenolphthalein as the indicator and titration with 0.1N NaOH to an endpoint of 8.2 to 10.0. The combined acid is the difference between the total acidity and the free acid.

There are two common procedures used to determine the gastric acidity using this concept. The first of these is called the one-dish method. As the name implies, the free, combined, and total acid values are found using only one dish. To begin the procedure, place an aliquot of gastric material in an evaporating dish. Add a drop of Töpfer's reagent and titrate to the endpoint with 0.1N NaOH. Note the number of milliliters of base required to reach the endpoint. This titration allows the calculation of the free acid.

Now add a drop of phenolphthalein to the sample and continue to titrate. There are two ways to continue the test, depending on how the base is handled. If the NaOH is contained in a relatively large pipette or buret, continue to titrate from the endpoint of Töpfer's reagent to the endpoint of phenolphthalein. Record the total quantity of NaOH used. This is the number of milliliters of 0.1N NaOH required for the total acid titration. To find the combined acid value, subtract the number of milliliters of NaOH required for the free acid titration from the number required for the total acid titration.

If a small pipette is used, refill it with base when the phenolphthalein is added to the test material, and titrate to an endpoint. This titration will produce the value for the combined acid. Add these two titrations to get the number of milliliters of NaOH required for the total acid.

The second method is called the two-dish method and makes use of two evaporating dishes, one to titrate the free acid and the other to titrate the total acid. To begin this procedure place an aliquot of gastric contents into each dish. Add a drop of Töpfer's reagent to the first dish and titrate with 0.1N NaOH. The number of milliliters of NaOH required to reach the endpoint is used to calculate the value for the free acid.

Add a drop of phenolphthalein to the gastric material in the second dish. Titrate with 0.1N NaOH to the endpoint and record the amount of base used. This amount is used to calculate the value for total acid. The combined acid is found by subtraction of the value for free acid from the value for total acid.

Remember that the free acid produces the pH values of less than 3.5; the combined acid produces the pH from 3.5 to approximately 8.2; and the total acid is responsible for pH values from 0 to approximately 8.2

In recent years, several studies have indicated that the concept of free and combined acid is not entirely correct. Because of this it has been suggested that these terms be abandoned and the term **titratable acidity** be used for all gastric acidity. Common procedures for the determination of titratable acidity involve the titration of a sample of gastric material with 0.1N NaOH to a pH of 7.0 using a pH meter. If a meter is not available, use phenol red as the indicator (pH 7.0 to 7.4).

SECTION 13.2 CALCULATIONS FOR GASTRIC ACIDITY

Regardless of which concept is used in the test procedures, the calculations of the concentration of HCl from the titration results are the same.

Units of Gastric Acidity

Three units are used for reporting the concentration of gastric acidity. The oldest of these is degrees of acidity per 100 milliliters of gastric material (written with a degree sign, °, and also called clinical units). The newer units are milliequivalents of acid per liter (mEq/L) and millimoles of acid per liter (mmol/L). When used for gastric acidity, all three units result in the same numerical value for the acidity of a given sample.

DEGREES OF ACIDITY PER 100 ML. The degrees of acidity equals the number of milliliters of 0.1N NaOH necessary to titrate 100 milliliters of gastric material to the endpoint. If a gastric sample of 100 milliliters is used for the test, there is no need for any calculation. Simply report the number of milliliters of NaOH used for the titration. However, since most gastric samples have less than 100 milliliters, calculation is usually necessary. This calculation is a simple ratio and proportion.

EXAMPLE 13-1: Five milliliters of gastric material is available for determination of free acid; 1.2 ml of 0.1N NaOH is required for the titration. What is the number of degrees of acidity of the sample?

Set up a ratio and proportion. If it takes 1.2 ml NaOH to titrate 5 ml of gastric contents, it will take x ml to titrate 100 ml.

$$\frac{1.2}{5} = \frac{x}{100}$$

$$5x = 1.2 \times 100$$

$$5x = 120$$

$$x = 24$$

It would take 24 ml of 0.1N NaOH for 100 ml of gastric material. Hence, the free acid equals 24° of acidity, or 24 clinical units.

The answer may also be calculated using a factor. If 5 milliliters of gastric material were used instead of 100 milliliters, that is $5/100$ or $1/20$ of the amount required. The factor to correct for this would be 20. **RECALL:** Divide by what is used and multiply by what should have been used. Hence, multiply the number of milliliters of 0.1N NaOH by the factor 20.

$$1.2 \times 20 = 24° \text{ free HCl}$$

EXAMPLE 13-2: A gastric sample contains 2 ml. The Töpfer's endpoint required 0.8 ml 0.1N NaOH, and the combined acid titration required 0.5 ml NaOH. Give degrees free acid, degrees combined acid, and degrees total acid.

The factor for 2 ml of gastric material would be  $\frac{100}{2}$ or 50.

$$\text{Free acid} = 0.8 \times 50 = 40° \text{ free acid}$$

$$\text{Combined acid} = 0.5 \times 50 = 25° \text{ combined acid}$$

$$\text{Total acid} = 1.3 \times 50 = 65° \text{ total acid}$$

MILLIEQUIVALENTS PER LITER. The normality of a solution is defined as the number of equivalents per liter. Hence, this unit of gastric acidity is a statement of one thousandth of the normality of the gastric sample.

EXAMPLE 13-3: A gastric sample contains 20 ml. Titration with phenol red required 3.2 ml of 0.1N NaOH. Find the titratable acidity in milliequivalents per liter.

Determine the normality of this sample using $V_1 \times C_1 = V_2 \times C_2$.

$$V_1 \times C_1 = V_2 \times C_2$$

$$3.2 \text{ ml} \times 0.1\text{N} = 20 \text{ ml} \times x$$

$$20x = 3.2 \times 0.1$$

$$20x = 0.32$$

$$x = 0.016\text{N}$$

The sample is 0.016N. In other words, the sample contains 0.016 eq of acid/L. Since 1 eq/L equals 1,000 mEq/L, there are 16 mEq/L in the sample ($0.016 \times 1,000 = 16$).

MILLIMOLES PER LITER. The recommended SI unit of gastric acidity is millimoles of acid per liter of gastric material. This is determined by multiplying the molarity of the sample by 1,000. Since 1 equivalent of NaOH and HCl are both equal to 1 mole of the substance, the number of equivalents per liter is equal to the number of moles per liter. Hence, 0.1N NaOH is also 0.1M NaOH and will titrate the molarity of HCl. One can calculate the molarity of a solution from the titration data by use of the $V_1 \times C_1 = V_2 \times C_2$ equation.

EXAMPLE 13-4: If 2.1 ml of 0.1N NaOH are required to titrate 25 ml of gastric material, determine the titratable acidity in millimoles per liter.

$$0.1\text{N NaOH} = 0.1\text{M NaOH}$$

$$V_1 \times C_1 = V_2 \times C_2$$

$$2.1 \text{ ml} \times 0.1\text{M} = 25 \text{ ml} \times x\text{M}$$

$$25x = 2.1 \times 0.1$$

$$25x = 0.21$$

$$x = 0.0084\text{M}$$

Convert 0.0084 mol/L to millimoles per liter by multiplying by 1,000.

$$0.0084 \text{ mol/L} \times 1,000 = 8.4 \text{ mmol/L}$$

Another formula recommended for calculation of millimoles per liter of gastric acidity is:

$$\text{Acid in mmol/L} = \frac{\text{ml of 0.1M NaOH} \times 0.1 \times 1,000}{\text{ml of sample}}$$

EXAMPLE 13-5: Use the information from Example 13-4 in the formula above.

$$\text{Acid in mmol/L} = \frac{2.1 \times 0.1 \times 1,000}{25}$$

$$= \frac{210}{25}$$

$$= 8.4 \text{ mmol/L titratable acidity}$$

As stated earlier, all three units of gastric acidity have the same numerical value for a given sample. The calculation of the same sample using each of the units will demonstrate this.

EXAMPLE 13-6: A 20 ml sample of gastric material required 2.6 ml of 0.1N NaOH to titrate to an endpoint of pH 7.0. What is the titratable acidity in degrees of acidity per 100 ml, millie-quivalents per liter, and millimoles per liter?

1. Gastric acidity in degrees per 100 ml

$$\frac{2.6}{20} = \frac{x}{100}$$

$$20x = 2.6 \times 100$$

$$20x = 260$$

$$x = 13 \text{ ml of } 0.1\text{N NaOH, hence, } \boxed{13° \text{ } acidity}$$

2. Gastric acidity in milliequivalents per liter

$$V_1 \times C_1 = V_2 \times C_2$$

$$2.6 \times 0.1\text{N} = 20 \text{ ml} \times x\text{N}$$

$$20x = 0.26$$

$$x = 0.013\text{N} = 0.013 \text{ Eq/L}$$

$$0.013 \text{ Eq/L} \times 1,000 = \boxed{13 \text{ } mEq/L}$$

3. Gastric acidity in millimoles per liter

$$V_1 \times C_1 = V_2 \times C_2$$

$$2.6 \text{ ml} \times 0.1\text{M} = 20 \text{ ml} \times x\text{M}$$

$$20x = 0.26$$

$$x = 0.013\text{M} = 0.013 \text{ mol/L}$$

$$0.013 \text{ mol/L} \times 1,000 = \boxed{13 \text{ } mmol/L}$$

Or:

$$\text{Acidity in mmol/L} = \frac{2.6 \times 0.1 \times 1,000}{20}$$

$$= \frac{260}{20}$$

$$= \boxed{13 \text{ } mmol/L}$$

SECTION 13.3 DETERMINATION OF FREE ACID OUTPUT

Free acid output by the stomach is described in three ways according to the condition of the patient during the time of acid secretion. The **basal acid output (BAO)** is the production of stomach acid while the patient is not receiving any stimuli that will influence gastric acidity. In other words, the BAO is acid output during the basal state without gastric stimulation. Free acid output after gastric stimulation is called the **maximum acid output (MAO).** This is usually reported as the average of four gastric samples taken 15 minutes apart after the stimulation of secretion. The **peak acid output (PAO)** is the average of the two greatest values used for the MAO.

The BAO, MAO, and PAO are usually reported as the amount of free acid output per hour regardless of the length of time used for the test.

SECTION 13.4 CALCULATION OF FREE ACID OUTPUT

To calculate an acid output, first calculate the concentration of gastric acidity in millimoles per liter.

$$\text{Free acid in mmol/L} = \frac{\text{ml of 0.1M NaOH} \times 0.1 \times 1,000}{\text{ml of sample}}$$

Then:

$$\text{Free acid in mmol/hr} = \frac{\text{mmol free acid/L} \times \text{tot. vol. of spec. (ml)}}{1,000} \times \frac{60}{\text{collection per. of spec. (min)}}$$

CALCULATION OF BAO. Place aliquot of gastric sample in evaporating dish. Analyze for free HCl using Töpfer's reagent. Calculate the BAO per hour by using the formulas given above.

CALCULATION OF MAO. Analyze samples using Töpfer's reagent. Calculate the free acid output of each of the 15-minute samples in millimoles per hour using the formulas given above. Average the acid output for all four specimens. This value is the MAO per hour.

CALCULATION OF PAO. Select the two specimens with the highest acid output from the MAO calculations. Take the average of the two. This is the PAO per hour.

CALCULATION OF BAO/MAO RATIO.

$$\frac{\text{BAO}}{\text{MAO}} \times 100 = \text{percent BAO/MAO}$$

EXAMPLE 13-7: A 30-minute basal secretion sample required 1.5 ml 0.1N NaOH to titrate 5 ml gastric material to the Töpfer's endpoint. The total volume of the sample was 25 ml. What would be the BAO?

$$\text{Free acid in mmol/L} = \frac{1.5 \times 0.1 \times 1,000}{5}$$

$$= \frac{150}{5}$$

$$= 30 \text{ mmol free acid/L}$$

$$\text{Free acid in mmol/hr} = \frac{30 \times 25}{1,000} \times \frac{60}{30}$$

$$= \frac{750}{1,000} \times \frac{60}{30}$$

$$= \frac{45,000}{30,000}$$

$$= 1.5 \text{ mmol free acid/hr (BAO/hr)}$$

EXAMPLE 13-8: Calculate the MAO and PAO for the following information:

Sample	Total volume (ml)	Amount titrated (ml)	Amount 0.1N NaOH (ml)	Collection time (min)
1	20	5	2.3	15
2	15	5	2.6	15
3	15	5	3.1	15
4	25	5	1.8	15

Sample 1:

$$\text{Free acid in mmol/L} = \frac{2.3 \times 0.1 \times 1{,}000}{5}$$

$$= \frac{230}{5}$$

$$= 46 \text{ mmol/L}$$

$$\text{Free acid in mmol/hr} = \frac{46 \times 20}{1{,}000} \times \frac{60}{15}$$

$$= \frac{920}{1{,}000} \times \frac{60}{15}$$

$$= \frac{55{,}200}{15{,}000}$$

$$= \boxed{3.7 \text{ mmol/hr}}$$

Sample 2:

$$\text{Free acid in mmol/L} = \frac{2.6 \times 0.1 \times 1{,}000}{5}$$

$$= \frac{260}{5}$$

$$= 52 \text{ mmol/L}$$

$$\text{Free acid in mmol/hr} = \frac{52 \times 15}{1{,}000} \times \frac{60}{15}$$

$$= \frac{780}{1{,}000} \times \frac{60}{15}$$

$$= \frac{46{,}800}{15{,}000}$$

$$= \boxed{3.1 \text{ mmol/hr}}$$

Sample 3:

$$\text{Free acid in mmol/L} = \frac{3.1 \times 0.1 \times 1{,}000}{5}$$

$$= \frac{310}{5}$$

$$= 62 \text{ mmol/L}$$

$$\text{Free acid in mmol/hr} = \frac{62 \times 15}{1{,}000} \times \frac{60}{15}$$

$$= \frac{930}{1{,}000} \times \frac{60}{15}$$

$$= \frac{55{,}800}{15{,}000}$$

$$= \boxed{3.7 \text{ mmol/hr}}$$

Sample 4:   Free acid in mmol/L $= \dfrac{1.8 \times 0.1 \times 1{,}000}{5}$

$= \dfrac{180}{5}$

$= 36$ mmol/L

Free acid in mmol/hr $= \dfrac{36 \times 25}{1{,}000} \times \dfrac{60}{15}$

$= \dfrac{900}{1{,}000} \times \dfrac{60}{15}$

$= \dfrac{54{,}000}{15{,}000}$

$= \boxed{3.6 \text{ mmol/hr}}$

Now average the output values for all four specimens for the MAO per hour.

$$\frac{3.7 + 3.1 + 3.7 + 3.6}{4} = 3.5 \text{ MAO/hr}$$

Average the two highest output values for the PAO per hour.

$$\frac{3.7 + 3.7}{2} = 3.7 \text{ PAO/hr}$$

APPENDIXES RELATED TO THIS CHAPTER

Q Formulas Presented in this Book

PRACTICE PROBLEMS

Calculate the answer for each problem. Understand each portion of the calculation and determine whether the answer is logical. *Just because an answer can be calculated does not mean that it is reasonable.*

1. If a sample of 3.0 ml of gastric contents is used in the titration of gastric acidity, 1.0 ml of 0.1N NaOH is necessary to titrate to Töpfer's endpoint, and an additional 2.2 ml of NaOH is required to reach the phenolphthalein endpoint, what is the total acid in degrees?
   a. 6.4   d. 128
   b. 12.8   e. none of these
   c. 64
2. A one-dish titration is performed on a 10-ml sample of gastric contents. The first titration required 1.5 ml of 0.1N NaOH, and the second required 1.1 ml of NaOH. Give the free, combined, and total acid concentrations in degrees and millimoles per liter.
3. A one-dish titration is performed on a 5 ml sample of gastric contents. The first titration required 1.2 ml of 0.1N NaOH and the second titration required 0.8 ml of NaOH. Give the free, combined, and total acid concentrations in degrees and millimoles per liter.
4. The total acid for a gastric sample is 70°. The free acid concentration for the same sample is 30°. What is the combined acid value?
5. A 5-ml sample of gastric juice is titrated to pH 7.4 with phenol red. The titration required 6.1 ml of 0.1N NaOH. What is the acid concentration in millimoles per liter?

6. Five milliliters of gastric contents are titrated with 0.1N NaOH. The first titration required 0.48 ml of 0.1N NaOH. The total titration required 1.6 ml of 0.1N NaOH. Give the free, combined, and total acid concentrations in degrees and in millimoles per liter.

7. Calculate the BAO, MAO, and PAO from the following information:

Sample	Total volume (ml)	Amount titrated (ml)	Amount 0.1N NaOH (ml)	Collection time (min)
Fasting	30	10	3.2	30
15 min	15	5	2.8	15
30 min	20	5	3.5	15
45 min	18	5	3.6	15
60 min	15	5	1.9	15

14
Renal Tests

EDUCATIONAL OBJECTIVES

To have successfully learned the material in this chapter, the student should be able to do the following properly:

- Calculate the renal clearance of creatinine in terms of milliliters of plasma cleared per minute.
- Calculate the renal clearance in a percent of normal.
- Determine the body surface of an individual by using a nomogram and by calculation.
- Adjust a renal clearance for body surface.
- Determine an amount of test substance per total volume in a timed urine specimen.
- Determine the amount of a test substance per given time in a timed urine specimen.

SECTION 14.1 RENAL CLEARANCE TESTS

Renal clearance is the value assigned to the rate at which the kidneys remove material from the plasma or the blood. This is a quantitative expression of the rate at which a substance is excreted by the kidneys in relation to the concentration of the same substance in the plasma. For example, if plasma passing through the kidneys contains 0.1 gram of a substance per 100 milliliters and 0.1 gram of this substance passed into the urine each minute, then 100 milliliters of plasma are *cleared* of this substance per minute. Renal clearances of material are usually expressed as milliliters of plasma cleared per minute.

EXAMPLE 14-1: The blood level of creatinine is 10 mg/dl, and the quantity of creatinine that passes into the urine per minute is 6 mg. What is the clearance of creatinine?

Set up a ratio and proportion: 100 ml of blood contains 10 mg; therefore x ml would contain 6 mg.

$$\frac{100}{10} = \frac{x}{6}$$

$$10x = 600$$

$$x = 60$$

Therefore 60 ml of blood contains 6 mg of creatinine; hence, 60 ml of blood are *cleared* of that amount of creatinine per minute.

Most clearances could be figured in this manner; however, a general formula based on the preceding relationship is usually used. This formula is:

$$C = \frac{U}{P} \times V$$

where C is the plasma clearance in milliliters per minute; U is the concentration of the substance in the urine; P is the concentration of the substance in the plasma or blood; and V is the volume of urine in milliliters per minute.

The concentration of the substance in the blood and in the urine must be expressed in the same units. This formula is usually more convenient to use than the ratio-proportion setup, because the concentration of the material in the blood and urine must be determined before any total amounts of the material can be obtained.

EXAMPLE 14-2: A patient of average size was found to have a creatinine concentration in the blood of 12 mg/dl and a urine concentration of 550 mg/dl. The patient produced 3 ml of urine/min. Determine the renal clearance for creatinine.

$$C = \frac{U}{P} \times V$$

$$C = \frac{550}{12} \times 3$$

$$C = 137.5 \text{ ml/min}$$

This means that 137.5 ml of blood would be cleared of creatinine per minute.

The formula:

$$C = \frac{U}{P} \times V$$

would apply to individuals who have an average body surface. All other factors being equal, the clearance rate is roughly proportional to the size of the kidney and the body surface area of the individual. To compensate for variations in body surface area, the formula is modified thus:

$$C = \frac{U}{P} \times V \times \frac{1.73 \text{ m}^2}{A}$$

The average body surface area for an adult human is 1.73 m^2. The value A in the formula is the body surface area of the patient. This body surface area may be obtained from a nomogram (see Appendix R). It may also be calculated using the following formula:

$$\log A = (0.425 \times \log W) + (0.725 \times \log H) - 2.144$$

where A is the body surface in square meters; W is the patient's weight (mass) in kilograms; and H is the patient's height in centimeters.

EXAMPLE 14-3: A creatinine clearance was performed on a male patient who is 1.5 m tall and weighs 65 kg. His blood contained 2.5 mg/dl creatinine. The urine creatinine was 50 mg/dl and the urine volume was 300 ml/4 hr. What is the creatinine clearance for this man?

Using the formula:

$$C = \frac{U}{P} \times V \times \frac{1.73}{A}$$

Determine the body surface area of the patient.

$$\log A = (0.425 \times \log W) + (0.725 \times \log H) - 2.144$$
$$\log A = (0.425 \times \log 65) + (0.725 \times \log 150) - 2.144$$
$$\log A = (0.425 \times 1.812) + (0.725 \times 2.176) - 2.144$$
$$\log A = 0.770 + 1.5776 - 2.144$$
$$\log A = 0.2036$$
$$A = 1.598 \text{ or } 1.6 \text{ m}^2$$

Convert 300 ml/4 hr urine production to milliliters per minute.

$$300 \text{ ml}/240 \text{ min} = 1.25 \text{ ml/min}$$

$$C = \frac{U}{P} \times V \times \frac{1.73}{A}$$

$$C = \frac{50}{2.5} \times 1.25 \times \frac{1.73}{1.6}$$

Do not confuse the body surface of the patient with the correction factor resulting when the body surface is divided into the average body surface. In this case the correction factor would be $1.73/1.6 = 1.08$.

$$C = \frac{50}{2.5} \times 1.25 \times 1.08 \text{ (correction factor for body surface)}$$

$$C = 20 \times 1.25 \times 1.08$$

$$C = 27 \text{ ml/min}$$

The substances for which renal clearance tests are most often made are urea, creatinine, and inulin. The use of each of these in such tests is beyond the scope of the book. However, when urea clearance is measured, the amount of urine produced must be considered in a slightly different light. This is due to the tendency of the kidney tubule to reabsorb some of the urea filtered by the glomeruli. The rate of this reabsorption of urea depends on the rate of the reabsorption of water. Adjustment for this is made by the use of a modified formula when a small amount of urine is produced. The production of a urine volume of 2.0 milliliters per minute or more is termed maximum clearance. Under maximum clearance conditions, the same formula is used for urea that is used for creatinine; that is,

$$C = \frac{U}{P} \times V \times \frac{1.73}{A}$$

If less than 2.0 milliliters per minute of urine is produced, this is called standard clearance, and the following formula is used:

$$C = \frac{U}{P} \times \sqrt{V} \times \frac{1.73}{A}$$

The square root of the volume of urine produced is used to compensate for the reabsorption of the urea by the renal tubules.

Because there are two sets of normal values for urea clearance, one for maximum clearance and one for standard, the urea clearance is often reported as *percent of normal*. This means the percent that the test values are of the normal range. The normal values for the maximum and standard clearances are as follows:

	Mean (ml/min)	Range (ml/min)	Range (% of normal)
Maximum	75	64 to 99	75 to 125
Standard	54	41 to 68	75 to 125

Note that the normal *range in percent of normal* is the same for both the maximum and standard clearance. To convert the clearance in milliliters per minute to percent of normal, it is necessary to expand the formulas as follows:

$$\text{Maximum } C\% \text{ of normal} = \frac{U}{P} \times V \times \frac{1.73}{A} \times \frac{100}{75}$$

$$\text{Standard } C\% \text{ of normal} = \frac{U}{P} \times \sqrt{V} \times \frac{1.73}{A} \times \frac{100}{54}$$

The numbers 75 and 54 represent the normal mean values for maximum and standard clearances, respectively.

SECTION 14.2 TIMED URINE VALUES

The calculated values for timed urine specimens may be reported in several ways. The most common methods are: (1) as the value taken directly from an instrument or standard curve, (2) as a quantity per total volume, and (3) as a quantity for a unit of time.

The least used of these methods is to report the values as they come from an instrument or standard curve. A total volume is not needed for this method. However, remember that it is poor laboratory procedure not to record the total volume and the duration of time over which the sample was produced. In this method the result is usually given as milligrams per deciliter, millimoles per liter, or as milliequivalents per liter. For example, a sodium determination is done for a urine sample. The sample is subjected to a urine sodium procedure. The result comes from the instrument as 160 millimoles per liter. This is the result to be reported. The value is not adjusted for the total volume or any other factor. In another example, a urine sample is subjected to a procedure for the determination of urine protein. The value resulting from this procedure is 40 milligrams per deciliter. This is the value to be reported.

Generally, this is not a desirable method for timed urine tests. The information desired from such tests is usually the total amount of a substance excreted or the amount of substance excreted in some period of time. The above method only gives the concentration of the substance in the urine sample tested.

The second method of reporting values of timed urine tests is as a quantity per total volume. In this method, a sample is subjected to some procedure and this result is adjusted for the total volume using ratio and proportion.

EXAMPLE 14-4: A procedure determined that a sample of urine had a sodium concentration of 160 mmol/L. The total volume of the sample was 2,400 ml. Determine the amount of sodium in the total volume.

$$\frac{160 \text{ mmol}}{1,000} = \frac{x \text{ mmol}}{2,400 \text{ ml}}$$

$$1,000x = 160 \times 2,400$$

$$x = \frac{384,000}{1,000}$$

$$x = 384 \text{ mmol}/2,400 \text{ ml}$$

EXAMPLE 14-5: It was found that a sample of 1,800 ml had a urine protein concentration of 40 mg/dl. Determine the amount of protein in the total volume of urine collected.

$$\frac{40 \text{ mg}}{100 \text{ ml}} = \frac{x \text{ mg}}{1,800 \text{ ml}}$$

$$100x = 40 \times 1,800$$

$$x = \frac{72,000}{100}$$

$$x = 720 \text{ mg}/1,800 \text{ ml}$$

The following formula may be used for this kind of calculation instead of the complete ratio and proportion procedure.

$$\frac{\text{Amount of substance}}{\text{per total vol.}} = \frac{\text{amount of substance}}{\text{reported from instrument}} \times \frac{\text{total vol. (ml)}}{\text{vol. reported from instrument}}$$

Using this formula to solve the above examples gives the following calculations.

EXAMPLE 14-6: Calculate the amount of sodium in 2,400 ml of urine having a sodium concentration of 160 mmol/L.

$$x \text{ mmol}/2,400 \text{ ml} = 160 \times \frac{2,400}{1,000}$$

$$x = \frac{384,000}{1,000}$$

$$x = 384$$

Hence, there are 384 mmol of sodium in 2,400 ml of this urine sample.

EXAMPLE 14-7: Calculate the amount of protein in 1,800 ml of urine having a concentration of 40 mg/dl.

$$x \text{ mg}/1,800 \text{ ml} = 40 \times \frac{1,800}{100}$$

$$x = \frac{72,000}{100}$$

$$x = 720$$

Hence, there are 720 mg of protein in 1,800 ml of this sample of urine.

A third method used to report the results of timed urine tests is to report the quantity of some component of the urine excreted in some period of time. The period of time is usually either the total time over which the sample was collected or 1 hour.

In reporting a result as a quantity per time of collection, one must first calculate the amount of the substance in the total volume of the sample. Since the total volume of the sample was collected during the total time of the test, the amount per total volume is the same as the amount per the time of collection. Hence, the value need not be changed. One only needs to substitute the length of time for the total volume in the reporting of the value.

EXAMPLE 14-8: A 4-hr urine sample contains 800 ml. It is subjected to a creatinine determination, and the instrument result is 15 mg/dl. Determine the amount of creatinine for the total sample by ratio and proportion.

$$\frac{15 \text{ mg}}{100 \text{ ml}} = \frac{x \text{ mg}}{800 \text{ ml}}$$

$$100x = 15 \times 800$$

$$100x = 12{,}000$$

$$x = 120 \text{ mg/800 ml}$$

Change the description of the value from total volume to the period of time of collection.

$$x = 120 \text{ mg/4 hr}$$

If the result desired is a quantity per 1 hour, one would simply have to divide the quantity per total volume by the number of hours over which the collection was made.

EXAMPLE 14-9: If a 4-hr urine sample was found to contain 120 mg of creatinine per 800 ml, this would also mean that 120 mg of creatinine was excreted in 4 hours. Hence:

$$\frac{x \text{ mg}}{1 \text{ hr}} = \frac{120 \text{ mg}}{4 \text{ hr}}$$

$$4x = 1 \times 120$$

$$4x = 120$$

$$x = 30 \text{ mg/hr}$$

If desired, the following formula can be used to calculate the amount of a urine component excreted per hour from a concentration of the component.

$$\text{Quantity per hour} = \frac{\text{amount of substance reported from instrument}}{\text{volume reported from instrument (in ml)}} \times \frac{\text{total volume (in ml)}}{\text{hours collected}}$$

Use the formula to solve Example 14-8 as follows:

$$x \text{ mg creatinine/hr} = \frac{15 \text{ mg}}{100 \text{ ml}} \times \frac{800}{4 \text{ hr}}$$

$$x = \frac{12{,}000}{400}$$

$$x = 30 \text{ mg/hr}$$

Hence, 30 mg of creatinine was excreted per hour during the duration of the collection.

Urine concentrations may be reported in several ways. This also applies to most other kinds of tests. Remember, a set of digits taken alone is meaningless. Any value is incomplete without some qualifying statement or units. For example, 46 alone has little meaning; 46 mg/24 hr has a great deal of meaning.

APPENDIXES RELATED TO THIS CHAPTER

F Four-Place Logarithms
H Square Root Chart
Q Formulas Presented in this Book
R Nomogram for the Determination of Body Surface Area

PRACTICE PROBLEMS

Calculate the answer for each problem. Understand each portion of the calculation and determine whether the answer is logical. *Just because an answer can be calculated does not mean that it is reasonable.*

Clearance tests

1. Patient data: height, 6 ft; weight, 145 lb; urine volume, 400 ml/4 hr; urine urea, 400 mg/dl; blood urea, 20 mg/dl. Give clearance in milliliters per minute and percent of normal.
2. A man weighs 195 lb and is 6 ft tall. Give the following:
   a. His body surface (two ways: nomogram and formula)
   b. The factor for correcting for his body surface
3. Patient data: height, 5 ft, 1 in; weight, 200 lbs; urine volume, 650 ml/3 hr; urine urea, 300 mg/3 hr; blood urea, 55 mg/dl. Give the clearance in milliliters per minute and percent of normal.
4. Give the creatinine clearance for the following: plasma creatinine, 1.8 mg/dl; urine creatinine, 40 mg/dl; urine volume, 600 ml/4 hr.
5. The following information is available for a urea clearance test: serum urea, 30 mg/dl; urine urea, 5,400 mg/24 hr; 24-hr total volume, 1,800 ml. The patient is 5 ft, 6 in tall and weighs 130 lb. Report the following:
   a. Patient's body surface
   b. Body surface correction factor
   c. Urea clearance in milliliters per minute uncorrected for body surface
   d. Urea clearance in milliliters per minute corrected for body surface
   e. Urea clearance in percent of normal corrected for body surface
   f. Urea clearance in percent of normal uncorrected for body surface
6. A urea clearance is performed on a male patient. The plasma urea is 22 mg/dl, the urine urea is 200 mg/dl, and the urine total volume is 150 ml/3 hr. Report as milliliters of plasma cleared per minute and as percent of normal.
7. Give the formula for finding the following:
   a. The factor to correct for body surface
   b. Maximum urea clearance in milliliters per minute, uncorrected
   c. Standard urea clearance in milliliters per minute, uncorrected
   d. Maximum urea clearance in percent of normal, corrected
   e. Standard urea clearance in percent of normal, corrected
   f. Creatinine clearance (correcting for size)
   g. For finding the bottom value in question *a*
8. The following information is available for a urea clearance test: serum urea, 40 mg/dl; urine urea, 2,400 mg/1,300 ml (24-hr specimen). The patient is 5 ft, 6 in tall and weighs 125 lb. Report the following:

    a. Patient's body surface
    b. Body surface correction factor
    c. Urea clearance in milliliters per minute uncorrected for body surface
    d. Urea clearance in milliliters per minute corrected for body surface
    e. Urea clearance in percent of normal corrected for body surface
    f. Urea clearance in percent of normal uncorrected for body surface

9. Patient data: height, 5 ft, 7 in; weight, 180 lb; urine volume, 700 ml/4 hr; urine urea, 300 mg/dl; blood urea, 10 mg/dl. Give the clearance in milliliters per minute and percent of normal.

10. Calculate the following urea clearance:
Report in milliliters per minute and percent of normal.
Patient's weight = 120 lb
Patient's height = 5 ft
Blood urea = 5 mg/dl
Urine urea = 2,000 mg/24 hr
Urine volume = 300 ml/24 hr

General renal tests

11. A 24-hr urine sample measuring 1,450 ml has a sodium concentration of 40 mEq/L. Express the amount of sodium in the 24-hr sample as:
    a. mg/dl
    b. mmol/L
    c. mg/24 hr
    d. In SI units

12. A 24-hr specimen with a total volume of 1,500 ml contains 100 mg/100 ml creatinine. How much creatinine is excreted in grams per day for this individual?

13. A 24-hr urine specimen having a volume of 2,100 ml and containing 12 g of protein is to be reported to the doctor in grams percent. What would be reported?

14. If 3.4 g% of albumin was found in a 24-hr urine specimen with a volume of 1,500 ml, how many grams per 24 hr did the patient excrete?

15. A spot urine sample with a total volume of 150 ml is found to have a creatinine concentration of 132 mg/dl. Express as:
    a. mg/total volume
    b. mg/ml

16. A 2-hr urine amylase is found to be 105 units/dl. The total volume is 255 ml. Report as:
    a. Units/2 hr
    b. Units/ml
    c. Units/255 ml

17. A 24-hr urine sample has a total volume of 1,800 ml. The sodium concentration is found to be 300 mEq/L. Report as:
    a. mg/dl
    b. g/d
    c. SI units
    d. mEq/24 hr

15
Quality Control

EDUCATIONAL OBJECTIVES

To have successfully learned the material in this chapter, the student should be able to do the following properly:

- Describe the need for quality control in the clinical laboratory.
- Differentiate between parameters and statistics.
- Calculate the mean, median, and mode of a set of variables.
- Calculate the standard deviation and coefficient of variation of a set of variables.
- Describe the organization of the normal distribution and the Levey-Jennings Chart in terms of the relationship between the mean and standard deviation of a set of data.
- Describe how a normal distribution is used to evaluate a series of laboratory results.
- Plot a set of test results with controls on a Levey-Jennings chart and determine whether the procedure is in or out of control.

SECTION 15.1 INTRODUCTION

The control of the quality of the analytical work of the laboratory is an integral part of the operation of every good laboratory. This part of the laboratory activities can be divided into three phases: (1) the establishment of accurate controls with which to compare production work, (2) the evaluation of the comparison of the work with the controls, and (3) the implementation of corrective measures to improve the quality of the laboratory work. Most of the first and last of these phases is beyond the scope of this book. The second phase is discussed in some detail in this chapter.

In the establishment of comparison of controls, several factors should be considered. The controls of similar laboratories, commercial suppliers, and the recommendations of associations, boards, congresses, and other cooperative groups are usually the most convenient sources of reliable controls. A reference control should reflect the phenomena for which the production test is being used to the highest degree of accuracy and precision possible. An individual laboratory may desire to develop a reference control. This is quite feasible, provided the personnel fully understand the phenomenon being evaluated and the theory and application of the test procedures.

The implementation of needed measures is the most important and often the most difficult phase of a quality control program. The most elaborate and complete evaluation of the work done by a laboratory is for naught unless some effective use is made of the information obtained.

The comparison of test results with control values and the evaluation of these comparisons usually involve the science of statistics. **Statistics** includes the mathematics involved with the estimation of the significance of deviations of test values from some theoretically correct value. Statistical methods must be used in combination with good logic and common sense. Quality control programs often fail to be beneficial when the laboratory personnel try to make statistics do their thinking.

Statistics is often the basis of accidental or designed errors. We actively condemn the purposeful use of statistics to create untrue implications or to support known lies. Statistics should be used as a tool to estimate a true situation!

A complete treatment of the mathematics of statistics is much beyond the scope of this book. This is a separate discipline of mathematics. There are many good books on the market that deal with statistics in general. However, there are fewer works that deal specifically with the statistics of the clinical and biological laboratory. Several are given in the bibliography. These cover the subject with much more depth than can be done here.

This chapter provides an introduction to the statistics likely to be used by almost all laboratory technologists. It does not pretend to be a comprehensive treatment of the subject.

Quality control programs should assist in increasing the accuracy and precision of the laboratory results. The terms *accuracy and precision* are often erroneously used to mean, or at least imply, the same thing. They both deal with quality, but each deals with a different property of quality.

Accuracy is used to describe the closeness of a test value to the actual value. **Precision** is used in two ways. In statistical use, it usually refers to the reproducibility of a test value, in which case it means the consistency of a series of test results. The term **reproducibility** is also often used in this manner. However, at times *precision* is used to denote the size of the increments used in the measure. For example, an object that has a mass of exactly 1.787 kilograms can be weighed in several ways. If it is weighed on a balance that only weighs to the nearest kilogram and is shown to have a mass of between 1 and 2 kilograms, this would be an accurate measurement of its mass. However, this would be a very low degree of precision. Another weighing of the object on another balance may show the mass to be 1.27489 kilograms. This value would be very precise but not accurate. Next, the mass of the object may be measured by five people using five different instruments. The values obtained could be 1.7870, 1.787, 1.8, 1.78700, and 1.78 kilograms. This series of measurements would all be accurate to different numbers of significant figures. The level of precision (reproducibility) of the series would also be high, and the fourth measurement would be extremely precise in itself.

A very definite possibility of measuring devices is that they can have precision and not accuracy. In words much used, "One is often precisely wrong. One may also be approximately accurate." The degree of accuracy or precision is relative to the situation. If one measures a distance of 5 kilometers to the nearest meter, this would probably be considered to be a high level of precision. However, if the width of a laboratory bench were measured to the nearest meter, this would be a very low degree of precision. The degree of precision necessary would depend on the situation in which the measurements are made. The term **reliability** is often used to describe the degree of accuracy and precision of a procedure.

In general, the evaluation of precision is easier than the evaluation of accuracy. In determining the precision of work, one needs only to calculate the *consistency* of the measurements or note the number of significant figures in the values. The degree of accuracy, however, must be determined by comparing the values obtained in the laboratory work with values known to be correct. The correct values are usually obtained from standardized test materials subjected to ideal test procedures and conditions.

SECTION 15.2 STATISTICAL TERMINOLOGY

Often the formulas and terminology found in statistics overwhelm the beginning student. This need not be the case if some effort is made to learn a basic language of statistics before attempting to analyze data.

Observations and Variables

Observations are the recognized characteristics of something. These observations can either be *qualitative* or *quantitative*. **Qualitative observations** are descriptions of such properties as color, texture, turbidity, and odor. These are nonnumerical in value. **Quantitative observations** are descriptions that utilize numerical values. The size of an object, the concentration of a solution, and the length of time required for some event are examples of quantitative observations. Observations that are not constant are called **variables,** and variables are the raw materials for statistical methods. Only quantitative variables can be treated by these methods. Some qualitative observations can be converted to quantitative values. For example, the wavelength of light reflected determines the color of a compound. Statistics can be used with a series of wavelengths, but they cannot be used with colors.

Quantitative variables may be continuous or discrete. **Continuous variables** are those for which any value within a particular range is possible. Examples of continuous variables include the diameter of red blood cells, the concentration of a solute in a solution, and the amount of uric acid excreted in a day. Continuous variables are limited only by the precision of the measurement. **Discrete variables** are those that can vary only in minimum increments. The number of tests completed in a day, the number of basophils in a differential blood count, and the number of heartbeats per minute are all examples of discrete variables. A series of related observations is usually referred to as **data** (singular, datum).

Populations and Samples

All possible values for a particular characteristic constitute a **population.** All these values do not have to be different, nor does their number have to be finite. Some populations are essentially infinite, such as the differential blood counts done in the past, present, and future. Some populations are relatively small, for example, the results of tests conducted by one laboratory during one particular month. A population can be anything it is defined to be.

A **sample** is any part of a population. Usually samples are small parts of large populations and are used to make inferences about populations. For this reason, samples should be chosen carefully so they are representative of the population. This is most important if the calculations of the observations in a sample are to accurately reflect the properties of the population. For a sample to be representative of a population, it has to be selected using procedures that ensure randomness. A **random sample** is one chosen so there is no preference given to any part of the population. There has been a great deal of experimentation showing that human beings cannot select a truly random sample without the use of some nonliving process. There are many such processes that may be used to generate a random sample. The drawing of a card from a shuffled deck, the roll of dice, and the toss of a balanced coin are all means of producing a random set of numbers. The statistician usually uses either a table of random numbers or a computer to produce the order of selection used to draw a random sample.

Parameters and Statistics

Calculations from data are either parameters or statistics, depending on the body of data used. If some calculation is made from an entire population, the results will be only one possible value. Such values are **parameters. Statistics** are calculated from samples of populations. Because different samples from the same populations can vary, statistics vary. Much of the work of the statistician involves the estimation of the extent of the variation of statistics.

SECTION 15.3 CALCULATED STATISTICAL VALUES

Most statistical calculations can be placed in one of two groups: measures of central tendency and measures of dispersion.

Measurements of Central Tendency

The most common measures of central tendency are the mean, the median, and the mode. The **mean** is the value usually referred to as the arithmetic average. This value is calculated by dividing the sum of all individual values by the number of values. When a mean is calculated from all values of a population, it is a parameter and is usually assigned the symbol μ. When the mean is calculated from a sample of a population, it is a statistic and is represented by symbol $\overline{X}$ (called X-bar),

$$\mu = \frac{\Sigma X}{N} \qquad \overline{X} = \frac{\Sigma X}{n}$$

where μ is the population mean; Σ means *the sum of;* X is the individual variables; N is the number of values in the population; $\overline{X}$ is the sample mean; the n is the number of variables in the sample.

The mean is the most used measure of central tendency. The value μ is a precise value for a population, whereas $\overline{X}$ is an estimate of μ based on a *sample* of that population.

The **median** is another measure of central tendency. This is the middle value of a body of data. If all the variables in the data are ranked in order of increasing magnitude, the median is that variable falling halfway between the highest and the lowest in position. In the case of a series containing an odd number of variables, the median will be the variable in the middle of the array. If the series contains an even number of observations, the median is the mean of the two middle values.

The **mode** is the most commonly occurring variable in a mass of data. This value may be any value within the body of data.

> EXAMPLE 15-1: Consider the following values for the number of eosinophils in seven differential blood counts: 3, 8, 5, 1, 3, 11, and 4. These counts would be a sample of a larger population unless otherwise defined. Hence, all values calculated from this body of data would be statistics.
>
> The *mean* of these values would be the sum of the values ($\Sigma X = 35$) divided by the total number of values ($n = 7$).

$$\overline{X} = \frac{\Sigma X}{n}$$

$$\overline{X} = \frac{35}{7}$$

$$\overline{X} = 5$$

The median would equal the middle value. To find the median, first rank the values according to magnitude: 1, 3, 3, 4, 5, 8, 11. There are seven values in this array. The median would be the middle value in the array. In an array of seven variables, the fourth variable from either end would be the median. In this case the median is the variable 4.

median
↓

1, 3, 3, ④, 5, 8, 11

The *mode* is the most frequently occurring value. In this array that value is 3, because it occurs twice.

mode

1, 3, 3, 4, 5, 8, 11

Measures of Dispersion

Measures of dispersion are calculated values that indicate the extent of variation of the observations. The most common measures of dispersion include the range, the variance, and the standard deviation. These may consider all observation of a particular kind, the entire population of observations, or they may consider a selected portion or sample of the population. The **range** (R), is the simplest and least useful measure of dispersion. It is simply the difference between the highest and lowest values considered. This is calculated by subtracting the lowest value from the highest.

EXAMPLE 15-2: Using the data from the sample of blood counts, calculate the range of the eosinophils in the sample. Remember that the observations are 3, 8, 5, 1, 3, 11, and 4.

The lowest value is 1, and the highest value is 11; hence, $11 - 1 = 10$. The range of this sample is 10.

The variance and standard deviation are the two most commonly used measures of dispersion. Abbreviations of these measures consider whether the body of data is a population or a sample. The population variance is abbreviated σ^2; the population standard deviation is σ, whereas s^2 and s are the abbreviations of the sample variance and sample standard deviation respectively. Almost all work in the laboratory involves samples of data. As implied from the abbreviations, the standard deviation is the square root of the variance. Hence, if the variance is known, the standard deviation can be easily calculated and vice versa. Both of these measures characterize the dispersion of the variables about the mean. The classic formula for the *variance* of a population sample is as follows:

$$s^2 = \frac{\Sigma(X - \overline{X})^2}{n - 1}$$

where s^2 is the variance of a sample; Σ means *the sum of*; X is the variables; $\overline{X}$ is the mean; and n is the number of variables in the sample. Consider the preceding example. The variables of the number of eosinophils from differential blood counts are 3, 8, 5, 1, 3, 11, and 4. The mean of these values is 5. To calculate the variance of the data, first calculate $X - \overline{X}$ for each variable.

X	$\overline{X}$	$X - \overline{X}$	$(X - \overline{X})^2$
3	5	-2	4
8	5	$+3$	9
5	5	0	0
1	5	-4	16
3	5	-2	4
11	5	$+6$	36
4	5	$\underline{-1}$	$\underline{1}$
		0	$70 = \Sigma(X - \overline{X})^2$

Note that the algebraic sum of $X - \overline{X}$ equals zero. This should be the case if the calculations are done correctly. This may vary slightly from zero if the values are rounded off. Also note that all $(X - \overline{X})^2$ values are positive, as a negative number times a negative number will yield a positive number.

Next divide $\Sigma(X - \overline{X})^2$ by the number of observations less one. One less than the number of observations is called the **degrees of freedom.**

The number of degrees of freedom is the number of variables in a sample or population that can be any value and still give the same result. In general, one degree of freedom is lost for every group of variables. In this case, all the variables are considered to be in one group. All the values but one could vary and still produce the same statistic. One variable must be one particular value to produce that particular statistic. Hence, all variables but one have freedom. The full implication of this concept requires a study of statistics beyond the scope of this book.

The calculation for the variance of the data above is:

$$s^2 = \frac{\Sigma(X - \overline{X})^2}{n - 1}$$

$$s^2 = \frac{70}{6}$$

$$s^2 = 11.67$$

The standard deviation is the square root of the variance; hence, the standard deviation of the preceding data is calculated as follows:

$$s = \sqrt{s^2} = \sqrt{\frac{\Sigma(X - \overline{X})^2}{n - 1}}$$

$$s = \sqrt{11.67}$$

$$s = 3.42$$

where s is the standard deviation.

Another formula that is commonly used to calculate the variance and standard deviation is as follows:

$$s^2 = \frac{\Sigma X^2 - \frac{(\Sigma X)^2}{n}}{n - 1}$$

Or:

$$s = \sqrt{\frac{\Sigma X^2 - \frac{(\Sigma X)^2}{n}}{n - 1}}$$

This formula is much easier to use with most calculators. For this reason, it is often referred to as the *machine formula*.

EXAMPLE 15-3: Consider the data used previously for the differential blood count: 3, 8, 5, 1, 3, 11, and 4. Calculate the variance and standard deviation using the machine formula.

X	X^2
3	9
8	64
5	25
1	1
3	9
11	121
4	16
$\Sigma X = 35$	$\Sigma X^2 = 245$

$$(\Sigma X)^2 = 1,225$$

$$s^2 = \frac{\Sigma X^2 - \frac{(\Sigma X)^2}{n}}{n - 1}$$

$$s^2 = \frac{245 - \frac{(35)^2}{7}}{6}$$

$$s^2 = \frac{245 - \frac{1,225}{7}}{6}$$

$$s^2 = \frac{245 - 175}{6}$$

$$s^2 = \frac{70}{6}$$

$$s^2 = 11.67$$

$$s = \sqrt{s^2}$$

$$s = \sqrt{11.67}$$

$$s = 3.42$$

The statistics or parameters, *variance* and *standard deviation,* are measures of the dispersion of a set of data around the mean. This gives an estimate of the degree of uniformity of the data. All large standard deviations in relation to the mean would indicate that the data are not very uniform. A lower standard deviation means that the data are more uniform.

Coefficient of Variation

The statistics *variance* and *standard deviation* vary with the data considered, so it is not accurate to compare the standard deviations of two samples without also considering the mean. The **coefficient of variation (CV)** is used to make such a comparison. This is equal to the standard deviation divided by the mean.

$$CV = \frac{s}{\overline{X}}$$

The coefficient of variation of the preceding example is calculated as follows:

$$CV = \frac{3.42}{5}$$

$$CV = 0.68$$

This value is often given as a percentage.

$$\%CV = \frac{s}{\overline{X}} \times 100$$

$$\%CV = \frac{3.42}{5} \times 100$$

$$\%CV = 68\%$$

The coefficient of variation can be used in many ways. It is useful in the comparison of the dispersion of two similar sets of data. It can be useful in comparing one day's work with a similar day, or it may compare test results in one laboratory with the same type of results from another laboratory.

It is not wise to use the coefficient of variation to compare situations that have several varying conditions. A coefficient of variation of 68% may be considered good for one body of data but very poor for another. As with all statistics and parameters, this should be used with care and common sense.

SECTION 15.4 NORMAL DISTRIBUTION

One common way of organizing the values of the observations of a population or sample is to construct a frequency distribution from the values of the variables. A **frequency distribution** represents a comparison of the magnitude of the variables with how frequently each particular value occurs. The usual method used to present a frequency distribution is a graph. The possible values in the population are usually arranged in increasing magnitude along the horizontal axis, whereas the number of times a particular value (that is, its frequency) occurs in the population or sample is arranged along the vertical axis. The frequency of each value is plotted on the graph. The pattern of the resulting curve indicates how the values are distributed throughout the range.

Many populations form a particular kind of frequency distribution, commonly called a **normal distribution,** or Gaussian distribution. This is usually presented as a curve on a graph, as described previously. Fig. 15-1 shows this curve. The curve of a normal distribution shows the frequency of values increasing until the mean is reached and then decreasing with the same slope. The curve of the normal distribution is often referred to as a *bell-shaped curve*. This relationship applies to a theoretical population distributed completely at random. In such a theoretical population the mean, median, and mode will be the same.

The normal distribution is useful in statistical calculations because of the large number of populations that either form this type of frequency distribution or approach it. Also, a completely random sample drawn from such a population will have a frequency distribution very close to a normal distribution.

If a particular sample does not form a normal distribution and the population is assumed to have a normal distribution, there is a probability that the sample is not random and that the observations result from conditions different from the population from which it was thought to have been drawn.

In a **normal distribution** *a constant relationship exists between the shape of the distribution curve and the standard deviation of the data.* This is true because both are functions of the dispersion of the data around the mean. A detailed discussion of this relationship is necessary to understand the basis of its use in quality control systems.

The curve of the normal distribution can be used to estimate the probability of a particular value occurring in a random sample. Stated very simply, **probability** is the chance of some event occurring. In this situation the probability is the chance of some particular value occurring in a sample. The probability of a particular value being chosen in a sample varies from zero to 1. If a value could never occur in a sample, its probability would be zero. If a

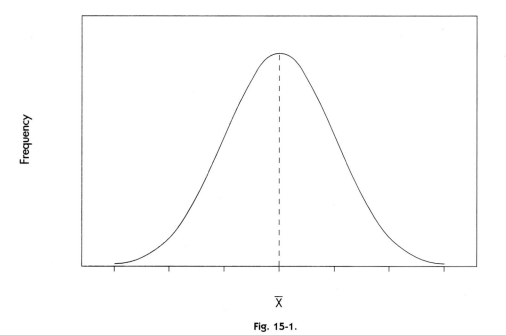

Fig. 15-1.

value were chosen every time in the selection of a sample, its probability would be 1. If a value occurred some of the time but not every time, its probability would be between zero and 1. This, of course, would be a fraction. Probability may be expressed in percentage. The probability values would then range from 0% to 100%. Percentage is usually more easily understood, so this will be the way in which probability is discussed here.

The curve of the frequency distribution of a population includes all the observations of the population. The area of the graph between the curve and the horizontal axis is analogous to the probability of some observation having a value between and including the lowest and the highest value in the population; this probability is 100%.

The probability of a particular observation having a value between any two points on the horizontal axis equals the proportion of the area under the curve between two vertical lines drawn from the curve to the horizontal axis at these points.

This same general relationship is true for the frequency distribution of a random sample drawn from a population. There is one difference, however. The probability of a value falling within the range of a sample will theoretically always be a little less than 100%. This will not significantly affect the considerations here, but it needs to be recognized if a more extensive study of statistics is undertaken.

Again, in a normal distribution there is a constant relationship between the standard deviation and the probability of values occurring in a population or sample.

The mean of a normally distributed body of data will be equal to the most frequently occurring value; hence, the mean will correspond to the highest point on the curve of a normal distribution.

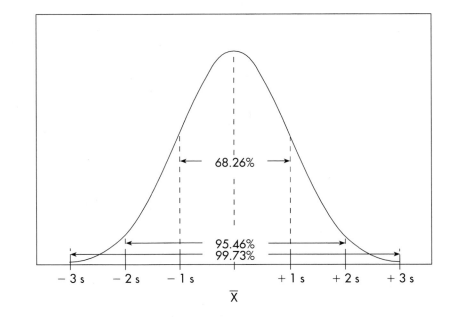

Fig. 15-2.

The probability of some observation having a value between the mean and one standard deviation ($1s$) greater than the mean is 34.13%. This is a constant value owing to the method of calculation of the standard deviation and the construction of the normal distribution curve. As the curve is symmetrical, the same probability exists for a value between $1s$ less than the mean and the mean value. Hence, the probability of some value from a population or sample being within one standard deviation on either side of the mean ($\pm 1s$) is 68.26% (2×34.13).

Study Fig. 15-2. Note that 68.26% of the area under the curve is between one standard deviation less than the mean ($-1s$) and one standard deviation greater than the mean ($+1s$). The probability of an observation having a value within $\pm 2s$ of the mean is 95.46%, whereas the probability of a value being within $\pm 3s$ of the mean is 99.73%.

This relationship between the frequency distribution curve and the standard deviation applies only to normal distributions. Not all populations will form a normal distribution. The reason for this can be found in more complete references on statistics. Be careful when using the procedures involving the standard deviations and the normal curve.

SECTION 15.5 $\overline{X}$ OR LEVEY-JENNINGS CHART

The most common system of quality control in the medical laboratory involves the use of the $\overline{X}$ or Levey-Jennings chart. In general, this system uses the mean and standard deviation of a series of control tests conducted during some previous time period. The $\overline{X}$ chart is an extension of points along the horizontal axis of the graph of the normal distribution. The graph is usually turned on its side for convenience so the horizontal axis becomes the vertical axis in this manner of presentation. Study Fig. 15-3.

The major lines of the chart are placed at the points on the axis corresponding to the mean and $\pm 1s$ and $\pm 2s$ from the mean. The probability of a control substance producing a test value within $1s$ of the mean is about 68.3%. The probability of the test results of a control being within $2s$ is about 95.5%. This means that every test result of the control solution has a 68.3% chance of being within $\pm 1s$ of the mean established for this particular test. The chance of being within $\pm 2s$ of the established mean is about 95.5%. This also means that each test result has a 31.7% chance of varying more than $\pm 1s$ from the mean or a 4.5% chance of varying more than $\pm 2s$ from the mean owing to random error alone.

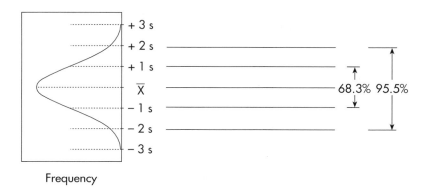

Fig. 15-3.

Therefore one would expect about 1 in 22 test values to vary more than $\pm$ 2s from the established mean, even if the test conditions are acceptable.

The mean and standard deviations used on an $\overline{X}$ chart are determined from a series of tests on control solutions done by the laboratory. In most situations, at least one test is made per day using the control. The mean and standard deviations are calculated from the test results of the controls over a given period of time. There should be at least 20 and preferably 30 test results used in the preparation of a chart.

The mean and standard deviations calculated from the test results of the laboratory are the values that should be used for the $\overline{X}$ and s values of that laboratory.

The most common source of controls is from commercial suppliers. These companies establish the mean and acceptable range of the control using results from several reference laboratories. These reference laboratories should have the most accurate and precise equipment, supplies, and personnel available. These values are to be used as a guide in a quality control program of a working laboratory. They are not the values to be used on the charts of the laboratory. The results of the daily tests of the control solution within the particular laboratory are the ones to be used in the establishment of the values on the chart. The mean of the laboratory tests should be within the acceptable range provided by the suppliers, however.

The procedure used to obtain the results on the control solutions should be as nearly like the procedure used with the patient samples as possible. If possible, the analyst conducting the test should not know which sample is the control. The control tests should be conducted at random within the normal routine of the laboratory. If more than one person conducts a particular type of test, each person involved should do some of the tests on the controls during each time period. Every control test result should be recorded on the quality control charts. This includes tests that may have been repeated for one reason or another.

The preceding considerations are necessary if a quality control program is to accurately reflect the work production of the laboratory.

A quality control program will aid in the evaluation of the conditions under which the control tests are conducted. If the conditions of the general laboratory work are different from the conditions of the control tests, the quality control program is not evaluating the work of the laboratory; it is evaluating the conditions used to run the controls! This situation occurs much too often. Many quality control programs are conducted to satisfy some regulatory or public relations requisite and not to determine the quality of the work done in the laboratory. This is very short sighted. It can only result in a false impression of the laboratory work and probably result in patient test results of lower reliability than should be tolerated.

A different $\overline{X}$ chart is set up for each procedure included in the quality control program. The magnitude of the mean and standard deviations is established using the results of the tests on the control solutions as described earlier in this chapter.

When the mean and standard deviations are calculated, the major lines of the $\overline{X}$ chart can be established.

The results of future tests on the control will then be plotted on the chart. The pattern formed by these points can be easily studied to determine whether the particular test procedure is *in control* or *out of control*. The terms **in control** and **out of control** are used to describe the acceptability of the reliability of the test procedures. A test under technical control at the bench level is said to be *in control* and has enough accuracy and precision to be used for patient testing. A test is *out of control* when the error associated with the procedure is too great to produce results of sufficient reliability to be used in patient diagnosis.

Since the pattern of the control test results is used to determine whether a test procedure is in or out of control, this requires careful interpretation.

The limits of variation normally considered allowable for the control test results have been established as $\pm 2s$ from the mean. If a test procedure is operating correctly, 95.5% of the control values will fall within this range. This also means that 4.5% of the values can fall outside this range as a result of acceptable error alone. Any interpretation of an $\overline{X}$ chart should be made using a series of test values. One value should never be used in any determination of the reliability of a test. Each value should be used in context with the other values in the series. In general, if a series of control results forms a random pattern between $+2s$ and $-2s$ on the $\overline{X}$ chart with only an occasional value falling outside this range, it is assumed that all technical phases of the test procedure are equal for all samples and that there is a high degree of probability that the patient values are correct and can be relied on in the formation of a diagnosis. However, this does not preclude the possibility that a particular patient sample may be tested so as to produce an erroneous result. As with all phases of laboratory technique, careful work and good logic are very necessary.

An occasional value falling outside the $\pm 2s$ limit may or may not be significant. One common practice in this situation is to repeat the control test. If the repeat result is within the $\pm 2s$ limit, it can be assumed that the wide-ranging value was due to chance alone and not to some problem with the procedure. If the second repeat test produces a value outside the accepted limits, the test procedure should be examined to determine the cause of the aberrant results. Patient values should not be reported until the problem is found and corrected. In either case, all results of the tests of the control should be plotted on the chart, except those caused by known errors.

Another generalization in the interpretation of the control values is that if six successive plots fall on the mean line or on one side of the mean line, the procedure is considered out of control. This condition is known as a **shift.** The mean of these tests has shifted from the established mean. The procedure should be examined to identify the problem and correct it. The placement of six plots on one side of the mean has been established as the most practical for the majority of clinical laboratories.

Another common situation seen on the $\overline{X}$ chart is that referred to as a trend. A **trend** is indicated by six successive plots being distributed in one general direction on the chart. This is another condition indicating that the test is out of control. Again, the test procedure should be examined and adjusted as with a shift.

Study the following examples, which include some common types of situations found in the quality control programs of the clinical laboratory.

Fig. 15-4 shows an $\overline{X}$ chart for the BUN procedure of a particular laboratory for the month of April. The mean and standard deviations used for this chart were calculated from the control values for the month of March. Fig. 15-5 shows these values for March with the calculations. This type of work sheet is provided by several companies. Many laboratories make their own. It helps to organize the calculations, and this type of chart may prove helpful for some people.

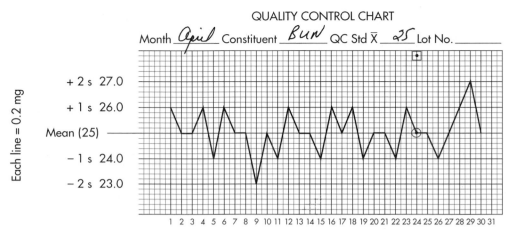

Fig. 15-4.

The chart in Fig. 15-4 shows that the test procedure is in control. The results of the control tests are distributed along each side of the mean in a random manner. Note the plot □ at day 24. This value was outside the ± 2s limit of the chart. The control test was repeated, and the plot ⊙ resulted. The second value fell within the acceptable limits, so the outlying value is considered to be due to random error and is acceptable. All values on this chart, including the outlier, should be used to calculate the mean and standard deviation for the chart to be used during the next test period.

The values of the April chart were used to calculate the mean and standard deviation for the May chart shown in Fig. 15-6.

The May chart shows a common situation in this type of quality control program. The control test for day 7 gave a result outside the ±2s limit (plot △). The test was repeated and gave the plot □. The second value for day 7 was also outside the acceptable limits, indicating an out-of-control situation. The reagents used in the procedure were examined and were found to be contaminated. These were replaced, and a third control test was conducted. The results of this test gave plot ⊙, and the test was back in control.

The values of the May test are used to calculate the mean and standard deviation used on the June chart. This raises the question as to whether or not to use the control values that detected an out-of-control situation. On this particular chart, this would include the first two control values for day seven. However, since the $\overline{X}$ chart is based on a normal distribution, it is recommended that only those values that are part of a randomly distributed set of control values should be used in the determination of the mean and standard deviations to be used on a quality control chart. Since the results of the first two control tests for day 7 were not part of the random distribution of the values for May, they should not be used in the calculation of the statistics for the June chart. However, they should *appear* on the May chart.

An example of a $\overline{X}$ chart showing a *shift* is presented in Fig. 15-7. The shift is in the control values from day 17 through day 22. The sixth consecutive value above the mean (plot ⊙) confirmed an out-of-control situation. The procedure was examined, and the problem was corrected. The plots of days 23 through 30 show the procedure to be back in control.

DATE	ANALYST	DETERMINATION	TRUE VALUE	AVERAGE
March		BUN	25	25

Procedure for Calculating Average and Standard Deviation:

1. Record each observation in colume "*X*".

2. Add the values in colume "*X*" and divide by the number of observations.

3. Calculate and record the differences between the average value and each individual observation in column "$X - \bar{X}$".

4. Square each individual difference and record in column "$(X - \bar{X})^2$".

5. Add the squared differences "$\Sigma(X - \bar{X})^2$".

6. Calculate Standard Deviation (s) using formula.

Calculations

1. Average $(\bar{X}) = \frac{\Sigma X}{n} = \frac{775}{31} = 25$

   where Σ = sum of

   X = each individual observation

   n = total number of observations = 31

2. Standard Deviation (s) = $\sqrt{\frac{\Sigma(X-\bar{X})^2}{n-1}}$ $\sqrt{\frac{30}{30}} = \sqrt{1} = 1$

   where s = standard deviation = 1.0

   Σ = sum of

   X = each individual observation

   n = total number of observations

   $\bar{X}$ = average value = 25

	X	$X - \bar{X}$	$(X - \bar{X})^2$
1.	25	0	
2.	25	0	
3.	24	1	1
4.	25	0	
5.	26	1	1
6.	27	2	4
7.	25	0	
8.	26	1	1
9.	23	2	4
10.	25	0	
11.	24	1	1
12.	24	1	1
13.	26	1	1
14.	25	0	
15.	27	2	4
16.	25	0	
17.	25	0	
18.	24	1	1
19.	25	0	
20.	26	1	1
21.	25	0	
22.	26	1	1
23.	26	1	1
24.	25	0	
25.	24	1	1
26.	25	0	
27.	24	1	1
28.	26	1	1
29.	25	0	
30.	24	1	1
31.	23	2	4
	25 $\bar{X}$		30 $\Sigma(X-\bar{X})^2$

Fig. 15-5. Standard deviation work sheet.

QUALITY CONTROL CHART

Month _May_ Constituent _BUN_ QC Std X̄ _25_ Lot No. _____

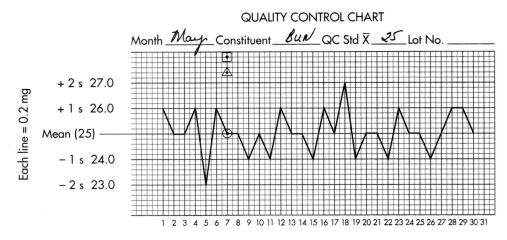

Fig. 15-6.

QUALITY CONTROL CHART

Month _____ Constituent _____ QC Std X̄ _____ Lot No. _____

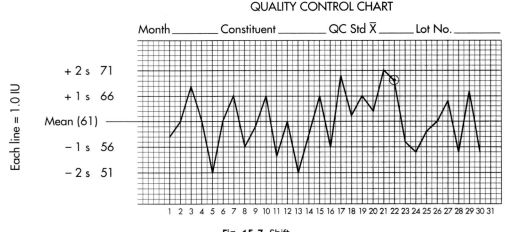

Fig. 15-7. Shift.

Fig. 15-8 shows a chart demonstrating a *trend*. The values from day 17 through 22 show a series of increasing values. The procedure for glucose determination was examined and the problem was corrected, as seen by the position of the plots for days 23 through 30.

When using the values on both of these charts to calculate the statistics for the next chart, one should not use the values that indicate the shift and the trend. These values were subject to conditions not common to the values indicating that the procedure was in control. Many technologists use these values as a matter of course. This practice results in a change of the mean and the standard deviations of the next month's chart, and the change is due to values that indicated an out-of-control condition. These values are bias and are not part of a random sample.

QUALITY CONTROL CHART

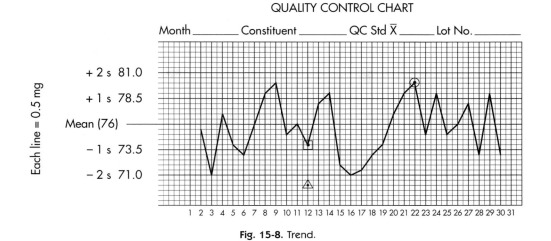

Month _____ Constituent _____ QC Std $\overline{X}$ _____ Lot No. _____

Fig. 15-8. Trend.

In Fig. 15-8 a control value fell outside the $\pm 2s$ limit at day 12 (plot △). Another control test was made and resulted in plot ⊡. The first plot was due to random error and did not indicate an out-of-control situation.

The foregoing discussion is useful for the day-to-day quality control programs of the clinical laboratory. It is a limited discussion of the use of statistics. The science of statistics includes much more than what is discussed here. This area of mathematics is so extensive that even a beginning study requires much more detail material than would be appropriate in this book. Several good books exist for most any program of the study of statistics. If more information is desired in this area, the reader should refer to more complete statistical works.

APPENDIXES RELATED TO THIS CHAPTER

H Square Root Chart
Q Formulas Presented in this Book

PRACTICE PROBLEMS

Calculate the answer for each problem. Understand each portion of the calculation and determine whether the answer is logical. *Just because an answer can be calculated does not mean that it is reasonable.*

1. When establishing 95% confidence limits for a particular method for a quality control program, one would expect how many test results to fall beyond the limits of allowable variation by chance?
   a. 1 in 95
   b. 1 in 5
   c. 1 in 10
   d. 1 in 20
   e. None

2. The following results were obtained for the three procedures listed below. Calculate the following for each procedure:

a. s

b. Range to include $\pm 2s$

c. CV

White blood cells (WBC)	BUN	Hemoglobin (Hb)
5,000	25	13.2
7,500	21	13.6
8,500	20	13.5
10,000	22	13.4
7,000	24	13.3
6,000	23	13.4
7,800	21	13.6
8,500	25	13.5
7,500	25	13.5
6,000	23	13.4
11,000	22	13.2
8,000	24	13.5
5,000	26	13.4
9,500	22	13.6
10,000	21	13.6
8,000	22	13.3
6,000	24	13.2
10,500	23	13.5

APPENDIXES

Appendix A
GREEK ALPHABET

Name of Greek letters	Capital letters	Lowercase letters	English translation
Alpha	A	α	a (ä)
Beta	B	β	b
	B (medial or terminal)	б (medial or terminal)	b
Gamma	Γ	γ	g
Delta	Δ	δ	d
Epsilon	E	ε	e (ě)
		ε (variant)	e (ě)
Zeta	Z	ζ	z
Eta	H	η	ē
Theta	Θ	θ	th
		ϑ (variant)	th
Iota	I	ι	i
Kappa	K	κ	k, c (Latin)
		ϰ (variant)	k, c (Latin)
Lambda	Λ	λ	l
Mu	M	μ	m
Nu	N	ν	n
Xi	Ξ	ξ	x (ks)
Omicron	O	o	o (ŏ)
Pi	Π	π	p
		ϖ (variant)	p
Rho	P	ρ	r, rh
		ϱ (variant)	r, rh
Sigma	Σ	σ	s
	Σ (terminal)	ς (terminal)	s
		ς (variant)	s
Tau	T	τ	t
Upsilon	Υ	υ	y (ü), u ($\overline{oo}$)
	Υ (variant)		y (ü), u ($\overline{oo}$)
Phi	Φ	φ	ph (f)
		φ (variant)	ph (f)
Chi	X	χ	ch (k)
Psi	Ψ	ψ	ps
Omega	Ω	ω	ō
		ϖ (variant)	ō

From Campbell JB, Campbell JM: *Mosby's survival guide to medical abbreviations and acronyms, prefixes and suffixes, symbols, greek alphabet,* St. Louis, 1995, Mosby.

Appendix B
SYMBOLS

Symbol	Common meaning	Symbol	Common meaning
$<$	Less than	$\not\approx$	Not approximately equal
$\not<$	Not less than	$=$	Equal to
$\leq, \leqq, \lesssim$	Less than or equal to	$\neq$	Not equal to
$\nleqq$	Neither less than nor equal	$\equiv$	Identical with
$\lesssim$	Less than or equivalent to	$\not\equiv$	Not identical with
$\ll$	Much less than	$'$	Prime, minute, feet
$\lll$	Much much less than	$''$	Double prime, second, inches
$\prec$	Precedes	$\triangle$	Change in, increment
$\not\prec$	Does not precede	$\triangleq$	Defined as
$\preceq$	Precedes or equals	$\triangleq$	Corresponds to
$\not\preceq$	Neither precedes nor equals	$+$	Plus, add
$>$	Greater than	$\pm$	Plus or minus
$\not>$	Not greater than	$-$	Minus, subtract
$\geq, \geqq, \gtrsim$	Greater than or equal to	$\times$	Multiply
$\ngeqq$	Neither greater than nor equal	$\div$	Divided by
$\gtrsim$	Greater than or equivalent to	$*$	Multiply, birth, presumed
$\gg$	Much greater than	$\dagger$	Death
$\ggg$	Much much greater than	$\#$	Number, pound
$\succ$	Follows	$\%$	Percent (per 100)
$\not\succ$	Does not follow	$\%o$	Per milli (per 1,000)
$\succeq$	Follows or equals	$\circ$	Degree
$\not\succeq$	Neither follows nor equals	$\propto$	Proportional
$<>$	Not equal to	∞	Infinity
$\rightarrow$	Yields, approaches	$(\ )$	Parenthesis
$\uparrow$	Diluted up to, given off	$[\ ]$	Brackets
$\sqrt{\ }$	Square root of	$\{\ \}$	Braces
$\because$	Because	$/$	Not (slash)
$\therefore$	Therefore	$\not/$	Does not divide
$::$	Proportion, as, varies directly as	$\parallel$	Parallel
$:$	Ratio, is to	$\nparallel$	Not parallel
$\sim$	Similar	$|\ |$	Absolute value
$\not\sim$	Not similar	$\overline{X}$	Arithmetic mean
$\simeq$	Similar or equal	Σ	Sum
$\not\simeq$	Not similar or equal	σ	Standard deviation (of population)
$\approx$	Approximately equal		

Appendix C
CARDINAL NUMBERS: ARABIC AND ROMAN

Name	Arabic symbol	Roman symbol
Naught, zero, or cipher	0	
One	1	I
Two	2	II
Three	3	III
Four	4	IV
Five	5	V
Six	6	VI
Seven	7	VII
Eight	8	VIII
Nine	9	IX
Ten	10	X
Eleven	11	XI
Twelve	12	XII
Thirteen	13	XIII
Fourteen	14	XIV
Fifteen	15	XV
Sixteen	16	XVI
Seventeen	17	XVII
Eighteen	18	XVIII
Nineteen	19	XIX
Twenty	20	XX
Twenty-one	21	XXI
Twenty-two	22	XXII
Twenty-three	23	XXIII
Twenty-four	24	XXIV
Twenty-five	25	XXV
Twenty-six	26	XXVI
Twenty-seven	27	XXVII
Twenty-eight	28	XXVIII
Twenty-nine	29	XXIX
Thirty	30	XXX
Thirty-one	31	XXXI
Forty	40	XL
Forty-one	41	XLI
Fifty	50	L
Sixty	60	LX

Continued.

CARDINAL NUMBERS: ARABIC AND ROMAN—cont'd

Name	Arabic symbol	Roman symbol
Seventy	70	LXX
Eighty	80	LXXX
Ninety	90	XC
One hundred	100	C
One hundred one	101	CI
Two hundred	200	CC
Three hundred	300	CCC
Four hundred	400	CD
Five hundred	500	D
Six hundred	600	DC
Seven hundred	700	DCC
Eight hundred	800	DCCC
Nine hundred	900	CM
One thousand or ten hundred	1,000	M
Two thousand	2,000	MM
Five thousand	5,000	$\overline{V}$
Ten thousand	10,000	$\overline{X}$
One hundred thousand	100,000	$\overline{C}$
One million	1,000,000	$\overline{M}$

Appendix D
ORDINAL NUMBERS

Name	Symbol
First	1st
Second	2d or 2nd
Third	3d or 3rd
Fourth	4th
Fifth	5th
Sixth	6th
Seventh	7th
Eighth	8th
Ninth	9th
Tenth	10th
Eleventh	11th
Twelfth	12th
Thirteenth	13th
Fourteenth	14th
Fifteenth	15th
Sixteenth	16th
Seventeenth	17th
Eighteenth	18th
Nineteenth	19th
Twentieth	20th
Twenty-first	21st
Twenty-second	22d or 22nd
Twenty-third	23d or 23rd
Twenty-fourth	24th
Twenty-fifth	25th
Twenty-sixth	26th
Twenty-seventh	27th
Twenty-eighth	28th
Twenty-ninth	29th
Thirtieth	30th
Thirty-first	31st
Thirty-second	32d or 32nd
Fortieth	40th
Forty-first	41st
Forty-second	42d or 42nd
Fiftieth	50th
Sixtieth	60th
Seventieth	70th
Eightieth	80th
Ninetieth	90th
Hundredth	100th
Hundred and first	101st

Continued.

ORDINAL NUMBERS—cont'd

Name	Symbol
Hundred and second	102d or 102nd
Two hundredth	200th
Three hundredth	300th
Four hundredth	400th
Five hundredth	500th
Six hundredth	600th
Seven hundredth	700th
Eight hundredth	800th
Nine hundredth	900th
Thousandth	1,000th
Two thousandth	2,000th
Ten thousandth	10,000th
Hundred thousandth	100,000th
Millionth	1,000,000th

Appendix E
DENOMINATIONS ABOVE ONE MILLION

Name	Value in powers of 10	Number of zeros
American system		
Billion	10^9	9
Trillion	10^{12}	12
Quadrillion	10^{15}	15
Quintillion	10^{18}	18
Sextillion	10^{21}	21
Septillion	10^{24}	24
Octillion	10^{27}	27
Nonillion	10^{30}	30
Decillion	10^{33}	33
Undecillion	10^{36}	36
Duodecillion	10^{39}	39
Tredecillion	10^{42}	42
Quattuordecillion	10^{45}	45
Quindecillion	10^{48}	48
Sexdecillion	10^{51}	51
Septendecillion	10^{54}	54
Octodecillion	10^{57}	57
Novemdecillion	10^{60}	60
Vigintillion	10^{63}	63
Centillion	10^{303}	303
British system		
Milliard	10^9	9
Billion	10^{12}	12
Trillion	10^{18}	18
Quadrillion	10^{24}	24
Quintillion	10^{30}	30
Sextillion	10^{36}	36
Septillion	10^{42}	42
Octillion	10^{48}	48
Nonillion	10^{54}	54
Decillion	10^{60}	60
Undecillion	10^{66}	66
Duodecillion	10^{72}	72
Tredecillion	10^{78}	78
Quattuordecillion	10^{84}	84
Quindecillion	10^{90}	90
Sexdecillion	10^{96}	96
Septendecillion	10^{102}	102
Octodecillion	10^{108}	108
Novemdecillion	10^{114}	114
Vigintillion	10^{120}	120
Centillion	10^{600}	600

Appendix F
FOUR-PLACE LOGARITHMS

N	0	1	2	3	4	5	6	7	8	9	Proportional Parts* 1 2 3 4 5 6 7 8 9
10	0000	0043	0086	0128	0170	0212	0253	0294	0334	0374	4 8 12 17 21 25 29 33 37
11	0414	0453	0492	0531	0569	0607	0645	0682	0719	0755	4 8 11 15 19 23 26 30 34
12	0792	0828	0864	0899	0934	0969	1004	1038	1072	1106	3 7 10 14 17 21 24 28 31
13	1139	1173	1206	1239	1271	1303	1335	1367	1399	1430	3 6 10 13 16 19 23 26 29
14	1461	1492	1523	1553	1584	1614	1644	1673	1703	1732	3 6 9 12 15 18 21 24 27
15	1761	1790	1818	1847	1875	1903	1931	1959	1987	2014	3 6 8 11 14 17 20 22 25
16	2041	2068	2095	2122	2148	2175	2201	2227	2253	2279	3 5 8 11 13 16 18 21 24
17	2304	2330	2355	2380	2405	2430	2455	2480	2504	2529	2 5 7 10 12 15 17 20 22
18	2553	2577	2601	2625	2648	2672	2695	2718	2742	2765	2 5 7 9 12 14 16 19 21
19	2788	2810	2833	2856	2878	2900	2923	2945	2967	2989	2 4 7 9 11 13 16 18 20
20	3010	3032	3054	3075	3096	3118	3139	3160	3181	3201	2 4 6 8 11 13 15 17 19
21	3222	3243	3263	3284	3304	3324	3345	3365	3385	3404	2 4 6 8 10 12 14 16 18
22	3424	3444	3464	3483	3502	3522	3541	3560	3579	3598	2 4 6 8 10 12 14 15 17
23	3617	3636	3655	3674	3692	3711	3729	3747	3766	3784	2 4 6 7 9 11 13 15 17
24	3802	3820	3838	3856	3874	3892	3909	3927	3945	3962	2 4 5 7 9 11 12 14 16
25	3979	3997	4014	4031	4048	4065	4082	4099	4116	4133	2 3 5 7 9 10 12 14 15
26	4150	4166	4183	4200	4216	4232	4249	4265	4281	4298	2 3 5 7 8 10 11 13 15
27	4314	4330	4346	4362	4378	4393	4409	4425	4440	4456	2 3 5 6 8 9 11 13 14
28	4472	4487	4502	4518	4533	4548	4564	4579	4594	4609	2 3 5 6 8 9 11 12 14
29	4624	4639	4654	4669	4683	4698	4713	4728	4742	4757	1 3 4 6 7 9 10 12 13
30	4771	4786	4800	4814	4829	4843	4857	4871	4886	4900	1 3 4 6 7 9 10 11 13
31	4914	4928	4942	4955	4969	4983	4997	5011	5024	5038	1 3 4 6 7 8 10 11 12
32	5051	5065	5079	5092	5105	5119	5132	5145	5159	5172	1 3 4 5 7 8 9 11 12
33	5185	5198	5211	5224	5237	5250	5263	5276	5289	5302	1 3 4 5 6 8 9 10 12
34	5315	5328	5340	5353	5366	5378	5391	5403	5416	5428	1 3 4 5 6 8 9 10 11
35	5441	5453	5465	5478	5490	5502	5514	5527	5539	5551	1 2 4 5 6 7 9 10 11
36	5563	5575	5587	5599	5611	5623	5635	5647	5658	5670	1 2 4 5 6 7 8 10 11
37	5682	5694	5705	5717	5729	5740	5752	5763	5775	5786	1 2 3 5 6 7 8 9 10
38	5798	5809	5821	5832	5843	5855	5866	5877	5888	5899	1 2 3 5 6 7 8 9 10
39	5911	5922	5933	5944	5955	5966	5977	5988	5999	6010	1 2 3 4 5 7 8 9 10
40	6021	6031	6042	6053	6064	6075	6085	6096	6107	6117	1 2 3 4 5 6 8 9 10
41	6128	6138	6149	6160	6170	6180	6191	6201	6212	6222	1 2 3 4 5 6 7 8 9
42	6232	6243	6253	6263	6274	6284	6294	6304	6314	6325	1 2 3 4 5 6 7 8 9
43	6335	6345	6355	6365	6375	6385	6395	6405	6415	6425	1 2 3 4 5 6 7 8 9
44	6435	6444	6454	6464	6474	6484	6493	6503	6513	6522	1 2 3 4 5 6 7 8 9
45	6532	6542	6551	6561	6571	6580	6590	6599	6609	6618	1 2 3 4 5 6 7 8 9
46	6628	6637	6646	6656	6665	6675	6684	6693	6702	6712	1 2 3 4 5 6 7 7 8
47	6721	6730	6739	6749	6758	6767	6776	6785	6794	6803	1 2 3 4 5 5 6 7 8
48	6812	6821	6830	6839	6848	6857	6866	6875	6884	6893	1 2 3 4 4 5 6 7 8
49	6902	6911	6920	6928	6937	6946	6955	6964	6972	6981	1 2 3 4 4 5 6 7 8
50	6990	6998	7007	7016	7024	7033	7042	7050	7059	7067	1 2 3 3 4 5 6 7 8
51	7076	7084	7093	7101	7110	7118	7126	7135	7143	7152	1 2 3 3 4 5 6 7 8
52	7160	7168	7177	7185	7193	7202	7210	7218	7226	7235	1 2 2 3 4 5 6 7 7
53	7243	7251	7259	7267	7275	7284	7292	7300	7308	7316	1 2 2 3 4 5 6 6 7
54	7324	7332	7340	7348	7356	7364	7372	7380	7388	7396	1 2 2 3 4 5 6 6 7
N	0	1	2	3	4	5	6	7	8	9	1 2 3 4 5 6 7 8 9

*Interpolation in this section of the table may not be accurate.

N	0	1	2	3	4	5	6	7	8	9	Proportional Parts *								
											1	2	3	4	5	6	7	8	9
55	7404	7412	7419	7427	7435	7443	7451	7459	7466	7474	1	2	2	3	4	5	5	6	7
56	7482	7490	7497	7505	7513	7520	7528	7536	7543	7551	1	2	2	3	4	5	5	6	7
57	7559	7566	7574	7582	7589	7597	7604	7612	7619	7627	1	2	2	3	4	5	5	6	7
58	7634	7642	7649	7657	7664	7672	7679	7686	7694	7701	1	1	2	3	4	4	5	6	7
59	7709	7716	7723	7731	7738	7745	7752	7760	7767	7774	1	1	2	3	4	4	5	6	7
60	7782	7789	7796	7803	7810	7818	7825	7832	7839	7846	1	1	2	3	4	4	5	6	6
61	7853	7860	7868	7875	7882	7889	7896	7903	7910	7917	1	1	2	3	4	4	5	6	6
62	7924	7931	7938	7945	7952	7959	7966	7973	7980	7987	1	1	2	3	3	4	5	6	6
63	7993	8000	8007	8014	8021	8028	8035	8041	8048	8055	1	1	2	3	3	4	5	5	6
64	8062	8069	8075	8082	8089	8096	8102	8109	8116	8122	1	1	2	3	3	4	5	5	6
65	8129	8136	8142	8149	8156	8162	8169	8176	8182	8189	1	1	2	3	3	4	5	5	6
66	8195	8202	8209	8215	8222	8228	8235	8241	8248	8254	1	1	2	3	3	4	5	5	6
67	8261	8267	8274	8280	8287	8293	8299	8306	8312	8319	1	1	2	3	3	4	5	5	6
68	8325	8331	8338	8344	8351	8357	8363	8370	8376	8382	1	1	2	3	3	4	4	5	6
69	8388	8395	8401	8407	8414	8420	8426	8432	8439	8445	1	1	2	2	3	4	4	5	6
70	8451	8457	8463	8470	8476	8482	8488	8494	8500	8506	1	1	2	2	3	4	4	5	6
71	8513	8519	8525	8531	8537	8543	8549	8555	8561	8567	1	1	2	2	3	4	4	5	5
72	8573	8579	8585	8591	8597	8603	8609	8615	8621	8627	1	1	2	2	3	4	4	5	5
73	8633	8639	8645	8651	8657	8663	8669	8675	8681	8686	1	1	2	2	3	4	4	5	5
74	8692	8698	8704	8710	8716	8722	8727	8733	8739	8745	1	1	2	2	3	4	4	5	5
75	8751	8756	8762	8768	8774	8779	8785	8791	8797	8802	1	1	2	2	3	3	4	5	5
76	8808	8814	8820	8825	8831	8837	8842	8848	8854	8859	1	1	2	2	3	3	4	5	5
77	8865	8871	8876	8882	8887	8893	8899	8904	8910	8915	1	1	2	2	3	3	4	4	5
78	8921	8927	8932	8938	8943	8949	8954	8960	8965	8971	1	1	2	2	3	3	4	4	5
79	8976	8982	8987	8993	8998	9004	9009	9015	9020	9025	1	1	2	2	3	3	4	4	5
80	9031	9036	9042	9047	9053	9058	9063	9069	9074	9079	1	1	2	2	3	3	4	4	5
81	9085	9090	9096	9101	9106	9112	9117	9122	9128	9133	1	1	2	2	3	3	4	4	5
82	9138	9143	9149	9154	9159	9165	9170	9175	9180	9186	1	1	2	2	3	3	4	4	5
83	9191	9196	9201	9206	9212	9217	9222	9227	9232	9238	1	1	2	2	3	3	4	4	5
84	9243	9248	9253	9258	9263	9269	9274	9279	9284	9289	1	1	2	2	3	3	4	4	5
85	9294	9299	9304	9309	9315	9320	9325	9330	9335	9340	1	1	2	2	3	3	4	4	5
86	9345	9350	9355	9360	9365	9370	9375	9380	9385	9390	1	1	2	2	3	3	4	4	5
87	9395	9400	9405	9410	9415	9420	9425	9430	9435	9440	0	1	1	2	2	3	3	4	4
88	9445	9450	9455	9460	9465	9469	9474	9479	9484	9489	0	1	1	2	2	3	3	4	4
89	9494	9499	9504	9509	9513	9518	9523	9528	9533	9538	0	1	1	2	2	3	3	4	4
90	9542	9547	9552	9557	9562	9566	9571	9576	9581	9586	0	1	1	2	2	3	3	4	4
91	9590	9595	9600	9605	9609	9614	9619	9624	9628	9633	0	1	1	2	2	3	3	4	4
92	9638	9643	9647	9652	9657	9661	9666	9671	9675	9680	0	1	1	2	2	3	3	4	4
93	9685	9689	9694	9699	9703	9708	9713	9717	9722	9727	0	1	1	2	2	3	3	4	4
94	9731	9736	9741	9745	9750	9754	9759	9763	9768	9773	0	1	1	2	2	3	3	4	4
95	9777	9782	9786	9791	9795	9800	9805	9809	9814	9818	0	1	1	2	2	3	3	4	4
96	9823	9827	9832	9836	9841	9845	9850	9854	9859	9863	0	1	1	2	2	3	3	4	4
97	9868	9872	9877	9881	9886	9890	9894	9899	9903	9908	0	1	1	2	2	3	3	4	4
98	9912	9917	9921	9926	9930	9934	9939	9943	9948	9952	0	1	1	2	2	3	3	4	4
99	9956	9961	9965	9969	9974	9978	9983	9987	9991	9996	0	1	1	2	2	3	3	3	4
N	0	1	2	3	4	5	6	7	8	9	1	2	3	4	5	6	7	8	9

*Interpolation in this section of the table may not be accurate.

Appendix G
ANTILOGARITHMS

	0	1	2	3	4	5	6	7	8	9	Proportional Parts * 1 2 3 4 5 6 7 8 9
.00	1000	1002	1005	1007	1009	1012	1014	1016	1019	1021	0 0 1 1 1 1 2 2 2
.01	1023	1026	1028	1030	1033	1035	1038	1040	1042	1045	0 0 1 1 1 1 2 2 2
.02	1047	1050	1052	1054	1057	1059	1062	1064	1067	1069	0 0 1 1 1 1 2 2 2
.03	1072	1074	1076	1079	1081	1084	1086	1089	1091	1094	0 0 1 1 1 1 2 2 2
.04	1096	1099	1102	1104	1107	1109	1112	1114	1117	1119	0 1 1 1 1 2 2 2 2
.05	1122	1125	1127	1130	1132	1135	1138	1140	1143	1146	0 1 1 1 1 2 2 2 2
.06	1148	1151	1153	1156	1159	1161	1164	1167	1169	1172	0 1 1 1 1 2 2 2 2
.07	1175	1178	1180	1183	1186	1189	1191	1194	1197	1199	0 1 1 1 1 2 2 2 2
.08	1202	1205	1208	1211	1213	1216	1219	1222	1225	1227	0 1 1 1 1 2 2 2 3
.09	1230	1233	1236	1239	1242	1245	1247	1250	1253	1256	0 1 1 1 1 2 2 2 3
.10	1259	1262	1265	1268	1271	1274	1276	1279	1282	1285	0 1 1 1 1 2 2 2 3
.11	1288	1291	1294	1297	1300	1303	1306	1309	1312	1315	0 1 1 1 2 2 2 3 3
.12	1318	1321	1324	1327	1330	1334	1337	1340	1343	1346	0 1 1 1 2 2 2 3 3
.13	1349	1352	1355	1358	1361	1365	1368	1371	1374	1377	0 1 1 1 2 2 2 3 3
.14	1380	1384	1387	1390	1393	1396	1400	1403	1406	1409	0 1 1 1 2 2 2 3 3
.15	1413	1416	1419	1422	1426	1429	1432	1435	1439	1442	0 1 1 1 2 2 2 3 3
.16	1445	1449	1452	1455	1459	1462	1466	1469	1472	1476	0 1 1 1 2 2 2 3 3
.17	1479	1483	1486	1489	1493	1496	1500	1503	1507	1510	0 1 1 1 2 2 2 3 3
.18	1514	1517	1521	1524	1528	1531	1535	1538	1542	1545	0 1 1 1 2 2 3 3 3
.19	1549	1552	1556	1560	1563	1567	1570	1574	1578	1581	0 1 1 1 2 2 3 3 3
.20	1585	1589	1592	1596	1600	1603	1607	1611	1614	1618	0 1 1 2 2 2 3 3 3
.21	1622	1626	1629	1633	1637	1641	1644	1648	1652	1656	0 1 1 2 2 2 3 3 3
.22	1660	1663	1667	1671	1675	1679	1683	1687	1690	1694	0 1 1 2 2 2 3 3 3
.23	1698	1702	1706	1710	1714	1718	1722	1726	1730	1734	0 1 1 2 2 2 3 3 4
.24	1738	1742	1746	1750	1754	1758	1762	1766	1770	1774	0 1 1 2 2 2 3 3 4
.25	1778	1782	1786	1791	1795	1799	1803	1807	1811	1816	0 1 1 2 2 2 3 3 4
.26	1820	1824	1828	1832	1837	1841	1845	1849	1854	1858	0 1 1 2 2 3 3 3 4
.27	1862	1866	1871	1875	1879	1884	1888	1892	1897	1901	0 1 1 2 2 3 3 3 4
.28	1905	1910	1914	1919	1923	1928	1932	1936	1941	1945	0 1 1 2 2 3 3 4 4
.29	1950	1954	1959	1963	1968	1972	1977	1982	1986	1991	0 1 1 2 2 3 3 4 4
.30	1995	2000	2004	2009	2014	2018	2023	2028	2032	2037	0 1 1 2 2 3 3 4 4
.31	2042	2046	2051	2056	2061	2065	2070	2075	2080	2084	0 1 1 2 2 3 3 4 4
.32	2089	2094	2099	2104	2109	2113	2118	2123	2128	2133	0 1 1 2 2 3 3 4 4
.33	2138	2143	2148	2153	2158	2163	2168	2173	2178	2183	0 1 1 2 2 3 3 4 4
.34	2188	2193	2198	2203	2208	2213	2218	2223	2228	2234	1 1 2 2 3 3 4 4 5
.35	2239	2244	2249	2254	2259	2265	2270	2275	2280	2286	1 1 2 2 3 3 4 4 5
.36	2291	2296	2301	2307	2312	2317	2323	2328	2333	2339	1 1 2 2 3 3 4 4 5
.37	2344	2350	2355	2360	2366	2371	2377	2382	2388	2393	1 1 2 2 3 3 4 4 5
.38	2399	2404	2410	2415	2421	2427	2432	2438	2443	2449	1 1 2 2 3 3 4 4 5
.39	2455	2460	2466	2472	2477	2483	2489	2495	2500	2506	1 1 2 2 3 3 4 5 5
.40	2512	2518	2523	2529	2535	2541	2547	2553	2559	2564	1 1 2 2 3 4 4 5 5
.41	2570	2576	2582	2588	2594	2600	2606	2612	2618	2624	1 1 2 2 3 4 4 5 5
.42	2630	2636	2642	2649	2655	2661	2667	2673	2679	2685	1 1 2 3 3 4 4 5 6
.43	2692	2698	2704	2710	2716	2723	2729	2735	2742	2748	1 1 2 3 3 4 4 5 6
.44	2754	2761	2767	2773	2780	2786	2793	2799	2805	2812	1 1 2 3 3 4 4 5 6
.45	2818	2825	2831	2838	2844	2851	2858	2864	2871	2877	1 1 2 3 3 4 5 5 6
.46	2884	2891	2897	2904	2911	2917	2924	2931	2938	2944	1 1 2 3 3 4 5 5 6
.47	2951	2958	2965	2972	2979	2985	2992	2999	3006	3018	1 1 2 3 3 4 5 5 6
.48	3020	3027	3034	3041	3048	3055	3062	3069	3076	3083	1 1 2 3 4 4 5 6 6
.49	3090	3097	3105	3112	3119	3126	3133	3141	3148	3155	1 1 2 3 4 4 5 6 6
	0	1	2	3	4	5	6	7	8	9	1 2 3 4 5 6 7 8 9

*Interpolation in this section of the table may not be accurate.

	0	1	2	3	4	5	6	7	8	9	Proportional Parts*								
											1	2	3	4	5	6	7	8	9
.50	3162	3170	3177	3184	3192	3199	3206	3214	3221	3228	1	1	2	3	4	4	5	6	7
.51	3236	3243	3251	3258	3266	3273	3281	3289	3296	3304	1	2	2	3	4	5	5	6	7
.52	3311	3319	3327	3334	3342	3350	3357	3365	3373	3381	1	2	2	3	4	5	5	6	7
.53	3388	3396	3404	3412	3420	3428	3436	3443	3451	3459	1	2	2	3	4	5	6	6	7
.54	3467	3475	3483	3491	3499	3508	3516	3524	3532	3540	1	2	2	3	4	5	6	6	7
.55	3548	3556	3565	3573	3581	3589	3597	3606	3614	3622	1	2	2	3	4	5	6	7	7
.56	3631	3639	3648	3656	3664	3673	3681	3690	3698	3707	1	2	3	3	4	5	6	7	8
.57	3715	3724	3733	3741	3750	3758	3767	3776	3784	3793	1	2	3	3	4	5	6	7	8
.58	3802	3811	3819	3828	3837	3846	3855	3864	3873	3882	1	2	3	4	4	5	6	7	8
.59	3890	3899	3908	3917	3926	3936	3945	3954	3963	3972	1	2	3	4	5	5	6	7	8
.60	3981	3990	3999	4009	4018	4027	4036	4046	4055	4064	1	2	3	4	5	6	6	7	8
.61	4074	4083	4093	4102	4111	4121	4130	4140	4150	4159	1	2	3	4	5	6	7	8	9
.62	4169	4178	4188	4198	4207	4217	4227	4236	4246	4256	1	2	3	4	5	6	7	8	9
.63	4266	4276	4285	4295	4305	4315	4325	4335	4345	4355	1	2	3	4	5	6	7	8	9
.64	4365	4375	4385	4395	4406	4416	4426	4436	4446	4457	1	2	3	4	5	6	7	8	9
.65	4467	4477	4487	4498	4508	4519	4529	4539	4550	4560	1	2	3	4	5	6	7	8	9
.66	4571	4581	4592	4603	4613	4624	4634	4645	4656	4667	1	2	3	4	5	6	7	9	10
.67	4677	4688	4699	4710	4721	4732	4742	4753	4764	4775	1	2	3	4	5	7	8	9	10
.68	4786	4797	4808	4819	4831	4842	4853	4864	4875	4887	1	2	3	4	6	7	8	9	10
.69	4898	4909	4920	4932	4943	4955	4966	4977	4989	5000	1	2	3	5	6	7	8	9	10
.70	5012	5023	5035	5047	5058	5070	5082	5093	5105	5117	1	2	4	5	6	7	8	9	11
.71	5129	5140	5152	5164	5176	5188	5200	5212	5224	5236	1	2	4	5	6	7	8	10	11
.72	5248	5260	5272	5284	5297	5309	5321	5333	5346	5358	1	2	4	5	6	7	9	10	11
.73	5370	5383	5395	5408	5420	5433	5445	5458	5470	5483	1	3	4	5	6	8	9	10	11
.74	5495	5508	5521	5534	5546	5559	5572	5585	5598	5610	1	3	4	5	6	8	9	10	12
.75	5623	5636	5649	5662	5675	5689	5702	5715	5728	5741	1	3	4	5	7	8	9	10	12
.76	5754	5768	5781	5794	5808	5821	5834	5848	5861	5875	1	3	4	5	7	8	9	11	12
.77	5888	5902	5916	5929	5943	5957	5970	5984	5998	6012	1	3	4	5	7	8	10	11	12
.78	6026	6039	6053	6067	6081	6095	6109	6124	6138	6152	1	3	4	6	7	8	10	11	13
.79	6166	6180	6194	6209	6223	6237	6252	6266	6281	6295	1	3	4	6	7	9	10	11	13
.80	6310	6324	6339	6353	6368	6383	6397	6412	6427	6442	1	3	4	6	7	9	10	12	13
.81	6457	6471	6486	6501	6516	6531	6546	6561	6577	6592	2	3	5	6	8	9	11	12	14
.82	6607	6622	6637	6653	6668	6683	6699	6714	6730	6745	2	3	5	6	8	9	11	12	14
.83	6761	6776	6792	6808	6823	6839	6855	6871	6887	6902	2	3	5	6	8	9	11	13	14
.84	6918	6934	6950	6966	6982	6998	7015	7031	7047	7063	2	3	5	6	8	10	11	13	15
.85	7079	7096	7112	7129	7145	7161	7178	7194	7211	7228	2	3	5	7	8	10	12	13	15
.86	7244	7261	7278	7295	7311	7328	7345	7362	7379	7396	2	3	5	7	8	10	12	13	15
.87	7413	7430	7447	7464	7482	7499	7516	7534	7551	7568	2	3	5	7	9	10	12	14	16
.88	7586	7603	7621	7638	7656	7674	7691	7709	7727	7745	2	4	5	7	9	11	12	14	16
.89	7762	7780	7798	7816	7834	7852	7870	7889	7907	7925	2	4	5	7	9	11	13	14	16
.90	7943	7962	7980	7998	8017	8035	8054	8072	8091	8110	2	4	6	7	9	11	13	15	17
.91	8128	8147	8166	8185	8204	8222	8241	8260	8279	8299	2	4	6	8	9	11	13	15	17
.92	8318	8337	8356	8375	8395	8414	8433	8453	8472	8492	2	4	6	8	10	12	14	15	17
.93	8511	8531	8551	8570	8590	8610	8630	8650	8670	8690	2	4	6	8	10	12	14	16	18
.94	8710	8730	8750	8770	8790	8810	8831	8851	8872	8892	2	4	6	8	10	12	14	16	18
.95	8913	8933	8954	8974	8995	9016	9036	9057	9078	9099	2	4	6	8	10	12	15	17	19
.96	9120	9141	9162	9183	9204	9226	9247	9268	9290	9311	2	4	6	8	11	13	15	17	19
.97	9333	9354	9376	9397	9419	9441	9462	9484	9506	9528	2	4	7	9	11	13	15	17	20
.98	9550	9572	9594	9616	9638	9661	9683	9705	9727	9750	2	4	7	9	11	13	16	18	20
.99	9772	9795	9817	9840	9863	9886	9908	9931	9954	9977	2	5	7	9	11	14	16	18	20
	0	1	2	3	4	5	6	7	8	9	1	2	3	4	5	6	7	8	9

*Interpolation in this section of the table may not be accurate.

Appendix H
SQUARE ROOT CHART

The columns designated with the square root sign ($\sqrt{}$) are the numbers for which the square root is to be determined. The columns to the right contain the numbers that are the square root values. For example, the square root of 1.2 is 1.09 ($1.09 \times 1.09 = 1.2$). The square root of 5 is 2.24, the square root of 10.8 is 3.29.

To determine square roots of numbers from 0.01 to 0.099 and from 0.10 to 0.99:
1. Move the decimal point (of the number for which you want the square root) two places to the right (0.02 becomes 2.0).
2. Move the decimal point of the number in the column to the right of the square root column one place to the left (1.41 becomes 0.141).

EXAMPLE: What is the square root of 0.02?
   1. Move the decimal point two places to the right to get 2.0.
   2. Opposite 2.0, find the square root number 1.41.
   3. Move the decimal point one place to the left (1.41 becomes 0.141).
   4. The square root of 0.02 ($\sqrt{0.02}$) is 0.141.

EXAMPLE: What is the square root of 0.96?
   1. Move the decimal point two places to the right (0.96 becomes 96).
   2. Opposite 96 is 9.80.
   3. Move the decimal point one place to the left (9.80 becomes 0.98).
   4. The square root of 0.96 ($\sqrt{0.96}$) is 0.98.

Square Roots of Numbers from 1 to 100 in Steps of 0.2

$\sqrt{1.0}$	1.00	$\sqrt{11.0}$	3.32	$\sqrt{21.0}$	4.58	$\sqrt{31.0}$	5.57	$\sqrt{41.0}$	6.40
1.2	1.09	11.2	3.35	21.2	4.60	31.2	5.59	41.2	6.42
1.4	1.18	11.4	3.38	21.4	4.63	31.4	5.60	41.4	6.43
1.6	1.26	11.6	3.41	21.6	4.65	31.6	5.62	41.6	6.45
1.8	1.34	11.8	3.44	21.8	4.67	31.8	5.64	41.8	6.47
2.0	1.41	12.0	3.46	22.0	4.69	32.0	5.66	42.0	6.48
2.2	1.48	12.2	3.49	22.2	4.71	32.2	5.67	42.2	6.50
2.4	1.55	12.4	3.52	22.4	4.73	32.4	5.69	42.4	6.51
2.6	1.61	12.6	3.55	22.6	4.75	32.6	5.71	42.6	6.53
2.8	1.67	12.8	3.58	22.8	4.77	32.8	5.73	42.8	6.54
3.0	1.73	13.0	3.61	23.0	4.80	33.0	5.74	43.0	6.56
3.2	1.79	13.2	3.63	23.2	4.82	33.2	5.76	43.2	6.57
3.4	1.84	13.4	3.66	23.4	4.84	33.4	5.78	43.4	6.59
3.6	1.90	13.6	3.69	23.6	4.86	33.6	5.80	43.6	6.60
3.8	1.95	13.8	3.71	23.8	4.88	33.8	5.81	43.8	6.62
4.0	2.00	14.0	3.74	24.0	4.90	34.0	5.83	44.0	6.63
4.2	2.05	14.2	3.77	24.2	4.92	34.2	5.85	44.2	6.65
4.4	2.10	14.4	3.79	24.4	4.94	34.4	5.87	44.4	6.66
4.6	2.14	14.6	3.82	24.6	4.96	34.6	5.88	44.6	6.68
4.8	2.19	14.8	3.85	24.8	4.98	34.8	5.90	44.8	6.69
5.0	2.24	15.0	3.87	25.0	5.00	35.0	5.92	45.0	6.71
5.2	2.28	15.2	3.90	25.2	5.02	35.2	5.93	45.2	6.72
5.4	2.32	15.4	3.92	25.4	5.04	35.4	5.95	45.4	6.74
5.6	2.37	15.6	3.95	25.6	5.06	35.6	5.97	45.6	6.75
5.8	2.41	15.8	3.97	25.8	5.08	35.8	5.98	45.8	6.77
6.0	2.45	16.0	4.00	26.0	5.10	36.0	6.00	46.0	6.78
6.2	2.49	16.2	4.02	26.2	5.12	36.2	6.02	46.2	6.80
6.4	2.53	16.4	4.05	26.4	5.14	36.4	6.03	46.4	6.81
6.6	2.57	16.6	4.07	26.6	5.16	36.6	6.05	46.6	6.83
6.8	2.61	16.8	4.10	26.8	5.18	36.8	6.07	46.8	6.84
7.0	2.65	17.0	4.12	27.0	5.20	37.0	6.08	47.0	6.86
7.2	2.68	17.2	4.15	27.2	5.22	37.2	6.10	47.2	6.87
7.4	2.72	17.4	4.17	27.4	5.23	37.4	6.12	47.4	6.88
7.6	2.76	17.6	4.20	27.6	5.25	37.6	6.13	47.6	6.90
7.8	2.79	17.8	4.22	27.8	5.27	37.8	6.15	47.8	6.91
8.0	2.83	18.0	4.24	28.0	5.29	38.0	6.16	48.0	6.93
8.2	2.86	18.2	4.27	28.2	5.31	38.2	6.18	48.2	6.94
8.4	2.90	18.4	4.29	28.4	5.33	38.4	6.20	48.4	6.96
8.6	2.93	18.6	4.31	28.6	5.35	38.6	6.21	48.6	6.97
8.8	2.97	18.8	4.34	28.8	5.37	38.8	6.23	48.8	6.99
9.0	3.00	19.0	4.36	29.0	5.39	39.0	6.24	49.0	7.00
9.2	3.03	19.2	4.38	29.2	5.40	39.2	6.26	49.2	7.01
9.4	3.07	19.4	4.40	29.4	5.42	39.4	6.28	49.4	7.03
9.6	3.10	19.6	4.43	29.6	5.44	39.6	6.29	49.6	7.04
9.8	3.13	19.8	4.45	29.8	5.46	39.8	6.31	49.8	7.06
10.0	3.16	20.0	4.47	30.0	5.48	40.0	6.32	50.0	7.07
10.2	3.19	20.2	4.49	30.2	5.50	40.2	6.34	50.2	7.09
10.4	3.22	20.4	4.52	30.4	5.51	40.4	6.36	50.4	7.10
10.6	3.26	20.6	4.54	30.6	5.53	40.6	6.37	50.6	7.11
10.8	3.29	20.8	4.56	30.8	5.55	40.8	6.39	50.8	7.13

Square Roots of Numbers from 1 to 100 in Steps of 0.2—cont'd

$\sqrt{51.0}$	7.14	$\sqrt{61.0}$	7.81	$\sqrt{71.0}$	8.43	$\sqrt{81.0}$	9.00	$\sqrt{91.0}$	9.54
51.2	7.16	61.2	7.82	71.2	8.44	81.2	9.01	91.2	9.55
51.4	7.17	61.4	7.84	71.4	8.45	81.4	9.02	91.4	9.56
51.6	7.18	61.6	7.85	71.6	8.46	81.6	9.03	91.6	9.57
51.8	7.20	61.8	7.86	71.8	8.47	81.8	9.04	91.8	9.58
52.0	7.21	62.0	7.87	72.0	8.49	82.0	9.06	92.0	9.59
52.2	7.22	62.2	7.89	72.2	8.50	82.2	9.07	92.2	9.60
52.4	7.24	62.4	7.90	72.4	8.51	82.4	9.08	92.4	9.61
52.6	7.25	62.6	7.91	72.6	8.52	82.6	9.09	92.6	9.62
52.8	7.27	62.8	7.92	72.8	8.53	82.8	9.10	92.8	9.63
53.0	7.28	63.0	7.94	73.0	8.54	83.0	9.11	93.0	9.64
53.2	7.29	63.2	7.95	73.2	8.56	83.2	9.12	93.2	9.65
53.4	7.31	63.4	7.96	73.4	8.57	83.4	9.13	93.4	9.66
53.6	7.32	63.6	7.97	73.6	8.58	83.6	9.14	93.6	9.67
53.8	7.33	63.8	7.99	73.8	8.59	83.8	9.15	93.8	9.68
54.0	7.35	64.0	8.00	74.0	8.60	84.0	9.17	94.0	9.70
54.2	7.36	64.2	8.01	74.2	8.61	84.2	9.18	94.2	9.71
54.4	7.38	64.4	8.02	74.4	8.63	84.4	9.19	94.4	9.72
54.6	7.39	64.6	8.04	74.6	8.64	84.6	9.20	94.6	9.73
54.8	7.40	64.8	8.05	74.8	8.65	84.8	9.21	94.8	9.74
55.0	7.42	65.0	8.06	75.0	8.66	85.0	9.22	95.0	9.75
55.2	7.43	65.2	8.07	75.2	8.67	85.2	9.23	95.2	9.76
55.4	7.44	65.4	8.09	75.4	8.68	85.4	9.24	95.4	9.77
55.6	7.46	65.6	8.10	75.6	8.69	85.6	9.25	95.6	9.78
55.8	7.47	65.8	8.11	75.8	8.71	85.8	9.26	95.8	9.79
56.0	7.48	66.0	8.12	76.0	8.72	86.0	9.27	96.0	9.80
56.2	7.50	66.2	8.14	76.2	8.73	86.2	9.28	96.2	9.81
56.4	7.51	66.4	8.15	76.4	8.74	86.4	9.30	96.4	9.82
56.6	7.52	66.6	8.16	76.6	8.75	86.6	9.31	96.6	9.83
56.8	7.54	66.8	8.17	76.8	8.76	86.8	9.32	96.8	9.84
57.0	7.55	67.0	8.19	77.0	8.77	87.0	9.33	97.0	9.85
57.2	7.57	67.2	8.20	77.2	8.79	87.2	9.34	97.2	9.86
57.4	7.58	67.4	8.21	77.4	8.80	87.4	9.35	97.4	9.87
57.6	7.59	67.6	8.22	77.6	8.81	87.6	9.36	97.6	9.88
57.8	7.60	67.8	8.23	77.8	8.82	87.8	9.37	97.8	9.89
58.0	7.62	68.0	8.25	78.0	8.83	88.0	9.38	98.0	9.90
58.2	7.63	68.2	8.26	78.2	8.84	88.2	9.39	98.2	9.91
58.4	7.64	68.4	8.27	78.4	8.85	88.4	9.40	98.4	9.92
58.6	7.66	68.6	8.28	78.6	8.87	88.6	9.41	98.6	9.93
58.8	7.67	68.8	8.29	78.8	8.88	88.8	9.42	98.8	9.94
59.0	7.68	69.0	8.31	79.0	8.89	89.0	9.43	99.0	9.95
59.2	7.69	69.2	8.32	79.2	8.90	89.2	9.44	99.2	9.96
59.4	7.71	69.4	8.33	79.4	8.91	89.4	9.46	99.4	9.97
59.6	7.72	69.6	8.34	79.6	8.92	89.6	9.47	99.6	9.98
59.8	7.73	69.8	8.35	79.8	8.93	89.8	9.48	99.8	9.99
60.0	7.75	70.0	8.37	80.0	8.94	90.0	9.49	100.00	10.00
60.2	7.76	70.2	8.38	80.2	8.96	90.2	9.50		
60.4	7.77	70.4	8.39	80.4	8.97	90.4	9.51		
60.6	7.78	70.6	8.40	80.6	8.98	90.6	9.52		
60.8	7.80	70.8	8.41	80.8	8.99	90.8	9.53		

Appendix I
SYMBOLS OF UNITS OF MEASURE

Unit	Symbol	Unit	Symbol
Angstrom	Å	Dram (US fluid)	fl dr
Atmosphere	atm	Exa-	E
Atto-	a	Exagram	Eg
Attogram	ag	Exaliter	El
Attoliter	al	Exameter	Em
Attometer	am	Femto-	f
Celsius, degree	°C	Femtogram	fg
Centi-	c	Femtoliter	fl
Centigram	cg	Femtometer	fm
Centiliter	cl	Foot	ft, '
Centimeter	cm	Gallon	gal
Cubic attometer	am^3	Giga-	G
Cubic centimeter	cm^3	Gigagram	Gg
Cubic decimeter	dm^3	Gigaliter	Gl
Cubic dekameter	dam^3	Gigameter	Gm
Cubic exameter	Em^3	Grain	gr
Cubic femtometer	fm^3	Gram	g
Cubic foot	ft^3	Hecto-	h
Cubic gigameter	Gm^3	Hectogram	hg
Cubic hectometer	hm^3	Hectoliter	hl
Cubic inch	in^3	Hectometer	hm
Cubic kilometer	km^3	Hour	h
Cubic megameter	Mm^3	Hundredweight	cwt
Cubic meter	m^3	Inch	in, "
Cubic micrometer	μm^3	Katal	kat
Cubic mile	mi^3	Kelvin, degree	K
Cubic millimeter	mm^3	Kilo-	k
Cubic nanometer	nm^3	Kilogram	kg
Cubic petameter	Pm^3	Kiloliter	kl
Cubic picometer	pm^3	Kilometer	km
Cubic terameter	Tm^3	Liter	l, L*
Cubic yard	yd^3	Mega-	M
Day	d	Megagram	Mg
Deci	d	Megaliter	Ml
Decigram	dg	Megameter	Mm
Deciliter	dl	Meter	m
Decimeter	dm	Micro-	μ
Deka-	da	Microgram	μg
Dekagram	dag	Microliter	μl
Dekaliter	dal	Micrometer	μm
Dekameter	dam	Mile	mi
Dram (apoth. or troy)	dr ap, ʒ	Milli-	m
Dram (avdp.)	dr avdp	Milliequivalent	mEq

*The capital "L" is recommended for liter to avoid confusion with the numeral "1".

Unit	Symbol	Unit	Symbol
Milligram	mg	Square centimeter	cm^2
Milliliter	ml	Square decimeter	dm^2
Millimeter	mm	Square dekameter	dam^2
Minum	♏	Square exameter	Em^2
Minute	min	Square femtometer	fm^2
Nano-	n	Square feet	ft^2
Nanogram	ng	Square gigameter	Gm^2
Nanoliter	nl	Square hectometer	hm^2
Nanometer	nm	Square inch	in^2
Ounce (apoth or troy)	oz ap, ℥	Square kilometer	km^2
Ounce (avdp)	oz avdp	Square megameter	Mm^2
Ounce (fluid)	fl oz	Square meter	m^2
Peta-	P	Square micrometer	μm^2
Petagram	Pg	Square miles	mi^2
Petaliter	Pl	Square millimeter	mm^2
Petameter	Pm	Square nanometer	nm^2
Pico-	p	Square petameter	Pm^2
Picogram	pg	Square picometer	pm^2
Picoliter	pl	Square terameter	Tm^2
Picometer	pm	Square yard	yd^2
Pint	pt	Tera-	T
Pound (apoth)	lb ap	Teragram	Tg
Pound (avoir)	lb avdp, #	Teraliter	Tl
Pound (troy)	lb tr	Terameter	Tm
Scruple	s ap, ℈	Tons (metric)	t
Second	s	Yard	yd
Square attometer	am^2	Year	a, yr

Appendix J
APOTHECARY, AVOIRDUPOIS, AND TROY SYSTEMS OF MEASURE

The grain is the same in all three systems: 1 grain = 64.8 milligrams = 0.0648 gram.

1. Apothecaries' weight: a system of weights used in compounding prescriptions, based on the grain (64.8 mg) and the minim (0.061610 ml).

Dry	**Liquid (US)**
Grain = 64.8 milligrams	Minim = 0.061610 milliliters
Scruple = 20 grains	Fluid dram = 60 minims
Dram = 3 scruples	Fluid ounce = 8 fluid drams
Ounce = 8 drams	Gill = 4 fluid ounces
Pound = 12 ounces	Pint = 4 gills
	Quart = 2 pints
	Gallon = 4 quarts

2. Avoirdupois weight: the system of weight commonly used for ordinary commodities in English-speaking countries.

Grain = 64.8 milligrams
Dram = 27.344 grains
Ounce = 16 drams
Pound = 16 ounces

3. Troy weight: a system of weights used by jewelers for gold and precious stones.

Grain = 64.8 milligrams
Pennyweight = 24 grains
Dram = 2.5 pennyweight = 60 grains
Ounce = 20 pennyweight = 8 drams
Pound = 12 ounces

Appendix K
CONVERSION FACTORS FOR UNITS OF MEASURE

To convert from unit	Abbreviation or symbol	Conventional units	
		To	Multiply by
Angstrom units	Å	Centimeters	1×10^{-8}
		Inches	3.9370079×10^{-9}
		Micrometers (microns)	0.0001
		Nanometers	0.1
Atmospheres, standard	atm	Bars	1.01325
		cm of Hg (0°C)	76
		cm of H_2O (4°C)	1033.26
		Feet of H_2O (39.2°F)	33.8995
		Grams/sq centimeter	1033.23
		Inches of Hg (32°F)	29.9213
		Kilograms/sq centimeter	1.03323
		mm of Hg (0°C)	760
		Pounds/sq inch	14.6960
		Torrs	760
Centigrams	cg	Grains	0.15432358
		Grams	0.01
Centiliters	cl	Cu centimeters	10
		Cu inches	0.6102545
		Liters	0.01
		Ounces (US fluid)	0.3381497
Centimeters	cm	Angström units	1×10^{8}
		Feet	0.032808399
		Inches	0.39370079
		Meters	0.01
		Microns	10,000
		Miles (naut., int.)	5.3995680×10^{-6}
		Miles (statute)	6.2137119×10^{-6}
		Millimeters	10
		Nanometers	1×10^{7}
		Rods	0.0019883878
		Yards	0.010936133
Cubic centimeters	cm^3	Cu feet	3.5314667×10^{-5}
		Cu inches	0.061023744
		Cu meters	1×10^{-6}
		Cu yards	1.3079506×10^{-6}
		Drams (US, fluid)	0.27051218

Modified from Weast, RC editor: *Handbook of chemistry and physics,* ed 54, Cleveland, Ohio, 1973, CRC Press.

Continued.

To convert from unit	Abbreviation or symbol	Conventional units	
		To	Multiply by
Cubic centimeters—cont'd		Gallons (Brit.)	0.0002199694
		Gallons (US, dry)	0.00022702075
		Gallons (US, liq.)	0.00026417205
		Gills (Brit.)	0.007039020
		Gills (US)	0.0084535058
		Liters	0.001
		Ounces (Brit., fluid)	0.03519510
		Ounces (US, fluid)	0.033814023
		Pints (US, dry)	0.0018161660
		Pints (US, liq.)	0.0021133764
		Quarts (Brit.)	0.0008798775
		Quarts (US, dry)	0.00090808298
		Quarts (US, liq.)	0.0010566882
Cubic decimeters	dm^3	Cu centimeters	1,000
		Cu feet	0.035316667
		Cu inches	61.023744
		Cu meters	0.001
		Cu yards	0.0013079506
		Liters	1
Cubic dekameters	dam^3	Cu decimeters	1×10^6
		Cu feet	35,314.667
		Cu inches	6.1023744×10^7
		Cu meters	1,000
		Liters	1,000,000
Cubic feet	ft^3	Cu centimeters	28,316.847
		Cu meters	0.028316847
		Gallons (US, dry)	6.4285116
		Gallons (US, liq.)	7.4805195
		Liters	28.316847
		Ounces (Brit., fluid)	996.6143
		Ounces (US, fluid)	957.50649
		Pints (US, liq.)	59.844156
		Quarts (US, dry)	25.714047
		Quarts (US, liq.)	29.922078
Cubic inches	in^3	Cu centimeters	16.387064
		Cu feet	0.00057870370
		Cu meters	1.6387064×10^{-5}
		Cu yards	2.1433470×10^{-5}
		Drams (US, fluid)	4.4329004
		Gallons (Brit.)	0.003604652
		Gallons (US, dry)	0.0037202035

To convert from unit	Abbreviation or symbol	Conventional units	
		To	Multiply by
Cubic inches—cont'd		Gallons (US, liq.)	0.0043290043
		Liters	0.016387064
		Milliliters	16.387064
		Ounces (Brit., fluid)	0.57674444
		Ounces (US, fluid)	0.55411255
		Pints (US, dry)	0.029761628
		Pints (US, liq.)	0.034632035
		Quarts (US, dry)	0.014880814
		Quarts (US, liq.)	0.017316017
Cubic meters	m^3	Cu centimeters	1×10^6
		Cu feet	35.314667
		Cu inches	61,023.74
		Cu yards	1.3079506
		Gallons (Brit.)	219.9694
		Gallons (US, liq.)	264.17205
		Liters	1,000
		Pints (US, liq.)	2,113.3764
		Quarts (US, liq.)	1,056.6882
Cubic millimeters	mm^3	Cu centimeters	0.001
		Cu inches	6.1023744×10^{-5}
		Cu meters	1×10^{-9}
		Minims (Brit.)	0.01689365
		Minims (US)	0.016230731
Decimeters	dm	Centimeters	10
		Feet	0.32808399
		Inches	3.9370079
		Meters	0.1
Degrees	°	Circles	0.0027777
		Minutes	60
		Quadrants	0.0111111
		Radians	0.017453293
		Seconds	3600
Degrees/centimeter		Radians/centimeter	0.017453293
Degrees/foot		Radians/centimeter	0.00057261458
Degrees/inch		Radians/centimeter	0.0068713750
Degrees/minute		Degrees/second	0.0166666
		Radians/second	0.00029088821
		Revolutions/second	4.629629×10^{-5}

Continued.

To convert from unit	Abbreviation or symbol	Conventional units	
		To	**Multiply by**
Degrees/second		Radians/second	0.017453293
		Revolutions/minute	0.166666
		Revolutions/second	0.0027777
Dekaliters	dal, dkl	Pecks (US)	1.135136
		Pints (US, dry)	18.16217
Dekameters	dam, dkm	Centimeters	1,000
		Feet	32.808399
		Inches	393.70079
		Kilometers	0.01
		Meters	10
		Yards	10.93613
Drachms (Brit., fluid)		Cu centimeters	3.551631
		Cu inches	0.2167338
		Drams (US, fluid)	0.9607594
		Milliliters	3.551531
Drams (apoth. or troy)	dr ap, ʒ	Drams (avdp.)	2.1942857
		Grains	60
		Grams	3.8879346
		Ounces (apoth. or troy)	0.125
		Ounces (avdp.)	0.13714286
		Scruples (apoth.)	3
Drams (avdp.)	dr avdp	Drams (apoth. or troy)	0.455729166
		Grains	27.34375
		Grams	1.7718452
		Ounces (apoth. or troy)	0.056966146
		Ounces (avdp.)	0.0625
		Pennyweights	1.1393229
		Pounds (apoth. or troy)	0.0047471788
		Pounds (avdp.)	0.00390625
		Scruples (apoth.)	1.3671875
Drams (US, fluid)	fl dr	Cu centimeters	3.6967162
		Cu inches	0.22558594
		Gills (US)	0.03125
		Milliliters	3.696588
		Minims (US)	60
		Ounces (US, fluid)	0.125
		Pints (US, liq.)	0.0078125

To convert from unit	Abbreviation or symbol	Conventional units	
		To	**Multiply by**
Feet	ft	Centimeters	30.48
		Inches	12
		Meters	0.3048
		Microns	304,800
		Miles (naut., int.)	0.00016457883
		Miles (statute)	0.000189393
		Rods	0.060606
		Yards	0.333333
Gallons (Brit.)	gal	Barrels (Brit.)	0.027777
		Cu centimeters	4546.087
		Cu feet	0.1605436
		Cu inches	277.4193
		Firkins (Brit.)	0.111111
		Gallons (US, liq.)	1.200949
		Gills (Brit.)	32
		Liters	4.545960
		Minims (Brit.)	76,800
		Ounces (Brit., fluid)	160
		Ounces (US, fluid)	153.7215
		Pecks (Brit.)	0.5
		Pounds of H_2O (62°F)	10
Gallons (US, dry)		Barrels (US, dry)	0.038095592
		Barrels (US, liq.)	0.036941181
		Cu centimeters	4,404.8828
		Cu feet	0.15555700
		Cu inches	268.8025
		Gallons (US, liq.)	1.16364719
		Liters	4.404760
Gallons (US, liq.)	gal	Barrels (US, liq.)	0.031746032
		Cu centimeters	3,785.4118
		Cu feet	0.133680555
		Cu inches	231
		Cu meters	0.0037854118
		Cu yards	0.0049511317
		Gallons (Brit.)	0.8326747
		Gallons (US, dry)	0.85936701
		Gallons (wine)	1
		Gills (US)	32
		Liters	3.7854118
		Minims (US)	61,440
		Ounces (US, fluid)	128
		Pints (US, liq.)	8
		Quarts (US, liq.)	4

Continued.

To convert from unit	Abbreviation or symbol	Conventional units	
		To	Multiply by
Gills (Brit.)		Cu centimeters	142.0652
		Gallons (Brit.)	0.03125
		Gills (US)	1.200949
		Liters	0.1420613
		Ounces (Brit., fluid)	5
		Ounces (US, fluid)	4.803764
		Pints (Brit.)	0.25
Gills (US)	gi	Cu centimeters	118.29412
		Cu inches	7.21875
		Drams (US, fluid)	32
		Gallons (US, liq.)	0.03125
		Gills (Brit.)	0.8326747
		Liters	0.1182908
		Minims (US)	1,920
		Ounces (US, fluid)	4
		Pints (US, liq.)	0.25
		Quarts (US, liq.)	0.125
Grains	gr	Carats (metric)	0.32399455
		Drams (apoth. or troy)	0.016666
		Drams (avdp.)	0.036571429
		Dynes	63.5460
		Grams	0.06479891
		Milligrams	64.79891
		Ounces (apoth. or troy)	0.0020833
		Ounces (avdp.)	0.0022857143
		Pennyweights	0.041666
		Pounds (apoth. or troy)	0.000173611
		Pounds (avdp.)	0.00014285714
		Scruples (apoth.)	0.05
Grams	g	Carats (metric)	5
		Decigrams	10
		Dekagrams	0.1
		Drams (apoth. or troy)	0.25720597
		Drams (avdp.)	0.56438339
		Grains	15.432358
		Kilograms	0.001
		Micrograms	1×10^6
		Myriagrams	0.0001
		Ounces (apoth. or troy)	0.032150737
		Ounces (avdp.)	0.035273962
		Pennyweights	0.64301493

To convert from unit	Abbreviation or symbol	Conventional units	
		To	Multiply by
Grams—cont'd		Poundals	0.0709316
		Pounds (apoth. or troy)	0.0026792289
		Pounds (avdp.)	0.0022046226
		Scruples (apoth.)	0.77161792
		Tons (metric)	1×10^{-6}
Hands		Centimeters	10.16
		Inches	4
Hectograms	hg	Grams	100
		Poundals	7.09316
		Pounds (apoth. or troy)	0.26792289
		Pounds (avdp.)	0.22046226
Hectoliters	hl	Bushels (Brit.)	2.749694
		Cu centimeters	1.00028×10^5
		Cu feet	3.531566
		Gallons (US, liq.)	26.41794
		Liters	100
		Ounces (US, fluid)	3,381.497
		Pecks (US)	11.35136
Hectometers	hm	Centimeters	10,000
		Decimeters	1,000
		Dekameters	10
		Feet	328.08399
		Meters	100
		Rods	19.883878
		Yards	109.3613
Inches	in	Angström units	2.54×10^8
		Centimeters	2.54
		Cubits	0.055555
		Fathoms	0.013888
		Feet	0.083333
		Meters	0.0254
		Mils	1,000
		Yards	0.027777
Inches of Hg (32°F)	in Hg	Atmospheres	0.0334211
		Bars	0.0338639
		Feet of air (1 atm, 60°F)	926.24
		Feet of H_2O (39.2°F)	1.132957
		Grams/sq centimeter	34.5316
		Kilograms/sq meter	345.316
		Millimeters of Hg (60°C)	25.4
		Ounces/sq inch	7.85847
		Pounds/sq foot	70.7262

Continued.

To convert from unit	Abbreviation or symbol	Conventional units	
		To	Multiply by
Kilograms	kg	Drams (apoth. or troy)	257.20597
		Drams (avdp.)	564.38339
		Grains	15,432.358
		Hundredweights (long)	0.019684131
		Hundredweights (short)	0.022046226
		Ounces (apoth. or troy)	32.150737
		Ounces (avdp.)	35.273962
		Pennyweights	643.01493
		Poundals	70.931635
		Pounds (apoth. or troy)	2.6792289
		Pounds (avdp.)	2.2046226
		Scruples (apoth.)	771.61792
		Tons (long)	0.00098420653
		Tons (metric)	0.001
		Tons (short)	0.0011023113
Kiloliters	kl	Cu centimeters	1×10^6
		Cu feet	35.31566
		Cu inches	61,025.45
		Cu meters	1.0
		Cu yards	1.307987
		Gallons (Brit.)	219.9755
		Gallons (US, dry)	227.0271
		Gallons (US, liq.)	264.1794
		Liters	1,000
Kilometers	km	Centimeters	100,000
		Feet	3,280.8399
		Light years	1.05702×10^{-13}
		Meters	1,000
		Miles (naut., int.)	0.53995680
		Miles (statute)	0.62137119
		Myriameters	0.1
		Rods	198.83878
		Yards	1,093.6133
Liters*	L	Bushels (Brit.)	0.02749617
		Bushels (US)	0.02837759
		Cu centimeters	1,000
		Cu feet	0.035314667
		Cu inches	61.023744
		Cu meters	0.001
		Cu yards	0.0013079506
		Drams (US, fluid)	270.51218

*It is recommended in the U.S. that the capital "L" be the accepted symbol for liter since most typescript gives insufficient distinction between "l" and the numeral "1" in the lower case.

To convert from unit	Abbreviation or symbol	Conventional units	
		To	Multiply by
Liters—cont'd		Gallons (Brit.)	0.2199694
		Gallons (US, dry)	0.22702075
		Gallons (US, liq.)	0.26417205
		Gills (Brit.)	7.039020
		Gills (US)	8.4535058
		Minims (US)	16,320.75
		Ounces (Brit., fluid)	35.19510
		Ounces (US, fluid)	33.814023
		Pints (Brit.)	1.795756
		Pints (US, dry)	1.8161660
		Pints (US, liq.)	2.1133764
		Quarts (Brit.)	0.8798775
		Quarts (US, dry)	0.90808298
		Quarts (US, liq.)	1.0566882
Meters	m	Angström units	1×10^{10}
		Centimeters	100
		Feet	3.2808399
		Inches	39.370079
		Kilometers	0.001
		Megameters	1×10^{-6}
		Miles (naut., Brit.)	0.00053961182
		Miles (naut., int.)	0.00053995680
		Miles (statute)	0.00062137119
		Millimeters	1,000
		Mils	39,370.079
		Nanometers	1×10^{9}
		Rods	0.19883878
		Yards	1.0936133
Meters of Hg (0°C)		Atmospheres	1.3157895
		Feet of H_2O (60°F)	44.6474
		Inches of Hg (32°F)	39.370079
		Kilograms/sq centimeter	1.35951
		Pounds/sq inch	19.3368
Micrograms	μg	Grams	1×10^{-6}
		Milligrams	0.001
Micrometers (microns)	μm	Angström units	10,000
		Centimeters	0.0001
		Feet	3.2808399×10^{-6}
		Inches	3.9370079×10^{-5}
		Meters	1×10^{-6}
		Millimeters	0.001
		Nanometers	1,000

Continued.

To convert from unit	Abbreviation or symbol	Conventional units	
		To	**Multiply by**
Miles (statute)	mi	Centimeters	160,934.4
		Feet	5,280
		Inches	63,360
		Kilometers	1.609344
		Meters	1,609.344
		Rods	320
		Yards	1,760
Milligrams	mg	Carats (1877)	0.004871
		Carats (metric)	0.005
		Drams (apoth. or troy)	0.00025720597
		Drams (advp.)	0.00056438339
		Grains	0.015432358
		Grams	0.001
		Ounces (apoth. or troy)	3.2150737×10^{-5}
		Ounces (avdp.)	3.5273962×10^{-5}
		Pennyweights	0.00064301493
		Pounds (apoth. or troy)	2.6792289×10^{-6}
		Pounds (avdp.)	2.2046226×10^{-6}
		Scruples (apoth.)	0.00077161792
Milliliters	ml	Cu centimeters	1
		Cu inches	0.06102545
		Drams (US, fluid)	0.2705198
		Gills (US)	0.008453742
		Liters	0.001
		Minims (US)	16.23119
		Ounces (Brit., fluid)	0.03519609
		Ounces (US, fluid)	0.03381497
		Pints (Brit.)	0.001759804
		Pints (US, liq.)	0.002113436
Millimeters	mm	Angström units	1×10^{7}
		Centimeters	0.1
		Decimeters	0.01
		Dekameters	0.0001
		Feet	0.0032808399
		Inches	0.039370079
		Meters	0.001
		Micrometers (microns)	1,000
		Mils	39.370079
Millimeters of Hg (0°C)	mm Hg	Atmospheres	0.0013157895
		Bars	0.00133322
		Dynes/sq centimeter	1,333.224

To convert from unit	Abbreviation or symbol	Conventional units	
		To	**Multiply by**
Millimeters of Hg (0°C)—cont'd		Grams/sq centimeter	1.35951
		Kilograms/sq meter	13.5951
		Pounds/sq foot	2.78450
		Pounds/sq inch	0.0193368
		Torrs	1
Minims (Brit.)	min	Cu centimeter	0.05919385
		Cu inches	0.003612230
		Milliliters	0.05919219
		Ounces (Brit., fluid)	0.0020833333
		Scruples (Brit., fluid)	0.05
Minims (US)	min, ℳ	Cu centimeters	0.061611520
		Cu inches	0.0037597656
		Drams (US, fluid)	0.0166666
		Gallons (US, liq.)	1.6276042×10^{-5}
		Gills (US)	0.0005208333
		Liters	6.160979×10^{-5}
		Milliliters	0.06160979
		Ounces (US, fluid)	0.002083333
		Pints (US, liq.)	0.0001302083
Minutes (angular)	′ (prime)	Degrees	0.0166666
		Quadrants	0.000185185
		Radians	0.00029088821
		Seconds (angular)	60
Minutes (mean solar)	min	Days (mean solar)	0.0006944444
		Days (sideral)	0.00069634577
		Hours (mean solar)	0.0166666
		Hours (sideral)	0.016712298
		Minutes (sideral)	1.00273791
Minutes (sideral)	min	Days (mean solar)	0.00069254831
		Minutes (mean solar)	0.99726957
		Months (mean solar)	2.2768712×10^{-5}
		Seconds (sideral)	60
Myriagrams		Grams	10,000
		Kilograms	10
		Pounds (avdp.)	22.046226
Nanometer	nm	Angström units	10
		Centimeters	1×10^{-7}
		Inches	3.9370079×10^{-8}
		Micrometers (microns)	0.001
		Millimeters	1×10^{-6}

Continued.

To convert from unit	Abbreviation or symbol	Conventional units	
		To	Multiply by
Newtons	N	Dynes	100,000
		Pounds	0.22480894
Ounces (apoth. or troy)	oz, ℥	Dekagrams	3.1103486
		Drams (apoth. or troy)	8
		Drams (avdp.)	17.554286
		Grains	480
		Grams	31.103486
		Milligrams	31,103.486
		Ounces (avdp.)	1.0971429
		Pennyweights	20
		Pounds (apoth. or troy)	0.0833333
		Pounds (avdp.)	0.068571429
		Scruples (apoth.)	24
Ounces (avpd.)	oz	Drams (apoth. or troy)	7.291666
		Drams (avdp.)	16
		Grains	437.5
		Grams	28.349523
		Hundredweights (long)	0.00055803571
		Hundredweights (short)	0.000625
		Ounces (apoth. or troy)	0.9114583
		Pennyweights	18.229166
		Pounds (apoth. or troy)	0.075954861
		Pounds (avdp.)	0.0625
		Scruples (apoth.)	21.875
Ounces (Brit., fluid)	oz	Cu centimeters	28.41305
		Cu inches	1.733870
		Drachms (Brit., fluid)	8
		Drams (US, fluid)	7.686075
		Gallons (Brit.)	0.00625
		Milliliters	28.41225
		Minims (Brit.)	480
		Ounces (US, fluid)	0.9607594
Ounces (US, fluid)	oz, fl oz	Cu centimeters	29.573730
		Cu inches	1.8046875
		Cu meters	2.9573730×10^{-5}
		Drams (US, fluid)	8
		Gallons (US, dry)	0.0067138047
		Gallons (US, liq.)	0.0078125
		Gills (US)	0.25
		Liters	0.029572702
		Minims (US)	480
		Ounces (Brit., fluid)	1.040843

To convert from unit	Abbreviation or symbol	Conventional units	
		To	Multiply by
Ounces (US, fluid)—cont'd		Pints (US, liq.)	0.0625
		Quarts (US, liq.)	0.03125
Parts per million[†]	ppm	Grains/gallon (Brit.)	0.07015488
		Grains/gallon (US)	0.05841620
		Grams/liter	0.001
		Milligrams/liter	1
Pennyweights	dwt, pwt	Drams (apoth. or troy)	0.4
		Drams (avdp.)	0.87771429
		Grains	24
		Grams	1.55517384
		Ounces (apoth. or troy)	0.05
		Ounces (avdp.)	0.054857143
		Pounds (apoth. or troy)	0.0041666
		Pounds (avdp.)	0.0034285714
Pints (Brit.)	pt	Cu centimeter	568.26092
		Gallons (Brit.)	0.125
		Gills (Brit.)	4
		Gills (US)	4.803797
		Liters	0.5682450
		Minims (Brit.)	9,600
		Ounces (Brit., fluid)	20
		Pints (US, dry)	1.032056
		Pints (US, liq.)	1.200949
		Quarts (Brit.)	0.5
		Scruples (Brit., fluid)	480
Pints (US, dry)	pt	Cu centimeters	550.61047
		Cu inches	33.6003125
		Gallons (US, dry)	0.125
		Gallons (US, liq.)	0.14545590
		Liters	0.5505951
		Quarts (US, dry)	0.5
Pints (US, liq.)	pt	Cu centimeters	473.17647
		Cu feet	0.016710069
		Cu inches	28.875
		Cu yards	0.00061889146
		Drams (US, fluid)	128
		Gallons (US, liq.)	0.125
		Gills (US)	4
		Liters	0.4731632
		Milliliters	473.1632
		Minims (US)	7,680

[†]Based on density of 1 g/ml for the solvent. (See also Chapter 6, section 6.4).   *Continued.*

To convert from unit	Abbreviation or symbol	Conventional units	
		To	**Multiply by**
Pints (US, liq.)—cont'd		Ounces (US, fluid)	16
		Pints (Brit.)	0.8326747
		Quarts (US, liq.)	0.5
Poundals		Dynes	13,825.50
		Grams	14.09808
		Pounds (avdp.)	0.0310810
Pounds (apoth. or troy)	lb ap	Drams (apoth. or troy)	96
		Drams (avdp.)	210.65143
		Grains	5,760
		Grams	373.24172
		Kilograms	0.37324172
		Ounces (apoth. or troy)	12
		Ounces (avdp.)	13.165714
		Pennyweights	240
		Pounds (avdp.)	0.8228571
		Scruples (apoth.)	288
		Tons (long)	0.00036734694
		Tons (metric)	0.00037324172
		Tons (short)	0.00041142857
Pounds (avdp.)	lb avdp, #	Drams (apoth. or troy)	116.6666
		Drams (avdp.)	256
		Grains	7,000
		Grams	453.59237
		Kilograms	0.45359237
		Ounces (apoth. or troy)	14.583333
		Ounces (avdp.)	16
		Pennyweights	291.6666
		Poundals	32.1740
		Pounds (apoth. or troy)	1.215277
		Scruples (apoth.)	350
		Slugs	0.0310810
		Tons (long)	0.00044642857
		Tons (metric)	0.00045359237
		Tons (short)	0.0005
Quarts (Brit.)	qt	Cu centimeters	1,136.522
		Cu inches	69.35482
		Gallons (Brit.)	0.25
		Gallons (US, liq.)	0.3002373
		Liters	1.136490
		Quarts (US, dry)	1.032056
		Quarts (US, liq.)	1.200949

To convert from unit	Abbreviation or symbol	Conventional units	
		To	**Multiply by**
Quarts (US, dry)	qt	Bushels (US)	0.03125
		Cu centimeters	1,101.2209
		Cu feet	0.038889251
		Cu inches	67.200625
		Gallons (US, dry)	0.25
		Gallons (US, liq.)	0.29091180
		Liters	1.1011901
		Pints (US, dry)	2
Quart (US, liq.)	qt	Cu centimeters	946.35295
		Cu feet	0.033420136
		Cu inches	57.75
		Drams (US, fluid)	256
		Gallons (US, dry)	0.21484175
		Gallons (US, liq.)	0.25
		Gills (US)	8
		Liters	0.9463264
		Ounces (US, fluid)	32
		Pints (US, liq.)	2
		Quarts (Brit.)	0.8326747
		Quarts (US, dry)	0.8593670
Quintals (metric)		Grams	100,000
		Hundredweights (long)	1.9684131
		Kilograms	100
		Pounds (avdp.)	220.46226
Scruples (apoth.)	s apoth, ℈	Drams (apoth. or troy)	0.333333
		Drams (avdp.)	0.73142857
		Grains	20
		Grams	1.2959782
		Ounces (apoth. or troy)	0.041666
		Ounces (avdp.)	0.045714286
		Pennyweights	0.833333
		Pounds (apoth. or troy)	0.003472222
		Pounds (avdp.)	0.0028571429
Scruples (Brit., fluid)		Minims (Brit.)	20
Square feet	ft^2	Sq centimeters	929.0304
		Sq inches	144
		Sq meters	0.09290304
		Sq miles	3.5870064×10^{-8}
		Sq rods	0.0036730946
		Sq yards	0.111111

Continued.

To convert from unit	Abbreviation or symbol	Conventional units	
		To	Multiply by
Square inches	in^2	Circular mils	1,273,239.5
		Sq centimeters	6.4516
		Sq decimeters	0.064516
		Sq feet	0.0069444
		Sq meters	0.00064516
		Sq miles	$2.4909767 \times 10^{-10}$
		Sq millimeters	645.16
		Sq mils	1×10^6
Square kilometers	km^2	Sq feet	1.0763910×10^7
		Sq inches	1.5500031×10^9
		Sq meters	1×10^6
		Sq miles	0.38610216
		Sq yards	1.1959900×10^{-6}
Square meters	m^2	Sq centimeters	10,000
		Sq feet	10.763910
		Sq inches	1,550.0031
		Sq kilometers	1×10^{-6}
		Sq miles	3.8610216×10^{-7}
		Sq millimeters	1×10^6
		Sq rods	0.039536861
		Sq yards	1.1959900
Square miles	mi^2	Sq feet	2.7878288×10^7
		Sq kilometers	2.5899881
		Sq meters	2,589,988.1
		Sq rods	102,400
		Sq yards	3.0976×10^6
Square millimeters	mm^2	Sq centimeters	0.01
		Sq inches	0.0015500031
		Sq meters	1×10^{-6}
Square yards	yd^2	Sq centimeters	8,361.2736
		Sq feet	9
		Sq feet (US survey)	8.9999640
		Sq inches	1,296
		Sq meters	0.83612736
		Sq miles	$3.228305785 \times 10^{-7}$
		Sq rods	0.033057851
Tons (long), British		Kilograms	1,016.0469
		Ounces (avdp.)	35,840
		Pounds (apoth. or troy)	2,722.22

To convert from unit	Abbreviation or symbol	Conventional units	
		To	Multiply by
Tons (long)—cont'd		Pounds (avdp.)	2,240
		Tons (metric)	1.0160469
		Tons (short)	1.12
Tons (metric)	t	Grams	1×10^6
		Hundredweights (short)	22.046226
		Kilograms	1,000
		Ounces (avdp.)	35,273.962
		Pounds (apoth. or troy)	2,679.2289
		Pounds (avdp.)	2,204.6226
		Tons (long)	0.98420653
		Tons (short)	1.1023113
Tons (short), US	sh tn	Hundredweights (short)	20
		Kilograms	907.18474
		Ounces (avdp.)	32,000
		Pounds (apoth. or troy)	2,430.555
		Pounds (avdp.)	2,000
		Tons (long)	0.89285714
		Tons (metric)	0.90718474
Yards	yd	Centimeters	91.44
		Cubits	2
		Fathoms	0.5
		Feet	3
		Feet (US survey)	2.9999940
		Inches	36
		Meters	0.9144
		Quarters (Brit., linear)	4
Years (calendar)	a, yr	Days (mean solar)	365
		Hours (mean solar)	8,760
		Minutes (mean solar)	525,600
		Months (lunar)	12.360065
		Months (mean calendar)	12
		Seconds (mean solar)	3.1536×10^7
		Weeks (mean calendar)	52.142857
		Years (sidereal)	0.99929814
		Years (tropical)	0.99933690

Appendix L
CONVERSION FACTORS FOR THE MORE COMMON ELECTROLYTES

Electrolyte	Unit reported in	×	Factor	=	Desired unit
Ca	mg/dl		0.5		mEq/L
Ca	mEq/L		2.0		mg/dl
Cl	mg/dl		0.282		mEq/L (as Cl)
Cl	mg/dl		0.282		mEq/L (as NaCl)
Cl	mEq/L		3.55		mg/dl (as Cl)
Cl	mEq/L		5.85		mg/dl (as NaCl)
Cl	mEq/L		0.0585		g/L (as NaCl)
CO_2	vol%		0.45		mEq/L
CO_2	mEq/L		2.226		vol%
K	mg/dl		0.256		mEq/L
K	mEq/L		3.91		mg/dl
K	mEq/L		0.0746		g/L (as KCl)
Na	mg/dl		0.435		mEq/L (as Na)
Na	mg/dl		0.435		mEq/L (as NaCl)
Na	mEq/L		2.3		mg/dl (as Na)
Na	mEq/L		5.85		mg/dl (as NaCl)
Na	mEq/L		0.0585		g/L (as NaCl)

Appendix M
CONVERSION FACTORS FOR CONVERTING CONVENTIONAL ENZYME UNITS TO INTERNATIONAL UNITS PER LITER (IU/L OR mU/ml)

Enzyme	One conventional unit	=	IU/L (mU/ml)
Acid phosphatase			
Bodansky	37°C, 1 mg P/hr/100 ml		5.37
Shinowara-Jones-Reinhart			5.37
King-Armstrong	37°C, 1 mg phenol/hr/100 ml		1.77
Kind-King			1.77
Bessey-Lowry-Brock	37°C, 1 mmole p-nitrophenol/hr/1,000 ml		16.67
Gutman-Gutman			1.77
Aldolase			
Sibley-Lehninger	1 μl (0.0446 μmole) fructose-1,6-diphosphate/hr/ml		0.74
Burns	37°C, 1 μl fructose-1,6-diphosphate/hr/ml		0.61
Schapira, et al.	37°C, 1 mg triosephosphate-p/min/1,000 ml		16.0
Alkaline phosphatase			
Bodansky	37°C, 1 mg P/hr/100 ml		5.37
Shinowara-Jones-Reinhart	37°C, 1 mg P/hr/100 ml		5.37
King-Armstrong	37°C, 1 mg phenol/15 min/100 ml		7.1
Kind-King	37°C, 1 mg phenol/15 min/100 ml		7.06
Bessey-Lowry-Brock	37°C, 1 mmole p-nitrophenol/hr/1,000 ml		16.67
Babson	1 μmole phenolphthalein/min/1,000 ml		1.0
Bowers-McComb	1 μmole p-nitrophenol/min/1,000 ml		1.0
Amylase			
Somogyi (saccharogenic)	40°C, 1 mg glucose/30 min/100 ml		1.85
Somogyi	37°C, 5 mg starch/15 min/100 ml		20.6
Cholinesterase			
de la Huerga	37°C, 1 μmole acetylcholine/hr/ml		16.7
Hydroxybutyric dehydrogenase			
Rosalki-Wilkinson	ΔA_{340} 0.001/min/ml (V_t, 3 ml) (NADH)		0.482
Isocitrate dehydrogenase			
Wolfson-Williams-Ashman	25°C, 1 nmole NADH/hr/ml		0.0167
Taylor-Friedman			0.0167
Lactate dehydrogenase			
Wroblewski-LaDue	ΔA_{340} 0.001/min/ml (V_t, 3 ml) (NADH)		0.482
Wroblewski-Gregory			0.482
Lipase			
Cherry-Crandall (Tietz-Fiereck)	50 μmoles of fatty acid/3 hr/ml		277.0
Malic dehydrogenase			
Wacker-Ulmer-Valee			0.482
Transaminase			
Reitman-Frankel			0.482
Karmen	25°C, ΔA_{340} 0.001/min/ml (V_t, 3 ml) (NADH)		0.482

Appendix N
TEMPERATURE CONVERSION TABLE

To °C	←°F or °C→	To °F	To °C	←°F or °C→	To °F	To °C	←°F or °C→	To °F
−190	−310		−167.78	−270	−454	−145.56	−230	−382
−189.44	−309	—	−167.22	−269	−452.2	−145	−229	−380.2
−188.89	−308	—	−166.67	−268	−450.4	−144.44	−228	−378.4
−198.33	−307	—	−166.11	−267	−448.6	−143.89	−227	−376.6
−187.78	−306	—	−165.56	−266	−446.8	−143.33	−226	−374.8
−187.22	−305	—	−165	−265	−445	−142.78	−225	−373
−186.67	−304	—	−164.44	−264	−443.2	−142.22	−224	−371.2
−186.11	−303	—	−163.89	−263	−441.4	−141.67	−223	−369.4
−185.56	−302	—	−163.33	−262	−439.6	−141.11	−222	−367.6
−185	−301	—	−162.78	−261	−437.8	−140.56	−221	−365.8
−184.44	−300	—	−162.22	−260	−436	−140	−220	−364
−183.89	−299	—	−161.67	−259	−434.2	−139.44	−219	−362.2
−183.33	−298	—	−161.11	−258	−432.4	−138.89	−218	−360.4
−182.78	−297	—	−160.56	−257	−430.6	−138.33	−217	−358.6
−182.22	−296	—	−160	−256	−428.8	−137.78	−216	−356.8
−181.67	−295	—	−159.44	−255	−427	−137.22	−215	−355
−181.11	−294	—	−158.89	−254	−425.2	−136.67	−214	−353.2
−180.56	−293	—	−158.33	−253	−423.4	−136.11	−213	−351.4
−180	−292	—	−157.78	−252	−421.6	−135.56	−212	−349.6
−179.44	−291	—	−157.22	−251	−419.8	−135	−211	−347.8
−178.89	−290	—	−156.67	−250	−418	−134.44	−210	−346
−178.33	−289	—	−156.11	−249	−416.2	−133.89	−209	−344.2
−177.78	−288	—	−155.56	−248	−414.4	−133.33	−208	−342.4
−177.22	−287	—	−155	−247	−412.6	−132.78	−207	−340.6
−176.67	−286	—	−154.44	−246	−410.8	−132.22	−206	−338.8
−176.11	−285	—	−153.89	−245	−409	−131.67	−205	−337
−175.56	−284	—	−153.33	−244	−407.2	−131.11	−204	−335.2
−175	−283	—	−152.78	−243	−405.4	−130.56	−203	−333.4
−174.44	−282	—	−152.22	−242	−403.6	−130	−202	−331.6
−173.89	−281	—	−151.67	−241	−401.8	−129.44	−201	−329.8
−173.33	−280	—	−151.11	−240	−400	−128.89	−200	−328
−172.78	−279	—	−150.56	−239	−398.2	−128.33	−199	−326.2
−172.22	−278	—	−150	−238	−396.4	−127.78	−198	−324.4
−171.67	−277	—	−149.44	−237	−394.6	−127.22	−197	−322.6
−171.11	−276	—	−148.89	−236	−392.8	−126.67	−196	−320.8
−170.56	−275	—	−148.33	−235	−391	−126.11	−195	−319
−170	−274		−147.78	−234	−389.2	−125.56	−194	−317.2
−169.53	−273.15	−459.67	−147.22	−233	−387.4	−125	−193	−315.4
−169.44	−273	−459.4	−146.67	−232	−385.6	−124.44	−192	−313.6
−168.89	−272	−457.6	−146.11	−231	−383.8	−123.89	−191	−311.8
−168.33	−271	−455.8						

Modified from Weast RC, editor: *Handbook of chemistry and physics,* ed 48, Cleveland, Ohio, 1967, CRC Press.

	To convert			To convert			To convert	
To °C	←°F or °C→	To °F	To °C	←°F or °C→	To °F	To °C	←°F or °C→	To °F
−123.33	−190	−310	−101.11	−150	−238	−78.89	−110	−166
−122.78	−189	−308.2	−100.56	−149	−236.2	−78.33	−109	−164.2
−122.22	−188	−306.4	−100	−148	−234.4	−77.78	−108	−162.4
−121.67	−187	−304.6	−99.44	−147	−232.6	−77.22	−107	−160.6
−121.11	−186	−302.8	−98.89	−146	−230.8	−76.67	−106	−158.8
−120.56	−185	−301	−98.33	−145	−229	−76.11	−105	−157
−120	−184	−299.2	−97.78	−144	−227.2	−75.56	−104	−155.2
−119.44	−183	−297.4	−97.22	−143	−225.4	−75	−103	−153.4
−118.89	−182	−295.6	−96.67	−142	−223.6	−74.44	−102	−151.6
−118.33	−181	−293.8	−96.11	−141	−221.8	−73.89	−101	−149.8
−117.78	−180	−292	−95.56	−140	−220	−73.33	−100	−148
−117.22	−179	−290.2	−95	−139	−218.2	−72.78	−99	−146.2
−116.67	−178	−288.4	−94.44	−138	−216.4	−72.22	−98	−144.4
−116.11	−177	−286.6	−93.89	−137	−214.6	−71.67	−97	−142.6
−115.56	−176	−284.8	−93.33	−136	−212.8	−71.11	−96	−140.8
−115	−175	−283	−92.78	−135	−211	−70.56	−95	−139
−114.44	−174	−281.2	−92.22	−134	−209.2	−70	−94	−137.2
−113.89	−173	−279.4	−91.67	−133	−207.4	−69.44	−93	−135.4
−113.33	−172	−277.6	−91.11	−132	−205.6	−68.89	−92	−133.6
−112.78	−171	−275.8	−90.56	−131	−203.8	−68.33	−91	−131.8
−112.22	−170	−274	−90	−130	−202	−67.78	−90	−130
−111.67	−169	−272.2	−89.44	−129	−200.2	−67.22	−89	−128.2
−111.11	−168	−270.4	−88.89	−128	−198.4	−66.67	−88	−126.4
−110.56	−167	−268.6	−88.33	−127	−196.6	−66.11	−87	−124.6
−110	−166	−266.8	−87.78	−126	−194.8	−65.56	−86	−122.8
−109.44	−165	−265	−87.22	−125	−193	−65	−85	−121
−108.89	−164	−263.2	−86.67	−124	−191.2	−64.44	−84	−119.2
−108.33	−163	−261.4	−86.11	−123	−189.4	−63.89	−83	−117.4
−107.78	−162	−259.6	−85.56	−122	−187.6	−63.33	−82	−115.6
−107.22	−161	−257.8	−85	−121	−185.8	−62.78	−81	−113.8
−106.67	−160	−256	−84.44	−120	−184	−62.22	−80	−112
−106.11	−159	−254.2	−83.89	−119	−182.2	−61.67	−79	−110.2
−105.56	−158	−252.4	−83.33	−118	−180.4	−61.11	−78	−108.4
−105	−157	−250.6	−82.78	−117	−178.6	−60.56	−77	−106.6
−104.44	−156	−248.8	−82.22	−116	−176.8	−60	−76	−104.8
−103.89	−155	−247	−81.67	−115	−175	−59.44	−75	−103
−103.33	−154	−245.2	−81.11	−114	173.2	−58.89	−74	−101.2
−102.78	−153	−243.4	−80.56	−113	−171.4	−58.33	−73	−99.4
−102.22	−152	−241.6	−80	−112	−169.6	−57.78	−72	−97.6
−101.67	−151	−239.8	−79.44	−111	−167.8	−57.22	−71	−95.8

Continued.

	To convert			To convert			To convert	
To °C	←°F or °C→	To °F	To °C	←°F or °C→	To °F	To °C	←°F or °C→	To °F
−56.67	−70	−94	−34.44	−30	−22	−12.22	10	50
−56.11	−69	−92.2	−33.89	−29	−20.2	−11.67	11	51.8
−55.56	−68	−90.4	−33.33	−28	−18.4	−11.11	12	53.6
−55	−67	−88.6	−32.78	−27	−16.6	−10.56	13	55.4
−54.44	−66	−86.8	−32.22	−26	−14.8	−10	14	57.2
−53.89	−65	−85	−31.67	−25	−13	−9.44	15	59
−53.33	−64	−83.2	−31.11	−24	−11.2	−8.89	16	60.8
−52.78	−63	−81.4	−30.56	−23	−9.4	−8.33	17	62.6
−52.22	−62	−79.6	−30	−22	−7.6	−7.78	18	64.4
−51.67	−61	−77.8	−29.44	−21	−5.8	−7.22	19	66.2
−51.11	−60	−76	−28.89	−20	−4	−6.67	20	68
−50.56	−59	−74.2	−28.33	−19	−2.2	−6.11	21	69.8
−50	−58	−72.4	−27.78	−18	−0.4	−5.56	22	71.6
−49.44	−57	−70.6	−27.22	−17	1.4	−5	23	73.4
−48.89	−56	−68.8	−26.67	−16	3.2	−4.44	24	75.2
−48.33	−55	−67	−26.11	−15	5	−3.89	25	77
−47.78	−54	−65.2	−25.56	−14	6.8	−3.33	26	78.8
−47.22	−53	−63.4	−25	−13	8.6	−2.78	27	80.6
−46.67	−52	−61.6	−24.44	−12	10.4	−2.22	28	82.4
−46.11	−51	−59.8	−23.89	−11	12.2	−1.67	29	84.2
−45.56	−50	−58	−23.33	−10	14	−1.11	30	86
−45	−49	−56.2	−22.78	−9	15.8	−0.56	31	87.8
−44.44	−48	−54.4	−22.22	−8	17.6	0.0	32	89.6
−43.89	−47	−52.6	−21.67	−7	19.4	0.56	33	91.4
−43.33	−46	−50.8	−21.11	−6	21.2	1.11	34	93.2
−42.78	−45	−49	−20.56	−5	23	1.67	35	95
−42.22	−44	−47.2	−20	−4	24.8	2.22	36	96.8
−41.67	−43	−45.4	−19.44	−3	26.6	2.78	37	98.6
−41.11	−42	−43.6	−18.89	−2	28.4	3.33	38	100.4
−40.56	−41	−41.8	−18.33	−1	30.2	3.89	39	102.2
−40	−40	−40	−17.78	0	32	4.44	40	104
−39.44	−39	−38.2	−17.22	1	33.8	5	41	105.8
−38.89	−38	−36.4	−16.67	2	35.6	5.56	42	107.6
−38.33	−37	−34.6	−16.11	3	37.4	6.11	43	109.4
−37.78	−36	−32.8	−15.56	4	39.2	6.67	44	111.2
−37.22	−35	−31	−15	5	41	7.22	45	113
−36.67	−34	−29.2	−14.44	6	42.8	7.78	46	114.8
−36.11	−33	−27.4	−13.89	7	44.6	8.33	47	116.6
−35.56	−32	−25.6	−13.33	8	46.4	8.89	48	118.4
−35	−31	−23.8	−12.78	9	48.2	9.44	49	120.2

	To convert			To convert			To convert	
To °C	←°F or °C→	To °F	To °C	←°F or °C→	To °F	To °C	←°F or °C→	To °F
10	50	122	32.22	90	194	54.44	130	266
10.56	51	123.8	32.78	91	195.8	55	131	267.8
11.11	52	125.6	33.33	92	197.6	55.56	132	269.6
11.67	53	127.4	33.89	93	199.4	56.11	133	271.4
12.22	54	129.2	34.44	94	201.2	56.67	134	273.2
12.78	55	131	35	95	203	57.22	135	275
13.33	56	132.8	35.56	96	204.8	57.78	136	276.8
13.89	57	134.6	36.11	97	206.6	58.33	137	278.6
14.44	58	136.4	36.67	98	208.4	58.89	138	280.4
15	59	138.2	37.22	99	210.2	59.44	139	282.2
15.56	60	140	37.78	100	212	60	140	284
16.11	61	141.8	38.33	101	213.8	60.56	141	285.8
16.67	62	143.6	38.89	102	215.6	61.11	142	287.6
17.22	63	145.4	39.44	103	217.4	61.67	143	289.4
17.78	64	147.2	40	104	219.2	62.22	144	291.2
18.33	65	149	40.56	105	221	62.78	145	293
18.89	66	150.8	41.11	106	222.8	63.33	146	294.8
19.44	67	152.6	41.67	107	224.6	63.89	147	296.6
20	68	154.4	42.22	108	226.4	64.44	148	298.4
20.56	69	156.2	42.78	109	228.2	65	149	300.2
21.11	70	158	43.33	110	230	65.56	150	302
21.67	71	159.8	43.89	111	231.8	66.11	151	303.8
22.22	72	161.6	44.44	112	233.6	66.67	152	305.6
22.78	73	163.4	45	113	235.4	67.22	153	307.4
23.33	74	165.2	45.56	114	237.2	67.78	154	309.2
23.89	75	167	46.11	115	239	68.33	155	311
24.44	76	168.8	46.67	116	240.8	68.89	156	312.8
25	77	170.6	47.22	117	242.6	69.44	157	314.6
25.56	78	172.4	47.78	118	244.4	70	158	316.4
26.11	79	174.2	48.33	119	246.2	70.56	159	318.2
26.67	80	176	48.89	120	248	71.11	160	320
27.22	81	177.8	49.44	121	249.8	71.67	161	321.8
27.78	82	179.6	50	122	251.6	72.22	162	323.6
28.33	83	181.4	50.56	123	253.4	72.78	163	325.4
28.89	84	183.2	51.11	124	255.2	73.33	164	327.2
29.44	85	185	51.67	125	257	73.89	165	329
30	86	186.8	52.22	126	258.8	74.44	166	330.8
30.56	87	188.6	52.78	127	260.6	75	167	332.6
31.11	88	190.4	53.33	128	262.4	75.56	168	334.4
31.67	89	192.2	53.89	129	264.2	76.11	169	336.2

Continued.

To convert			To convert			To convert		
To °C	←°F or °C→	To °F	To °C	←°F or °C→	To °F	To °C	←°F or °C→	To °F
76.67	170	338	98.89	210	410	121.11	250	482
77.22	171	339.8	99.44	211	411.8	121.67	251	483.8
77.78	172	341.6	100	212	413.6	122.22	252	485.6
78.33	173	343.4	100.56	213	415.4	122.78	253	487.4
78.89	174	345.2	101.11	214	417.2	123.33	254	489.2
79.44	175	347	101.67	215	419	123.89	255	491
80	176	348.8	102.22	216	420.8	124.44	256	492.8
80.56	177	350.6	102.78	217	422.6	125	257	494.6
81.11	178	352.4	103.33	218	424.4	125.56	258	496.4
81.67	179	354.2	103.89	219	426.2	126.11	259	498.2
82.22	180	356	104.44	220	428	126.67	260	500
82.78	181	357.8	105	221	429.8	127.22	261	501.8
83.33	182	359.6	105.56	222	431.6	127.78	262	503.6
83.89	183	361.4	106.11	223	433.4	128.33	263	505.4
84.44	184	363.2	106.67	224	435.2	128.89	264	507.2
85	185	365	107.22	225	437	129.44	265	509
85.56	186	366.8	107.78	226	438.8	130	266	510.8
86.11	187	368.6	108.33	227	440.6	130.56	267	512.6
86.67	188	370.4	108.89	228	442.4	131.11	268	514.4
87.22	189	372.2	109.44	229	444.2	131.67	269	516.2
87.78	190	374	110	230	446	132.22	270	518
88.33	191	375.8	110.56	231	447.8	132.78	271	519.8
88.89	192	377.6	111.11	232	449.6	133.33	272	521.6
89.44	193	379.4	111.67	233	451.4	133.89	273	523.4
90	194	381.2	112.22	234	453.2	134.44	274	525.2
90.56	195	383	112.78	235	455	135	275	527
91.11	196	384.8	113.33	236	456.8	135.56	276	528.8
91.67	197	386.6	113.89	237	458.6	136.11	277	530.6
92.22	198	388.4	114.44	238	460.4	136.67	278	532.4
92.78	199	390.2	115	239	462.2	137.22	279	534.2
93.33	200	392	115.56	240	464	137.78	280	536
93.89	201	393.8	116.11	241	465.8	138.33	281	537.8
94.44	202	395.6	116.67	242	467.6	138.89	282	539.6
95	203	397.4	117.22	243	469.4	139.44	283	541.4
95.56	204	399.2	117.78	244	471.2	140	284	543.2
96.11	205	401	118.33	245	473	140.56	285	545
96.67	206	402.8	118.89	246	474.8	141.11	286	546.8
97.22	207	404.6	119.44	247	476.6	141.67	287	548.6
97.78	208	406.4	120	248	478.4	142.22	288	550.4
98.33	209	408.2	120.56	249	480.2	142.78	289	552.2

	To convert			To convert			To convert	
To °C	←°F or °C→	To °F	To °C	←°F or °C→	To °F	To °C	←°F or °C→	To °F
143.33	290	554	165.56	330	626	187.78	370	698
143.89	291	555.8	166.11	331	627.8	188.33	371	699.8
144.44	292	557.6	166.67	332	629.6	188.89	372	701.6
145	293	559.4	167.22	333	631.4	189.44	373	703.4
145.56	294	561.2	167.78	334	633.2	190	374	705.2
146.11	295	563	168.33	335	635	190.56	375	707
146.67	296	564.8	168.89	336	636.8	191.11	376	708.8
147.22	297	566.6	169.44	337	638.6	191.67	377	710.6
147.78	298	568.4	170	338	640.4	192.22	378	712.4
148.33	299	570.2	170.56	339	642.2	192.78	379	714.2
148.89	300	572	171.11	340	644	193.33	380	716
149.44	301	573.8	171.67	341	645.8	193.89	381	717.8
150	302	575.6	172.22	342	647.6	194.44	382	719.6
150.56	303	577.4	172.78	343	649.4	195	383	721.4
151.11	304	579.2	173.33	344	651.2	195.56	384	723.2
151.67	305	581	173.89	345	653	196.11	385	725
152.22	306	582.8	174.44	346	654.8	196.67	386	726.8
152.78	307	584.6	175	347	656.6	197.22	387	728.6
153.33	308	586.4	175.56	348	658.4	197.78	388	730.4
153.89	309	588.2	176.11	349	660.2	198.33	389	732.2
154.44	310	590	176.67	350	662	198.89	390	734
155	311	591.8	177.22	351	663.8	199.44	391	735.8
155.56	312	593.6	177.78	352	665.6	200	392	737.6
156.11	313	595.4	178.33	353	667.4	200.56	393	739.4
156.67	314	597.2	178.89	354	669.2	201.11	394	741.2
157.22	315	599	179.44	355	671	201.67	395	743
157.78	316	600.8	180	356	672.8	202.22	396	744.8
158.33	317	602.6	180.56	357	674.6	202.78	397	746.6
158.89	318	604.4	181.11	358	676.4	203.33	398	748.4
159.44	319	606.2	181.67	359	678.2	203.89	399	750.2
160	320	608	182.22	360	680	204.44	400	752
160.56	321	609.8	182.78	361	681.8	205	401	753.8
161.11	322	611.6	183.33	362	683.6	205.56	402	755.6
161.67	323	613.4	183.89	363	685.4	206.11	403	757.4
162.22	324	615.2	184.44	364	687.2	206.67	404	759.2
162.78	325	617	185	365	689	207.22	405	761
163.33	326	618.8	185.56	366	690.8	207.78	406	762.8
163.89	327	620.6	186.11	367	692.6	208.33	407	764.6
164.44	328	622.4	186.67	368	694.4	208.89	408	766.4
165	329	624.2	187.22	369	696.2	209.44	409	768.2

Appendix O
FAHRENHEIT-CELSIUS CONVERSIONS: 96.0°F TO 108.0°F (IN TENTHS)

Fahrenheit	Celsius	Fahrenheit	Celsius	Fahrenheit	Celsius
96.0	35.6	100.1	37.8	104.1	40.1
96.1	35.6	100.2	37.9	104.2	40.1
96.2	35.7	100.3	37.9	104.3	40.2
96.3	35.7	100.4	38.0	104.4	40.2
96.4	35.8	100.5	38.1	104.5	40.3
96.5	35.8	100.6	38.1	104.6	40.3
96.6	35.9	100.7	38.2	104.7	40.4
96.7	35.9	100.8	38.2	104.8	40.4
96.8	36.0	100.9	38.3	104.9	40.5
96.9	36.1	101.0	38.3	105.0	40.6
97.0	36.1	101.1	38.4	105.1	40.6
97.1	36.2	101.2	38.4	105.2	40.7
97.2	36.2	101.3	38.5	105.3	40.7
97.3	36.3	101.4	38.6	105.4	40.8
97.4	36.3	101.5	38.6	105.5	40.8
97.5	36.4	101.6	38.7	105.6	40.9
97.6	36.4	101.7	38.7	105.7	40.9
97.7	36.5	101.8	38.8	105.8	41.0
97.8	36.6	101.9	38.8	105.9	41.1
97.9	36.6	102.0	38.9	106.0	41.1
98.0	36.7	102.1	38.9	106.1	41.2
98.1	36.7	102.2	39.0	106.2	41.2
98.2	36.8	102.3	39.1	106.3	41.3
98.3	36.8	102.4	39.1	106.4	41.3
98.4	36.9	102.5	39.2	106.5	41.4
98.5	36.9	102.6	39.2	106.6	41.4
98.6	37.0	102.7	39.3	106.7	41.5
98.7	37.1	102.8	39.3	106.8	41.6
98.8	37.1	102.9	39.4	106.9	41.6
98.9	37.2	103.0	39.4	107.0	41.7
99.0	37.2	103.1	39.5	107.1	41.7
99.1	37.3	103.2	39.6	107.2	41.8
99.2	37.3	103.3	39.6	107.3	41.8
99.3	37.4	103.4	39.7	107.4	41.9
99.4	37.4	103.5	39.7	107.5	41.9
99.5	37.5	103.6	39.8	107.6	42.0
99.6	37.6	103.7	39.8	107.7	42.1
99.7	37.6	103.8	39.9	107.8	42.1
99.8	37.7	103.9	39.9	107.9	42.2
99.9	37.7	104.0	40.0	108.0	42.2
100.0	37.8				

Appendix P
TRANSMISSION (%T)-OPTICAL DENSITY (OD) TABLE

%T	OD(A)	%T	OD(A)	%T	OD(A)	%T	OD(A)
1.0	2.000	22.0	0.658	43.0	0.367	64.0	0.194
1.5	1.824	22.5	0.648	43.5	0.362	64.5	0.191
2.0	1.699	23.0	0.638	44.0	0.357	65.0	0.187
2.5	1.602	23.5	0.629	44.5	0.352	65.5	0.184
3.0	1.523	24.0	0.620	45.0	0.347	66.0	0.181
3.5	1.456	24.5	0.611	45.5	0.342	66.5	0.177
4.0	1.398	25.0	0.602	46.0	0.337	67.0	0.174
4.5	1.347	25.5	0.594	46.5	0.332	67.5	0.171
5.0	1.301	26.0	0.585	47.0	0.328	68.0	0.168
5.5	1.260	26.5	0.577	47.5	0.323	68.5	0.164
6.0	1.222	27.0	0.569	48.0	0.319	69.0	0.161
6.5	1.187	27.5	0.561	48.5	0.314	69.5	0.158
7.0	1.155	28.0	0.553	49.0	0.310	70.0	0.155
7.5	1.126	28.5	0.545	49.5	0.305	70.5	0.152
8.0	1.097	29.0	0.538	50.0	0.301	71.0	0.149
8.5	1.071	29.5	0.530	50.5	0.297	71.5	0.146
9.0	1.046	30.0	0.523	51.0	0.292	72.0	0.143
9.5	1.022	30.5	0.516	51.5	0.288	72.5	0.140
10.0	1.000	31.0	0.509	52.0	0.284	73.0	0.137
10.5	0.979	31.5	0.502	52.5	0.280	73.5	0.134
11.0	0.959	32.0	0.495	53.0	0.276	74.0	0.131
11.5	0.939	32.5	0.488	53.5	0.272	74.5	0.128
12.0	0.921	33.0	0.482	54.0	0.268	75.0	0.125
12.5	0.903	33.5	0.475	54.5	0.264	75.5	0.122
13.0	0.886	34.0	0.469	55.0	0.260	76.0	0.119
13.5	0.870	34.5	0.462	55.5	0.256	76.5	0.116
14.0	0.854	35.0	0.456	56.0	0.252	77.0	0.114
14.5	0.838	35.5	0.450	56.5	0.248	77.5	0.111
15.0	0.824	36.0	0.444	57.0	0.244	78.0	0.108
15.5	0.810	36.5	0.438	57.5	0.240	78.5	0.105
16.0	0.796	37.0	0.432	58.0	0.237	79.0	0.102
16.5	0.782	37.5	0.426	58.5	0.233	79.5	0.100
17.0	0.770	38.0	0.420	59.0	0.229	80.0	0.097
17.5	0.757	38.5	0.414	59.5	0.226	80.5	0.094
18.0	0.745	39.0	0.409	60.0	0.222	81.0	0.092
18.5	0.733	39.5	0.403	60.5	0.218	81.5	0.089
19.0	0.721	40.0	0.398	61.0	0.215	82.0	0.086
19.5	0.710	40.5	0.392	61.5	0.211	82.5	0.084
20.0	0.699	41.0	0.387	62.0	0.208	83.0	0.081
20.5	0.688	41.5	0.382	62.5	0.204	83.5	0.078
21.0	0.678	42.0	0.377	63.0	0.201	84.0	0.076
21.5	0.668	42.5	0.372	63.5	0.197	84.5	0.073

Continued.

%T	OD(A)	%T	OD(A)	%T	OD(A)	%T	OD(A)
85.0	0.071	89.0	0.051	93.0	0.032	97.0	0.013
85.5	0.068	89.5	0.048	93.5	0.029	97.5	0.011
86.0	0.066	90.0	0.046	94.0	0.027	98.0	0.009
86.5	0.063	90.5	0.043	94.5	0.025	98.5	0.007
87.0	0.061	91.0	0.041	95.0	0.022	99.0	0.004
87.5	0.058	91.5	0.039	95.5	0.020	99.5	0.002
88.0	0.056	92.0	0.036	96.0	0.018	100.0	0.000
88.5	0.053	92.5	0.034	96.5	0.016		

Appendix Q
FORMULAS PRESENTED IN THIS BOOK

Systems of Measure (Chapter 2)

1. To convert one metric unit to another metric unit:

$$\frac{\text{Exponent of 10}}{\text{of existing unit}} - \frac{\text{exponent of 10}}{\text{of desired unit}} = \frac{\text{exponent of 10}}{\text{of the factor}}$$

Factor × number of existing units = number of desired units

2. To convert one square metric unit to another square metric unit:

$$\frac{\text{Exponent of 10}}{\text{of existing unit}} - \frac{\text{exponent of 10}}{\text{of desired unit}} \times 2 = \frac{\text{exponent of 10}}{\text{of the factor}}$$

Factor × number of existing units = number of desired units

3. To convert one cubic metric unit to another cubic metric unit:

$$\frac{\text{Exponent of 10}}{\text{of existing unit}} - \frac{\text{exponent of 10}}{\text{of desired unit}} \times 3 = \frac{\text{exponent of 10}}{\text{of factor}}$$

Factor × number of existing units = number of desired units

Temperature Conversions (Chapter 3)

1. To convert °C to K: $K = °C + 273$

2. To convert K to °C: $°C = K - 273$

3. To convert °C to °F:
   $°F = (°C \times \frac{9}{5}) + 32$
   $°F = (°C \times 1.8) + 32$
   $°F = [(°C + 40) \times \frac{9}{5}] - 40$
   $°F = [(°C + 40) \times 1.8] - 40$

4. To convert °F to °C:
   $°C = (°F - 32) \times \frac{5}{9}$
   $°C = (°F - 32) \times 0.556$
   $°C = [(°F + 40) \times \frac{5}{9}] - 40$
   $°C = [(°F + 40) \times 0.556] - 40$

5. To convert °C to °F or °F to °C: $9C = 5F - 160$

Conversion Factors (Chapter 4)

1. To correct when the drug being used as a standard is different from the one being measured:

$$\text{Conversion factor} = \frac{\text{mol wt of drug being measured}}{\text{mol wt of drug used as the standard}}$$

2. To correct for variations in procedure quantities:

$$\frac{\text{What should have been used or done}}{\text{What was used or done}} \times \text{answer from machine}$$

Dilutions (Chapter 5)

1. Original conc. $\times$ $\dfrac{\text{tube}}{\text{dilution 1}}$ $\times$ $\dfrac{\text{tube}}{\text{dilution 2}}$ $\times$ $\dfrac{\text{tube}}{\text{dilution 3}}$ $\times$ . . . . = final conc.

Solutions (Chapter 6)

Percent

1. To find the amount of solute to make a given volume of solution

$$\frac{\text{Percent} \times \text{desired volume}}{100} = \text{Grams (or milliliters) of solute to be diluted up to the desired volume}$$

2. To find the percent of a solution when the amount of solute and total volume of solution are known:

$$\frac{\text{Grams (or ml) of solute} \times 100}{\text{Volume of solution}} = \text{percent}$$

3. When changing concentration or performing titration procedures:

$$V_1 \times C_1 = V_2 \times C_2$$

4. When mixing two or more solutions together:

$$(V_1 \times C_1) + (V_2 \times C_2) + (V_3 \times C_3) + . . . = V_F \times C_F$$

Molarity

1. mol wt $\times$ M $=$ g/L

$$M = \frac{\text{g/L}}{\text{mol wt}}$$

$$\text{mmol/L} = \frac{\text{mg/L}}{\text{mol wt}}$$

Osmolarity

1. Osmolarity (osmol/L) $=$ M $\times$ particles per molecule resulting from ionization
2. Milliosmolarity (mOsmol/L) $=$ mmol/L $\times$ particles per molecule resulting from ionization

3. $\text{osmol/L} = \dfrac{\Delta \text{ temperature}}{1.86}$

$$\text{mOsmol/L} = \frac{\Delta \text{ temperature}}{0.00186}$$

Normality

1. eq wt $\times$ N $=$ g/L

$$N = \frac{\text{g/L}}{\text{eq wt}}$$

Specific Gravity

1. sp gr $\times$ % purity (as decimal) = grams of specific solute/ml

2.
$$\text{sp gr} = \frac{\text{Weight of solid or liquid}}{\text{Weight of equal volume of } H_2O \text{ at } 4°C}$$

Concentration Relationships

1. To convert $\%^{w/v}$ to molarity or molarity to $\%^{w/v}$:

$$M = \frac{\%^{w/v} \times 10}{\text{mol wt}}$$

2. To convert $\%^{w/v}$ to normality or normality to $\%^{w/v}$:

$$N = \frac{\%^{w/v} \times 10}{\text{eq wt}}$$

3. To convert mg/dl to mEq/L or mEq/L to mg/dl:

$$\text{mEq/L} = \frac{\text{mg/dl} \times 10}{\text{eq wt}}$$

4. To convert molarity to normality:

$$N = M \times \text{valence}$$

5. To convert normality to molarity:

$$M = \frac{N}{\text{valence}}$$

6. To convert vol% CO_2 to mmol/L CO_2: $\text{mmol/L} = \text{vol\%} \times 0.45$

7. To convert mmol/L CO_2 to vol% CO_2: $\text{vol\%} = \text{mmol/L} \times 2.226$

8. To convert one complex metric unit to another complex metric unit:

$$\text{Desired unit} = \text{original unit} \times \frac{\text{power of 10 to convert the top unit}}{\text{power of 10 to convert the bottom unit}}$$

Ionic Solutions (Chapter 8)

pH-pOH

1. $[H^+] \times [OH^-] = 1 \times 10^{-14}$

$pH + pOH = 14$

$N \times \%$ ionization $= [H^+]$

$$pH = \log \frac{1}{[H^+]}$$

$$pH = -\log [H^+]$$

$$pH = b - \log a \text{ (using } [H^+] \text{ expressed in scientific notation)}$$

$$pOH = \log \frac{1}{[OH^-]}$$

$$pOH = -\log [OH^-]$$

$$pOH = b - \log a \text{ (using } [OH^-] \text{ expressed in scientific notation)}$$

Henderson-Hasselbalch Equation

1. $pH = pK + \log \dfrac{[\text{salt}]}{[\text{acid}]}$

   $pH = pK + \log \dfrac{[HCO_3^-]}{[CO_2]}$

   $pH = pK + \log \dfrac{\text{Total } CO_2 - a \times P_{CO_2}}{a \times P_{CO_2}}$

2. $P_{CO_2} \text{ (mm Hg)} = \dfrac{\text{Total } CO_2 \text{ (mmol/L)}}{0.03 \, [\text{antilog } (pH - 6.1) + 1]}$

3. $\text{Total } CO_2 \text{ (mmol/L)} = 0.03 \, P_{CO_2} \, [\text{antilog } (pH - 6.1) + 1]$

Colorimetry (Chapter 9)

1. To calculate the concentration of an unknown that follows Beer's law:

$$C_u = \frac{A_u}{A_s} \times C_s$$

2. Relationship between absorbance and percent transmittance:

$$A = \log \frac{1}{T}$$
$$A = -\log T$$
$$A = 2 - \log \%T$$

3. Relationship between absorbance, molar absorptivity, and concentration:

$$A = \epsilon \times C \times d$$

Graphs (Chapter 10)

1. $\text{Slope} = \dfrac{\Delta y}{\Delta x}$

2. To calculate the concentration of a standard for a given test:

$$C_s = W_s \times D \times \frac{V_c}{V_t}$$

$$C_s = \text{ml } WS \times \frac{100}{\text{quantity of sample used}} \times \text{conc } WS/ml$$

Hematology Math (Chapter 11)

1. To calculate a final factor when using diluting pipettes and the counting chamber:

$$\text{Dilution factor} \times \text{depth factor} \times \frac{1}{\text{area counted (in mm}^2)} = \text{final factor}$$

$$\text{Dilution factor} \times \text{depth factor} \times \text{area factor} = \text{final factor}$$

$$\text{Dilution factor} \times \frac{1}{\text{volume counted (in mm}^3)} = \text{final factor}$$

$$\text{Dilution factor} \times \text{volume factor} = \text{final factor}$$

$$\frac{\text{Dilution factor} \times \text{depth factor}}{\text{Area counted (in } mm^2)} = \text{final factor}$$

2. To find the area factor:

$$\text{Area factor} = \frac{1}{\text{area counted (in } mm^2)}$$

3. To find the volume factor:

$$\text{Volume factor} = \frac{1}{\text{volume counted (in } mm^3)}$$

$$\text{Volume factor} = \text{depth factor} \times \text{area factor}$$

4. To find the mean corpuscular volume:

$$MCV = \frac{Hct \times 10}{RBC \text{ (in millions)}}$$

5. To find the mean corpuscular hemoglobin:

$$MCH = \frac{Hb \text{ (in grams)} \times 10}{RBC \text{ (in millions)}}$$

6. To find the mean corpuscular hemoglobin concentration:

$$MCHC = \frac{Hb \text{ (in grams)} \times 100}{Hct}$$

7. To find the concentration for a hemoglobin standard in a given procedure:

$$\frac{\text{Conc of std (assay)} \times \text{dilution factor}}{1{,}000} = g\%$$

Enzyme Calculations (Chapter 12)

1. To calculate international units per liter:

$$IU/L = \frac{\Delta A_{340}/\min \times V_t}{6.22 \times V_s} \times 1{,}000 \times \frac{1}{T}$$

$$IU/L = \frac{\Delta A_{334}/\min \times V_t}{6.0 \times V_s} \times 1{,}000 \times \frac{1}{T}$$

$$IU/L = \frac{\Delta A_{366}/\min \times V_t}{3.3 \times V_s} \times 1{,}000 \times \frac{1}{T}$$

$$IU/L = \mu mol/min/L$$

2. To calculate IU/ml:

$$IU/ml = \mu mol/min/ml$$

3. Calculations based on ϵ and the absorbance:

$$IU/L = \frac{A \text{ of sample}}{\epsilon \times d} \times 10^6 \times \frac{1}{T} \times \frac{V_t}{V_s}$$

4. Calculations based on a standard:

$$IU/L = \frac{A \text{ of sample}}{A \text{ of standard}} \times 10^6 \times \text{Standard conc (in moles/L)} \times \frac{1}{T} \times \frac{V_t}{V_s}$$

Gastric Acidity (Chapter 13)

1.
$$\text{Degrees of acidity} = \frac{\text{ml of 0.1N NaOH} \times 100}{\text{ml of sample}}$$

2.
$$\text{Total acid in mmol/L} = \frac{\text{ml of 0.1M NaOH} \times 0.1 \times 1,000}{\text{ml of sample}}$$

3.
$$\text{Free acid in mmol/L} = \frac{\text{ml of 0.1M NaOH} \times 0.1 \times 1,000}{\text{ml of sample}}$$

4. $$\text{Free acid in mmol/hr} = \frac{\text{mmol free acid/L} \times \text{tot vol of spec (ml)}}{1,000} \times \frac{60}{\text{collection time of spec (min)}}$$

5.
$$\text{BAO/MAO ratio} = \frac{\text{BAO}}{\text{MAO}}$$

6.
$$\text{Percent BAO/MAO} = \frac{\text{BAO}}{\text{MAO}} \times 100$$

Renal Tests (Chapter 14)

Creatinine Clearance
1. Uncorrected:

$$C = \frac{U}{P} \times V$$

2. Corrected for body surface:

$$C = \frac{U}{P} \times V \times \frac{1.73}{A}$$

Urea Clearance
1. Maximum, uncorrected:

$$C = \frac{U}{P} \times V$$

2. Maximum, corrected for body surface:

$$C = \frac{U}{P} \times V \times \frac{1.73}{A}$$

3. Maximum, corrected for body surface and reported in percent of normal:

$$C = \frac{U}{P} \times V \times \frac{1.73}{A} \times \frac{100}{75}$$

4. Standard, uncorrected:

$$C = \frac{U}{P} \times \sqrt{V}$$

5. Standard, corrected for body surface:

$$C = \frac{U}{P} \times \sqrt{V} \times \frac{1.73}{A}$$

6. Standard, corrected for body surface and reported in percent of normal:

$$C = \frac{U}{P} \times \sqrt{V} \times \frac{1.73}{A} \times \frac{100}{54}$$

Body Surface in Square Meters

1. $\log A = (0.425 \times \log W) + (0.725 \times \log H) - 2.144$

Timed Urine Tests

1. To calculate a quantity per total volume:

$$\frac{\text{Amount of substance}}{\text{per total volume}} = \frac{\text{amount of substance}}{\text{reported from instrument}} \times \frac{\text{total volume (in ml)}}{\text{volume reported from instrument (in ml)}}$$

2. To calculate a quantity per hour:

$$\text{Quantity per hour} = \frac{\text{amount of substance from instrument}}{\text{volume reported from instrument (in ml)}} \times \frac{\text{total volume (in ml)}}{\text{hours collected}}$$

Quality Control (Chapter 15)

1. Variance:

$$s^2 = \frac{\Sigma(X - \overline{X})^2}{n - 1}$$

2. Standard deviation:

$$s = \sqrt{s^2}$$

$$s = \sqrt{\frac{\Sigma(X - \overline{X})^2}{n - 1}}$$

3. Percent coefficient of variation:

$$\%CV = \frac{s}{\overline{X}} \times 100$$

Appendix R
NOMOGRAM FOR DETERMINATION OF BODY SURFACE AREA

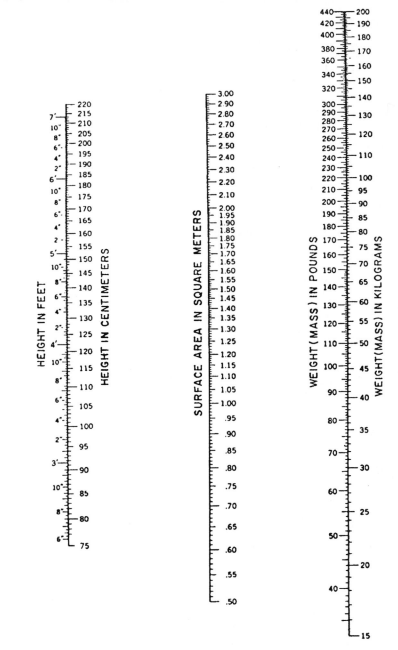

From Boothby W, Sandiford RB: Surface area nomogram (DuBois), *N Engl J Med* 185:337, 1921.

Appendix S
IEC RELATIVE CENTRIFUGAL FORCE NOMOGRAPH

Instructions

To determine the relative centrifugal force (rcf), place a straightedge on the nomograph connecting the known speed (rpm) and the known rotating radius. The point at which the straightedge intersects the rcf axis is the force.

For example, if the rotating radius is 10 cm and the speed is 3,000 rpm, the relative centrifugal force is 1,000 $\times$ g (gravity).

If the force and the radius are known, the corresponding speed can be determined.

To Calculate RCF

$RCF = .00001118 \times r \times N^2$
RCF = relative centrifugal force (gravities)
r = rotating radius (centimeters)
N = rotating speed (rev. per min. or rpm)

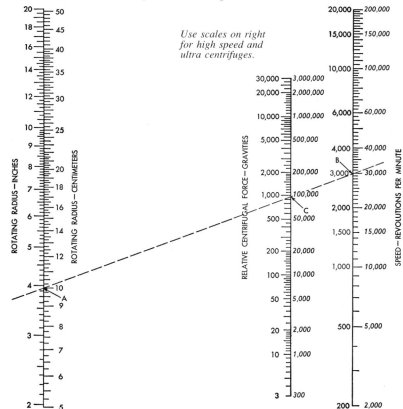

Modified from International Equipment Company, Needham Heights, Mass.

Appendix T
CONVERSIONS AMONG METRIC PREFIXES

		10^{18} exa (E)	10^{15} peta (P)	10^{12} tera (T)	10^{9} giga (G)	10^{6} mega (M)	10^{3} kilo (k)	10^{2} hecto (h)
10^{18}	exa (E)	1	10^{3}	10^{6}	10^{9}	10^{12}	10^{15}	10^{16}
10^{15}	peta (P)	10^{-3}	1	10^{3}	10^{6}	10^{9}	10^{12}	10^{13}
10^{12}	tera (T)	10^{-6}	10^{-3}	1	10^{3}	10^{6}	10^{9}	10^{10}
10^{9}	giga (G)	10^{-9}	10^{-6}	10^{-3}	1	10^{3}	10^{6}	10^{7}
10^{6}	mega (M)	10^{-12}	10^{-9}	10^{-6}	10^{-3}	1	10^{3}	10^{4}
10^{3}	kilo (k)	10^{-15}	10^{-12}	10^{-9}	10^{-6}	10^{-3}	1	10^{1}
10^{2}	hecto (h)	10^{-16}	10^{-13}	10^{-10}	10^{-7}	10^{-4}	10^{-1}	1
10^{1}	deka (da)	10^{-17}	10^{-14}	10^{-11}	10^{-8}	10^{-5}	10^{-2}	10^{-1}
10^{0}	primary unit L, gm, or m	10^{-18}	10^{-15}	10^{-12}	10^{-9}	10^{-6}	10^{-3}	10^{-2}
10^{-1}	deci (d)	10^{-19}	10^{-16}	10^{-13}	10^{-10}	10^{-7}	10^{-4}	10^{-3}
10^{-2}	centi (c)	10^{-20}	10^{-17}	10^{-14}	10^{-11}	10^{-8}	10^{-5}	10^{-4}
10^{-3}	milli (m)	10^{-21}	10^{-18}	10^{-15}	10^{-12}	10^{-9}	10^{-6}	10^{-5}
10^{-6}	micro (μ)	10^{-24}	10^{-21}	10^{-18}	10^{-15}	10^{-12}	10^{-9}	10^{-8}
10^{-9}	nano (n)	10^{-27}	10^{-24}	10^{-21}	10^{-18}	10^{-15}	10^{-12}	10^{-11}
10^{-12}	pico (p)	10^{-30}	10^{-27}	10^{-24}	10^{-21}	10^{-18}	10^{-15}	10^{-14}
10^{-15}	femto (f)	10^{-33}	10^{-30}	10^{-27}	10^{-24}	10^{-21}	10^{-18}	10^{-17}
10^{-18}	atto (a)	10^{-36}	10^{-33}	10^{-30}	10^{-27}	10^{-24}	10^{-21}	10^{-20}

To convert from one metric unit to another:
1. Find the prefix you have in the left-hand column.
2. Move from the left-hand column to the right in the same row until you locate the column headed by the desired prefix.
3. Locate the number where these two lines intersect.
4. Multiply the units of the prefix on hand by this number to get the equivalent number of units of the prefix desired.

EXAMPLE: 100 mg is equal to how many femtograms?

Locate *milli* in the left-hand column; move to the right in the same row until you locate the column headed by *femto*. At the point where the two lines intersect, you should see 10^{12}. Multiply 100 by 10^{12} to get 10^{14}. Hence, 100 mg = 10^{14} fg.

EXAMPLE: 28 dekaliters is equal to how many deciliters?

Locate *deka* in the left-hand column; find the point where this row intersects the row under *deci* (10^{-1}). At this point you should find 10^{2}. Multiply 28 by 10^{2} (28 × 100) to get 2,800. Hence, 28 dekaliters is equal to 2,800 deciliters.

10^1 deka (da)	10^0 primary unit L, gm, or m	10^{-1} deci (d)	10^{-2} centi (c)	10^{-3} milli (m)	10^{-6} micro (μ)	10^{-9} nano (n)	10^{-12} pico (p)	10^{-15} femto (f)	10^{-18} atto (a)
10^{17}	10^{18}	10^{19}	10^{20}	10^{21}	10^{24}	10^{27}	10^{30}	10^{33}	10^{36}
10^{14}	10^{15}	10^{16}	10^{17}	10^{18}	10^{21}	10^{24}	10^{27}	10^{30}	10^{33}
10^{11}	10^{12}	10^{13}	10^{14}	10^{15}	10^{18}	10^{21}	10^{24}	10^{27}	10^{30}
10^{8}	10^{9}	10^{10}	10^{11}	10^{12}	10^{15}	10^{18}	10^{21}	10^{24}	10^{27}
10^{5}	10^{6}	10^{7}	10^{8}	10^{9}	10^{12}	10^{15}	10^{18}	10^{21}	10^{24}
10^{2}	10^{3}	10^{4}	10^{5}	10^{6}	10^{9}	10^{12}	10^{15}	10^{18}	10^{21}
10^{1}	10^{2}	10^{3}	10^{4}	10^{5}	10^{8}	10^{11}	10^{14}	10^{17}	10^{20}
1	10^{1}	10^{2}	10^{3}	10^{4}	10^{7}	10^{10}	10^{13}	10^{16}	10^{19}
10^{-1}	1	10^{1}	10^{2}	10^{3}	10^{6}	10^{9}	10^{12}	10^{15}	10^{18}
10^{-2}	10^{-1}	1	10^{1}	10^{2}	10^{5}	10^{8}	10^{11}	10^{14}	10^{17}
10^{-3}	10^{-2}	10^{-1}	1	10^{1}	10^{4}	10^{7}	10^{10}	10^{13}	10^{16}
10^{-4}	10^{-3}	10^{-2}	10^{-1}	1	10^{3}	10^{6}	10^{9}	10^{12}	10^{15}
10^{-7}	10^{-6}	10^{-5}	10^{-4}	10^{-3}	1	10^{3}	10^{6}	10^{9}	10^{12}
10^{-10}	10^{-9}	10^{-8}	10^{-7}	10^{-6}	10^{-3}	1	10^{3}	10^{6}	10^{9}
10^{-13}	10^{-12}	10^{-11}	10^{-10}	10^{-9}	10^{-6}	10^{-3}	1	10^{3}	10^{6}
10^{-16}	10^{-15}	10^{-14}	10^{-13}	10^{-12}	10^{-9}	10^{-6}	10^{-3}	1	10^{3}
10^{-19}	10^{-18}	10^{-17}	10^{-16}	10^{-15}	10^{-12}	10^{-9}	10^{-6}	10^{-3}	1

Appendix U

CONVERSIONS AMONG SQUARE METRIC UNITS

		10^{18} exa (E)	10^{15} peta (P)	10^{12} tera (T)	10^{9} giga (G)	10^{6} mega (M)	10^{3} kilo (k)	10^{2} hecto (h)
10^{18}	exa (E)	1	10^{6}	10^{12}	10^{18}	10^{24}	10^{30}	10^{32}
10^{15}	peta (P)	10^{-6}	1	10^{6}	10^{12}	10^{18}	10^{24}	10^{26}
10^{12}	tera (T)	10^{-12}	10^{-6}	1	10^{6}	10^{12}	10^{18}	10^{20}
10^{9}	giga (G)	10^{-18}	10^{-12}	10^{-6}	1	10^{6}	10^{12}	10^{14}
10^{6}	mega (M)	10^{-24}	10^{-18}	10^{-12}	10^{-6}	1	10^{6}	10^{8}
10^{3}	kilo (k)	10^{-30}	10^{-24}	10^{-18}	10^{-12}	10^{-6}	1	10^{2}
10^{2}	hecto (h)	10^{-32}	10^{-26}	10^{-20}	10^{-14}	10^{-8}	10^{-2}	1
10^{1}	deka (da)	10^{-34}	10^{-28}	10^{-22}	10^{-16}	10^{-10}	10^{-4}	10^{-2}
10^{0}	primary unit (meter)	10^{-36}	10^{-30}	10^{-24}	10^{-18}	10^{-12}	10^{-6}	10^{-4}
10^{-1}	deci (d)	10^{-38}	10^{-32}	10^{-26}	10^{-20}	10^{-14}	10^{-8}	10^{-6}
10^{-2}	centi (c)	10^{-40}	10^{-34}	10^{-28}	10^{-22}	10^{-16}	10^{-10}	10^{-8}
10^{-3}	milli (m)	10^{-42}	10^{-36}	10^{-30}	10^{-24}	10^{-18}	10^{-12}	10^{-10}
10^{-6}	micro (μ)	10^{-48}	10^{-42}	10^{-36}	10^{-30}	10^{-24}	10^{-18}	10^{-16}
10^{-9}	nano (n)	10^{-54}	10^{-48}	10^{-42}	10^{-36}	10^{-30}	10^{-24}	10^{-22}
10^{-12}	pico (p)	10^{-60}	10^{-54}	10^{-48}	10^{-42}	10^{-36}	10^{-30}	10^{-28}
10^{-15}	femto (f)	10^{-66}	10^{-60}	10^{-54}	10^{-48}	10^{-42}	10^{-36}	10^{-34}
10^{-18}	atto (a)	10^{-72}	10^{-66}	10^{-60}	10^{-54}	10^{-48}	10^{-42}	10^{-40}

To convert from one square metric unit to another.
1. Find the prefix you have in the left-hand column.
2. Move from the left-hand column to the right in the same row until you locate the column headed by the desired prefix.
3. Locate the number where these two lines intersect.
4. Multiply the units of the prefix on hand by this number to get the equivalent number of units of the prefix desired.

EXAMPLE: 300 square meters is equal to how many square dekameters?

The known unit is meter; there is no prefix; the power of 10 is 10^{0}.
The desired unit is dekameter; the prefix is *deka;* the power of 10 is 10^{1}.

Locate *meter* (the known unit) or 10^{0} in the left hand column. Move to the right in the same row until you locate the column headed by *deka* (the desired unit). At the point where the two lines intersect, you should see 10^{-2}. Multiply 300 by 10^{-2} to get 3. Hence, 300 square meters is equal to 3 square dekameters.

10^1 deka (da)	10^0 primary unit (meter)	10^{-1} deci (d)	10^{-2} centi (c)	10^{-3} milli (m)	10^{-6} micro (μ)	10^{-9} nano (n)	10^{-12} pico (p)	10^{-15} femto (f)	10^{-18} atto (a)
10^{34}	10^{36}	10^{38}	10^{40}	10^{42}	10^{48}	10^{54}	10^{60}	10^{66}	10^{72}
10^{28}	10^{30}	10^{32}	10^{34}	10^{36}	10^{42}	10^{48}	10^{54}	10^{60}	10^{66}
10^{22}	10^{24}	10^{26}	10^{28}	10^{30}	10^{36}	10^{42}	10^{48}	10^{54}	10^{60}
10^{16}	10^{18}	10^{20}	10^{22}	10^{24}	10^{30}	10^{36}	10^{42}	10^{48}	10^{54}
10^{10}	10^{12}	10^{14}	10^{16}	10^{18}	10^{24}	10^{30}	10^{36}	10^{42}	10^{48}
10^{4}	10^{6}	10^{8}	10^{10}	10^{12}	10^{18}	10^{24}	10^{30}	10^{36}	10^{42}
10^{2}	10^{4}	10^{6}	10^{8}	10^{10}	10^{16}	10^{22}	10^{28}	10^{34}	10^{40}
1	10^{2}	10^{4}	10^{6}	10^{8}	10^{14}	10^{20}	10^{26}	10^{32}	10^{38}
10^{-2}	1	10^{2}	10^{4}	10^{6}	10^{12}	10^{18}	10^{24}	10^{30}	10^{36}
10^{-4}	10^{-2}	1	10^{2}	10^{4}	10^{10}	10^{16}	10^{22}	10^{28}	10^{34}
10^{-6}	10^{-4}	10^{-2}	1	10^{2}	10^{8}	10^{14}	10^{20}	10^{26}	10^{32}
10^{-8}	10^{-6}	10^{-4}	10^{-2}	1	10^{6}	10^{12}	10^{18}	10^{24}	10^{30}
10^{-14}	10^{-12}	10^{-10}	10^{-8}	10^{-6}	1	10^{6}	10^{12}	10^{18}	10^{24}
10^{-20}	10^{-18}	10^{-16}	10^{-14}	10^{-12}	10^{-6}	1	10^{6}	10^{12}	10^{18}
10^{-26}	10^{-24}	10^{-22}	10^{-20}	10^{-18}	10^{-12}	10^{-6}	1	10^{6}	10^{12}
10^{-32}	10^{-30}	10^{-28}	10^{-26}	10^{-24}	10^{-18}	10^{-12}	10^{-6}	1	10^{6}
10^{-38}	10^{-36}	10^{-34}	10^{-32}	10^{-30}	10^{-24}	10^{-18}	10^{-12}	10^{-6}	1

Appendix V
CONVERSIONS AMONG CUBIC METRIC UNITS

		10^{18} exa (E)	10^{15} peta (P)	10^{12} tera (T)	10^{9} giga (G)	10^{6} mega (M)	10^{3} kilo (k)	10^{2} hecto (h)
10^{18}	exa (E)	1	10^{9}	10^{18}	10^{27}	10^{36}	10^{45}	10^{48}
10^{15}	peta (P)	10^{-9}	1	10^{9}	10^{18}	10^{27}	10^{36}	10^{39}
10^{12}	tera (T)	10^{-18}	10^{-9}	1	10^{9}	10^{18}	10^{27}	10^{30}
10^{9}	giga (G)	10^{-27}	10^{-18}	10^{-9}	1	10^{9}	10^{18}	10^{21}
10^{6}	mega (M)	10^{-36}	10^{-27}	10^{-18}	10^{-9}	1	10^{9}	10^{12}
10^{3}	kilo (k)	10^{-45}	10^{-36}	10^{-27}	10^{-18}	10^{-9}	1	10^{3}
10^{2}	hecto (h)	10^{-48}	10^{-39}	10^{-30}	10^{-21}	10^{-12}	10^{-3}	1
10^{1}	deka (da)	10^{-51}	10^{-42}	10^{-33}	10^{-24}	10^{-15}	10^{-6}	10^{-3}
10^{0}	primary unit (meter)	10^{-54}	10^{-45}	10^{-36}	10^{-27}	10^{-18}	10^{-9}	10^{-6}
10^{-1}	deci (d)	10^{-57}	10^{-48}	10^{-39}	10^{-30}	10^{-21}	10^{-12}	10^{-9}
10^{-2}	centi (c)	10^{-60}	10^{-51}	10^{-42}	10^{-33}	10^{-24}	10^{-15}	10^{-12}
10^{-3}	milli (m)	10^{-63}	10^{-54}	10^{-45}	10^{-36}	10^{-27}	10^{-18}	10^{-15}
10^{-6}	micro (μ)	10^{-72}	10^{-63}	10^{-54}	10^{-45}	10^{-36}	10^{-27}	10^{-24}
10^{-9}	nano (n)	10^{-81}	10^{-72}	10^{-63}	10^{-54}	10^{-45}	10^{-36}	10^{-33}
10^{-12}	pico (p)	10^{-90}	10^{-81}	10^{-72}	10^{-63}	10^{-54}	10^{-45}	10^{-42}
10^{-15}	femto (f)	10^{-99}	10^{-90}	10^{-81}	10^{-72}	10^{-63}	10^{-54}	10^{-51}
10^{-18}	atto (a)	10^{-108}	10^{-99}	10^{-90}	10^{-81}	10^{-72}	10^{-63}	10^{-60}

To convert from one cubic metric unit to another.
1. Find the prefix you have in the left-hand column.
2. Move from the left-hand column to the right in the same row until you locate the column headed by the desired prefix.
3. Locate the number where these two lines intersect.
4. Multiply the units of the prefix on hand by this number to get the equivalent number of units of the prefix desired.

EXAMPLE: 10 cubic centimeters is equal to how many cubic millimeters?

> The known unit is centimeter; the prefix is centi; the power of 10 is 10^{-2}.
> The desired unit is millimeter; the prefix is milli; the power of 10 is 10^{-3}.

Locate *centi* (the known unit) or 10^{-2} in the left hand column. Move to the right in the same row until you locate the column headed by *milli* (the desired unit). At the point where the two lines intersect you should see 10^{3}. Multiply 10 by 10^{3} to get 10,000. Hence, 10 cubic centimeters is equal to 10,000 cubic millimeters.

10^1 deka (da)	10^0 primary unit (meter)	10^{-1} deci (d)	10^{-2} centi (c)	10^{-3} milli (m)	10^{-6} micro (μ)	10^{-9} nano (n)	10^{-12} pico (p)	10^{-15} femto (f)	10^{-18} atto (a)
10^{51}	10^{54}	10^{57}	10^{60}	10^{63}	10^{72}	10^{81}	10^{90}	10^{99}	10^{108}
10^{42}	10^{45}	10^{48}	10^{51}	10^{54}	10^{63}	10^{72}	10^{81}	10^{90}	10^{99}
10^{33}	10^{36}	10^{39}	10^{42}	10^{45}	10^{54}	10^{63}	10^{72}	10^{81}	10^{90}
10^{24}	10^{27}	10^{30}	10^{33}	10^{36}	10^{45}	10^{54}	10^{63}	10^{72}	10^{81}
10^{15}	10^{18}	10^{21}	10^{24}	10^{27}	10^{36}	10^{45}	10^{54}	10^{63}	10^{72}
10^{6}	10^{9}	10^{12}	10^{15}	10^{18}	10^{27}	10^{36}	10^{45}	10^{54}	10^{63}
10^{3}	10^{6}	10^{9}	10^{12}	10^{15}	10^{24}	10^{33}	10^{42}	10^{51}	10^{60}
1	10^{3}	10^{6}	10^{9}	10^{12}	10^{21}	10^{30}	10^{39}	10^{48}	10^{57}
10^{-3}	1	10^{3}	10^{6}	10^{9}	10^{18}	10^{27}	10^{36}	10^{45}	10^{54}
10^{-6}	10^{-3}	1	10^{3}	10^{6}	10^{15}	10^{24}	10^{33}	10^{42}	10^{51}
10^{-9}	10^{-6}	10^{-3}	1	10^{3}	10^{12}	10^{21}	10^{30}	10^{39}	10^{48}
10^{-12}	10^{-9}	10^{-6}	10^{-3}	1	10^{9}	10^{18}	10^{27}	10^{36}	10^{45}
10^{-21}	10^{-18}	10^{-15}	10^{-12}	10^{-9}	1	10^{9}	10^{18}	10^{27}	10^{36}
10^{-30}	10^{-27}	10^{-24}	10^{-21}	10^{-18}	10^{-9}	1	10^{9}	10^{18}	10^{27}
10^{-39}	10^{-36}	10^{-33}	10^{-30}	10^{-27}	10^{-18}	10^{-9}	1	10^{9}	10^{18}
10^{-48}	10^{-45}	10^{-42}	10^{-39}	10^{-36}	10^{-27}	10^{-18}	10^{-9}	1	10^{9}
10^{-57}	10^{-54}	10^{-51}	10^{-48}	10^{-45}	10^{-36}	10^{-27}	10^{-18}	10^{-9}	1

Appendix W
CONVERSIONS AMONG LITER UNITS AND CUBIC METRIC UNITS

		10^{18} exa (E)	10^{15} peta (P)	10^{12} tera (T)	10^{9} giga (G)	10^{6} mega (M)	10^{3} kilo (k)	10^{2} hecto (h)
10^{18}	exa (E)	10^{-39}	10^{-30}	10^{-21}	10^{-12}	10^{-3}	10^{6}	10^{9}
10^{15}	peta (P)	10^{-42}	10^{-33}	10^{-24}	10^{-15}	10^{-6}	10^{3}	10^{6}
10^{12}	tera (T)	10^{-45}	10^{-36}	10^{-27}	10^{-18}	10^{-9}	1	10^{3}
10^{9}	giga (G)	10^{-48}	10^{-39}	10^{-30}	10^{-21}	10^{-12}	10^{-3}	1
10^{6}	mega (M)	10^{-51}	10^{-42}	10^{-33}	10^{-24}	10^{-15}	10^{-6}	10^{-3}
10^{3}	kilo (k)	10^{-54}	10^{-45}	10^{-36}	10^{-27}	10^{-18}	10^{-9}	10^{-6}
10^{2}	hecto (h)	10^{-55}	10^{-46}	10^{-37}	10^{-28}	10^{-19}	10^{-10}	10^{-7}
10^{1}	deka (da)	10^{-56}	10^{-47}	10^{-38}	10^{-29}	10^{-20}	10^{-11}	10^{-8}
10^{0}	primary unit (liter)	10^{-57}	10^{-48}	10^{-39}	10^{-30}	10^{-21}	10^{-12}	10^{-9}
10^{-1}	deci (d)	10^{-58}	10^{-49}	10^{-40}	10^{-31}	10^{-22}	10^{-13}	10^{-10}
10^{-2}	centi (c)	10^{-59}	10^{-50}	10^{-41}	10^{-32}	10^{-23}	10^{-14}	10^{-11}
10^{-3}	milli (m)	10^{-60}	10^{-51}	10^{-42}	10^{-33}	10^{-24}	10^{-15}	10^{-12}
10^{-6}	micro (μ)	10^{-63}	10^{-54}	10^{-45}	10^{-36}	10^{-27}	10^{-18}	10^{-15}
10^{-9}	nano (n)	10^{-66}	10^{-57}	10^{-48}	10^{-39}	10^{-30}	10^{-21}	10^{-18}
10^{-12}	pico (p)	10^{-69}	10^{-60}	10^{-51}	10^{-42}	10^{-33}	10^{-24}	10^{-21}
10^{-15}	femto (f)	10^{-72}	10^{-63}	10^{-54}	10^{-45}	10^{-36}	10^{-27}	10^{-24}
10^{-18}	atto (a)	10^{-75}	10^{-66}	10^{-57}	10^{-48}	10^{-39}	10^{-30}	10^{-27}

Conversion can go in two directions: (1) from liquid measure to cubic volume measure, and (2) from cubic volume measure to liquid measure.

A. To convert from liquid measure to cubic volume measure
   1. Find the prefix you have in the left-hand column.
   2. Move from the left-hand column to the right in the same row until you locate the column headed by the desired prefix.
   3. Locate the number where these two lines intersect.
   4. Multiply the units of the prefix on hand by this number to get the equivalent number of units of the prefix desired.

   EXAMPLE: 10 centiliters is equal to how many cubic millimeters?

   > The known unit is centiliter; the prefix is centi; the power of 10 is 10^{-2}.
   > The desired unit is cubic millimter; the prefix is milli; the power of 10 is 10^{-3}.

   Locate *centi* (the known unit) or 10^{-2} in the left hand column. Move to the right in the same row until you locate the column headed by *milli* (the desired unit). At the point where the two lines intersect you should see 10^{4}. Multiply 10 by 10^{4} to get 100,000. Hence, 10 centiliters is equal to 100,000 cubic millimeters.

B. To convert from cubic volume measure to liquid measure
   This may be done in two ways:
   1. Multiply by the reverse power of 10.
   2. Divide by the power of 10 instead of multiplying.

10^1 deka (da)	10^0 primary unit (cubic meter)	10^{-1} deci (d)	10^{-2} centi (c)	10^{-3} milli (m)	10^{-6} micro (μ)	10^{-9} nano (n)	10^{-12} pico (p)	10^{-15} femto (f)	10^{-18} atto (a)
10^{12}	10^{15}	10^{18}	10^{21}	10^{24}	10^{33}	10^{42}	10^{51}	10^{60}	10^{69}
10^{9}	10^{12}	10^{15}	10^{18}	10^{21}	10^{30}	10^{39}	10^{48}	10^{57}	10^{66}
10^{6}	10^{9}	10^{12}	10^{15}	10^{18}	10^{27}	10^{36}	10^{45}	10^{54}	10^{63}
10^{3}	10^{6}	10^{9}	10^{12}	10^{15}	10^{24}	10^{33}	10^{42}	10^{51}	10^{60}
1	10^{3}	10^{6}	10^{9}	10^{12}	10^{21}	10^{30}	10^{39}	10^{48}	10^{57}
10^{-3}	1	10^{3}	10^{6}	10^{9}	10^{18}	10^{27}	10^{36}	10^{45}	10^{54}
10^{-4}	10^{-1}	10^{2}	10^{5}	10^{8}	10^{17}	10^{26}	10^{35}	10^{44}	10^{53}
10^{-5}	10^{-2}	10^{1}	10^{4}	10^{7}	10^{16}	10^{25}	10^{34}	10^{43}	10^{52}
10^{-6}	10^{-3}	1	10^{3}	10^{6}	10^{15}	10^{24}	10^{33}	10^{42}	10^{51}
10^{-7}	10^{-4}	10^{-1}	10^{2}	10^{5}	10^{14}	10^{23}	10^{32}	10^{41}	10^{50}
10^{-8}	10^{-5}	10^{-2}	10^{1}	10^{4}	10^{13}	10^{22}	10^{31}	10^{40}	10^{49}
10^{-9}	10^{-6}	10^{-3}	1	10^{3}	10^{12}	10^{21}	10^{30}	10^{39}	10^{48}
10^{-12}	10^{-9}	10^{-6}	10^{-3}	1	10^{9}	10^{18}	10^{27}	10^{36}	10^{45}
10^{-15}	10^{-12}	10^{-9}	10^{-6}	10^{-3}	10^{6}	10^{15}	10^{24}	10^{33}	10^{42}
10^{-18}	10^{-15}	10^{-12}	10^{-9}	10^{-6}	10^{3}	10^{12}	10^{21}	10^{30}	10^{39}
10^{-21}	10^{-18}	10^{-15}	10^{-12}	10^{-9}	1	10^{9}	10^{18}	10^{27}	10^{36}
10^{-24}	10^{-21}	10^{-18}	10^{-15}	10^{-12}	10^{-3}	10^{6}	10^{15}	10^{24}	10^{33}

Appendix X
X.1 CONVERSIONS BETWEEN CONVENTIONAL AND SI UNITS

	Conventional units	×	Factor	=	SI units
Gram	g/ml		$\dfrac{10^{15}}{mw}$		pmol/L
	g/100 ml		10		g/L
	g/100 ml		$\dfrac{10}{mw}$		mol/L
	g/100 ml		$\dfrac{10^4}{mw}$		mmol/L
	g/d		$\dfrac{1}{mw}$		mol/d
	g/d		$\dfrac{10^3}{mw}$		mmol/d
	g/d		$\dfrac{10^9}{mw}$		nmol/d
Microgram	μg/100 ml		$\dfrac{10}{mw}$		μmol/L
	μg/d		$\dfrac{1}{mw}$		μmol/d
	μg/d		$\dfrac{10^3}{mw}$		nmol/d
Micromicrogram (Nanogram)	$\mu\mu$g		$\dfrac{10^3}{mw}$		fmol
	$\mu\mu$g/ml		$\dfrac{10^3}{mw}$		pmol/L
Milliequivalent	mEq/L		$\dfrac{1}{valence}$		mmol/L
	mEq/kg		$\dfrac{1}{valence}$		mmol/kg
	mEq/d		$\dfrac{1}{valence}$		mmol/d

	Conventional units	×	Factor	=	SI units
Milligram	mg/100 ml		10^{-2}		g/L
	mg/100 ml		$\dfrac{10^{-2}}{mw}$		mol/L
	mg/100 ml		$\dfrac{10}{mw}$		mmol/L
	mg/100 ml		$\dfrac{10^4}{mw}$		μmol/L
	mg/100 g		10		mg/kg
	mg/100 g		$\dfrac{10}{mw}$		mmol/kg
	mg/d		$\dfrac{1}{mw}$		mmol/d
	mg/d		$\dfrac{10^3}{mw}$		μmol/d
Milliliter	ml/100 g		10		ml/kg
	ml/min		1.667×10^{-2}		ml/s
Millimeters of mercury	mm Hg		1.333		mbar
	mm Hg		0.133		kPa
Minute	min		60		s
	min		0.06		ks
Percent	%		10^{-2}		1 (unity)
	% (g/100 g)		10		g/kg
	% (g/100 g)		10^{-2}		kg/kg
	% (g/100 ml)		10		g/L
	% (g/100 ml)		$\dfrac{10}{mw}$		mol/L
	% (g/100 ml)		$\dfrac{10^4}{mw}$		mmol/L
	% (ml/100 ml)		10^{-2}		L/L

X.2 CONVERSION OF PARTIAL PRESSURE IN mm Hg to kPa
(mm Hg × 0.133 = kPa)

mm Hg	kPa	mm Hg	kPa	mm Hg	kPa	mm Hg	kPa	mm Hg	kPa
1	0.13	26	3.5	70	9.3	114	15.2	158	21.0
1.5	0.20	27	3.6	71	9.4	115	15.3	159	21.1
2.0	0.27	28	3.7	72	9.6	116	15.4	160	21.3
2.5	0.33	29	3.9	73	9.7	117	15.6	161	21.4
3.0	0.40	30	4.0	74	9.8	118	15.7	162	21.5
3.5	0.47	31	4.1	75	10.0	119	15.8	163	21.7
4.0	0.53	32	4.3	76	10.1	120	16.0	164	21.8
4.5	0.60	33	4.4	77	10.2	121	16.1	165	21.9
5.0	0.66	34	4.5	78	10.4	122	16.2	166	22.1
5.5	0.73	35	4.7	79	10.5	123	16.4	167	22.2
6.0	0.80	36	4.8	80	10.6	124	16.5	168	22.3
6.5	0.86	37	4.9	81	10.8	125	16.6	169	22.5
7.0	0.93	38	5.1	82	10.9	126	16.8	170	22.6
7.5	1.00	39	5.2	83	11.0	127	16.9	171	22.7
8.0	1.06	40	5.3	84	11.2	128	17.0	172	22.9
8.5	1.13	41	5.5	85	11.3	129	17.2	173	23.0
9.0	1.20	42	5.6	86	11.4	130	17.3	174	23.1
9.5	1.26	43	5.7	87	11.6	131	17.4	175	23.3
10.0	1.33	44	5.9	88	11.7	132	17.6	176	23.4
10.5	1.40	45	6.0	89	11.8	133	17.7	177	23.5
11.0	1.46	46	6.1	90	12.0	134	17.8	178	23.7
11.5	1.53	47	6.3	91	12.1	135	18.0	179	23.8
12.0	1.60	48	6.4	92	12.2	136	18.1	180	23.9
12.5	1.66	49	6.5	93	12.4	137	18.2	181	24.1
13.0	1.73	50	6.7	94	12.5	138	18.4	182	24.2
13.5	1.80	51	6.8	95	12.6	139	18.5	183	24.3
14.0	1.86	52	6.9	96	12.8	140	18.6	184	24.5
14.5	1.93	53	7.0	97	12.9	141	18.8	185	24.6
15.0	1.99	54	7.2	98	13.0	142	18.9	186	24.7
15.5	2.06	55	7.3	99	13.2	143	19.0	187	24.9
16.0	2.13	56	7.4	100	13.3	144	19.2	188	25.0
16.5	2.19	57	7.6	101	13.4	145	19.3	189	25.1
17.0	2.26	58	7.7	102	13.6	146	19.4	190	25.3
17.5	2.33	59	7.8	103	13.7	147	19.6	191	25.4
18.0	2.39	60	8.0	104	13.8	148	19.7	192	25.5
18.5	2.46	61	8.1	105	14.0	149	19.8	193	25.7
19.0	2.53	62	8.2	106	14.1	150	19.9	194	25.8
19.5	2.59	63	8.4	107	14.2	151	20.1	195	25.9
20.0	2.7	64	8.5	108	14.4	152	20.2	196	26.1
21	2.8	65	8.6	109	14.5	153	20.3	197	26.2
22	2.9	66	8.8	110	14.6	154	20.5	198	26.3
23	3.1	67	8.9	111	14.8	155	20.6	199	26.5
24	3.2	68	9.0	112	14.9	156	20.7	200	26.6
25	3.3	69	9.2	113	15.0	157	20.9	201	26.7

mm Hg	kPa	mm Hg	kPa	mm Hg	kPa	mm Hg	kPa	mm Hg	kPa
202	26.9	222	29.5	242	32.2	262	34.8	282	37.5
203	27.0	223	29.7	243	32.3	263	35.0	283	37.6
204	27.1	224	29.8	244	32.5	264	35.1	284	37.8
205	27.3	225	29.9	245	32.6	265	35.2	285	37.9
206	27.4	226	30.1	246	32.7	266	35.4	286	38.0
207	27.5	227	30.2	247	32.9	267	35.5	287	38.2
208	27.7	228	30.3	248	33.0	268	35.6	288	38.3
209	27.8	229	30.5	249	33.1	269	35.8	289	38.4
210	27.9	230	30.6	250	33.3	270	35.9	290	38.6
211	28.1	231	30.7	251	33.4	271	36.0	291	38.7
212	28.2	232	30.9	252	33.5	272	36.2	292	38.8
213	28.3	233	31.0	253	33.6	273	36.3	293	39.0
214	28.5	234	31.1	254	33.8	274	36.4	294	39.1
215	28.6	235	31.3	255	33.9	275	36.6	295	39.2
216	28.7	236	31.4	256	34.0	276	36.7	296	39.4
217	28.9	237	31.5	257	34.2	277	36.8	297	39.5
218	29.0	238	31.7	258	34.3	278	37.0	298	39.6
219	29.1	239	31.8	259	34.4	279	37.1	299	39.8
220	29.3	240	31.9	260	34.6	280	37.2	300	39.9
221	29.4	241	32.1	261	34.7	281	37.4		

X.3 CONVERSION OF pH TO cH (nmol/L)[*]

pH	cH	pH	cH	pH	cH
7.80	15.9	7.46	34.7	7.12	76
7.79	16.2	7.45	35.5	7.11	78
7.78	16.6	7.44	36.3	7.10	80
7.77	17.0	7.43	37.2	7.09	81
7.76	17.4	7.42	38.0	7.08	83
7.75	17.8	7.41	38.9	7.07	85
7.74	18.2	7.40	40	7.06	87
7.73	18.6	7.39	41	7.05	89
7.72	19.1	7.38	42	7.04	91
7.71	19.5	7.37	43	7.03	93
7.70	19.9	7.36	44	7.02	96
7.69	20.4	7.35	45	7.01	98
7.68	20.9	7.34	46	7.00	100
7.67	21.4	7.33	47	6.99	102
7.66	21.9	7.32	48	6.98	105
7.65	22.4	7.31	49	6.97	107
7.64	22.9	7.30	50	6.96	110
7.63	23.4	7.29	51	6.95	112
7.62	24.0	7.28	53	6.94	115
7.61	24.6	7.27	54	6.93	115
7.60	25.1	7.26	55	6.92	120
7.59	25.7	7.25	56	6.91	123
7.58	26.3	7.24	58	6.90	126
7.57	26.9	7.23	59	6.89	129
7.56	27.5	7.22	60	6.88	132
7.55	28.2	7.21	62	6.87	135
7.54	28.8	7.20	63	6.86	138
7.53	29.5	7.19	65	6.85	141
7.52	30.2	7.18	66	6.84	145
7.51	30.9	7.17	68	6.83	149
7.50	31.6	7.16	70	6.82	152
7.49	32.4	7.15	71	6.81	155
7.48	33.1	7.14	73	6.80	159
7.47	33.9	7.13	74		

[*]For conversion method see pp. 201-202.

$$cH\ (nmol/L) = Antilog\ (9 - pH)$$

EXAMPLE: Convert pH 7.31 to cH.

$$9 - 7.31 = 1.69$$

$$antilog\ 1.69 = 48.98 = 49$$

Hence, pH 7.31 = cH 49 nmol/L

Appendix Y

PERIODIC TABLE OF ELEMENTS

NON-METALS

METALS

KEY TO TABLE

1988 IUPAC notation	13
1970 IUPAC notation	IIIB
CAS notation	IIIA

..... Group

	Oxidation states
Atomic number	29	+1
Symbol	Cu	+2
1995 Atomic weight ...	63.546	
Electron configuration ...	-8-18-1	
of outer shells		

Transition Elements

PERIOD

Group 1 (IA / IA)

Z	Symbol	Atomic weight	Config	Oxidation
1	H	1.00794	1	+1, -1
3	Li	6.941	2-1	+1
11	Na	22.989768	2-8-1	+1
19	K	39.0983	-8-8-1	+1
37	Rb	85.4678	-18-8-1	+1
55	Cs	132.90543	-18-8-1	+1
87	Fr	(223)	-18-8-1	+1

Group 2 (IIA / IIA)

Z	Symbol	Atomic weight	Config	Oxidation
4	Be	9.012182	2-2	+2
12	Mg	24.3050	2-8-2	+2
20	Ca	40.078	-8-8-2	+2
38	Sr	87.62	-18-8-2	+2
56	Ba	137.327	-18-18-2	+2
88	Ra	(226)	-18-8-2	+2

Transition Elements

Group 3 (IIIA/IIIB)	Group 4 (IVA/IVB)	Group 5 (VA/VB)	Group 6 (VIA/VIB)	Group 7 (VIIA/VIIB)	Group 8 (VIIIA/VIIIB)	Group 9 (VIIIA/VIIIB)	Group 10	Group 11 (IB/IB)	Group 12 (IIB/IIB)
21 Sc 44.955910 -8-9-2 +3	22 Ti 47.867 -8-10-2 +2 +3 +4	23 V 50.9415 -8-11-2 +2 +3 +4 +5	24 Cr 51.9961 -8-13-1 +2 +3 +6	25 Mn 54.93805 -8-13-2 +2 +3 +4 +6 +7	26 Fe 55.845 -8-14-2 +2 +3	27 Co 58.93320 -8-15-2 +2 +3	28 Ni 58.6934 -8-16-2 +2 +3	29 Cu 63.546 -18-1 +1 +2	30 Zn 65.39 -8-18-2 +2
39 Y 88.90585 -18-9-2 +3	40 Zr 91.224 -18-10-2 +4	41 Nb 92.90638 -18-12-1 +3 +5	42 Mo 95.94 -18-13-1 +6	43 Tc (98) -18-13-2 +6 +7	44 Ru 101.07 -18-15-1 +3	45 Rh 102.90550 -18-16-1 +3	46 Pd 106.42 -18-18-0 +2 +4	47 Ag 107.8682 -18-18-1 +1	48 Cd 112.411 -18-18-2 +2
57-71 see Lantha-nides*	72 Hf 178.49 -32-10-2 +4	73 Ta 180.9479 -32-11-2 +5	74 W 183.84 -32-12-2 +6	75 Re 186.207 -32-13-2 +4 +6 +7	76 Os 190.2 -32-14-2 +3 +4 +6 +8	77 Ir 192.217 -32-15-2 +3 +4	78 Pt 195.078 -32-16-2 +2 +4	79 Au 196.96654 -32-18-1 +1 +3	80 Hg 200.59 -32-18-2 +1 +2
89-103 see Actinides**	104 Unq (261) -32-10-2	105 Unp (262) -32-11-2	106 Unh (263) -32-12-2	107 Uns (262) -32-13-2					

Group 13 (IIIB/IIIA)

Z	Symbol	Atomic weight	Config	Oxidation
5	B	10.811	2-3	+3
13	Al	26.981539	2-8-3	+3
31	Ga	69.723	-8-18-3	+3
49	In	114.818	-18-18-3	+3
81	Tl	204.3833	-32-18-3	+1 +3

Group 14 (IVB/IVA)

Z	Symbol	Atomic weight	Config	Oxidation
6	C	12.0107	2-4	+2 +4 -4
14	Si	28.0855	2-8-4	+2 +4 -4
32	Ge	72.61	-8-18-4	+2 +4
50	Sn	118.710	-18-18-4	+2 +4
82	Pb	207.2	-32-18-4	+2 +4

Group 15 (VB/VA)

Z	Symbol	Atomic weight	Config	Oxidation
7	N	14.00674	2-5	+1 +2 +3 +4 +5 -3
15	P	30.973762	2-8-5	+3 +5 -3
33	As	74.92159	-8-18-5	+3 +5 -3
51	Sb	121.760	-18-18-5	+3 +5
83	Bi	208.98037	-32-18-5	+3 +5

Group 16 (VIB/VIA)

Z	Symbol	Atomic weight	Config	Oxidation
8	O	15.9994	2-6	-2
16	S	32.066	2-8-6	+4 +6 -2
34	Se	78.96	-8-18-6	+4 +6 -2
52	Te	127.60	-18-18-6	+4 +6 -2
84	Po	(209)	-32-18-6	+2 +4

Group 17 (VIIB/VIIA)

Z	Symbol	Atomic weight	Config	Oxidation
9	F	18.9984032	2-7	-1
17	Cl	35.4527	2-8-7	+1 +5 +7 -1
35	Br	79.904	-8-18-7	+1 +5 -1
53	I	126.90447	-18-18-7	+1 +5 +7 -1
85	At	(210)	-32-18-7	

Group 18 (VIIIB/VIIIA) — INERT GASES

Z	Symbol	Atomic weight	Config	Oxidation	Shell
2	He	4.002602	2	0	K
10	Ne	20.1797	2-8	0	K-L
18	Ar	39.948	2-8-8	0	K-L-M
36	Kr	83.80	-8-18-8	0	L-M-N
54	Xe	131.29	-18-18-8	0	M-N-O
86	Rn	(222)	-32-18-8	0	N-O-P

* Lanthanides

Z	Symbol	Atomic weight	Config	Oxidation
57	La	138.9055	-18-9-2	+3
58	Ce	140.116	-20-8-2	+3 +4
59	Pr	140.90765	-21-8-2	+3 +4
60	Nd	144.24	-22-8-2	+3
61	Pm	(145)	-23-8-2	+3
62	Sm	150.36	-24-8-2	+2 +3
63	Eu	151.964	-25-8-2	+2 +3
64	Gd	157.25	-25-9-2	+3
65	Tb	158.92534	-27-8-2	+3
66	Dy	162.50	-28-8-2	+3
67	Ho	164.93032	-29-8-2	+3
68	Er	167.26	-30-8-2	+3
69	Tm	168.93421	-31-8-2	+3
70	Yb	173.04	-32-8-2	+2 +3
71	Lu	174.967	-32-9-2	+3

Shell O-P-Q / N-O-P

** Actinides

Z	Symbol	Atomic weight	Config	Oxidation
89	Ac	(277)	-18-9-2	+3
90	Th	232.0381	-18-10-2	+4
91	Pa	231.03588	-20-9-2	+4 +5
92	U	238.0289	-21-9-2	+3 +4 +5 +6
93	Np	(237)	-22-9-2	+3 +4 +5 +6
94	Pu	(244)	-24-8-2	+3 +4 +5 +6
95	Am	(243)	-25-8-2	+3 +4 +5 +6
96	Cm	(247)	-25-9-2	+3
97	Bk	(247)	-27-8-2	+3 +4
98	Cf	(251)	-28-8-2	+3
99	Es	(252)	-29-8-2	+3
100	Fm	(257)	-30-8-2	+3
101	Md	(258)	-31-8-2	+2 +3
102	No	(259)	-32-8-2	+2 +3
103	Lr	(262)	-32-9-2	+3

Shell N-O-P / O-P-Q

The 1988 IUPAC format numbers the groups from 1 to 18. The 1970 IUPAC numbering system and the system used by the Chemical Abstracts Service (CAS) are also shown. For radioactive elements that do not occur in nature, the mass number of the most stable isotope is given in parenthesis. Adapted from Leigh, 1990.

Appendix Z
STANDARD ATOMIC MASSES (IUPAC, 1993)

Atomic masses (which are equivalent to atomic weights) are given relative to the most common isotope of Carbon taken as 12.

By Atomic Number

Atomic no.	Name	Symbol	Atomic mass	Atomic no.	Name	Symbol	Atomic mass
1	Hydrogen	H	1.00794	55	Cesium	Cs	132.90543
2	Helium	He	4.002602	56	Barium	Ba	137.327
3	Lithium	Li	6.941	57	Lanthanum	La	138.9055
4	Beryllium	Be	9.012182	58	Cerium	Ce	140.116
5	Boron	B	10.811	59	Praseodymium	Pr	140.90765
6	Carbon	C	12.0107	60	Neodymium	Nd	144.24
7	Nitrogen	N	14.00674	61	Promethium	Pm	(145)
8	Oxygen	O	15.9994	62	Samarium	Sm	150.36
9	Fluorine	F	18.9984032	63	Europium	Eu	151.964
10	Neon	Ne	20.1797	64	Gadolinium	Gd	157.25
11	Sodium	Na (L. *natrium*)	22.989768	65	Terbium	Tb	158.92534
12	Magnesium	Mg	24.3050	66	Dysprosium	Dy	162.50
13	Aluminum	Al	26.981539	67	Holmium	Ho	164.93032
14	Silicon	Si	28.0855	68	Erbium	Er	167.26
15	Phosphorous	P	30.973762	69	Thulium	Tm	168.93421
16	Sulfur	S	32.066	70	Ytterbium	Yb	173.04
17	Chlorine	Cl	35.4527	71	Lutetium	Lu	174.967
18	Argon	Ar	39.948	72	Hafnium	Hf	178.49
19	Potassium	K (L. *kalium*)	39.0983	73	Tantalum	Ta	180.9479
20	Calcium	Ca	40.078	74	Tungsten	W (Ger. *Wolfram*)	183.84
21	Scandium	Sc	44.955910	75	Rhenium	Re	186.207
22	Titanium	Ti	47.867	76	Osmium	Os	190.23
23	Vanadium	V	50.9415	77	Iridium	Ir	192.217
24	Chromium	Cr	51.9961	78	Platinum	Pt	195.078
25	Manganese	Mn	54.93805	79	Gold	Au (L. *aurum*)	196.96654
26	Iron	Fe (L. *ferrum*)	55.845	80	Mercury	Hg (L. *hydrargyrum*)	200.59
27	Cobalt	Co	58.93320	81	Thallium	Tl	204.3833
28	Nickel	Ni	58.6934	82	Lead	Pb (L. *plumbum*)	207.2
29	Copper	Cu (L. *cuprum*)	63.546	83	Bismuth	Bi	208.98037
30	Zinc	Zn	65.39	84	Polonium	Po	(209)
31	Gallium	Ga	69.723	85	Astatine	At	(210)
32	Germanium	Ge	72.61	86	Radon	Rn	(222)
33	Arsenic	As	74.92159	87	Francium	Fr	(223)
34	Selenium	Se	78.96	88	Radium	Ra	(226)
35	Bromine	Br	79.904	89	Actinium	Ac	(227)
36	Krypton	Kr	83.80	90	Thorium	Th	232.0381
37	Rubidium	Rb	85.4678	91	Protactinium	Pa	231.03588
38	Strontium	Sr	87.62	92	Uranium	U	238.0289
39	Yttrium	Y	88.90585	93	Neptunium	Np	(237)
40	Zirconium	Zr	91.224	94	Plutonium	Pu	(244)
41	Niobium	Nb	92.90638	95	Americium	Am	(243)
42	Molybdenum	Mo	95.94	96	Curium	Cm	(247)
43	Technetium	Tc	(98)	97	Berkelium	Bk	(247)
44	Ruthenium	Ru	101.07	98	Californium	Cf	(251)
45	Rhodium	Rh	102.90550	99	Einsteinium	Es	(252)
46	Palladium	Pd	106.42	100	Fermium	Fm	(257)
47	Silver	Ag (L. *argentum*)	107.8682	101	Mendelevium	Md	(258)
48	Cadmium	Cd	112.411	102	Nobelium	No	(259)
49	Indium	In	114.818	103	Lawrencium	Lr	(262)
50	Tin	Sn (L. *stannum*)	118.710	104	Unnilquadium	Unq	(261)
51	Antimony	Sb (L. *stibium*)	121.760	105	Unnilpentium	Unp	(262)
52	Tellurium	Te	127.60	106	Unnihexium	Unh	(263)
53	Iodine	I	126.90447	107	Unnilseptium	Uns	(262)
54	Xenon	Xe	131.29				

For radioactive elements that do not occur in nature, the mass number of the most stable isotope is given in parentheses.

By Element Name

Atomic no.	Name	Symbol	Atomic mass	Atomic no.	Name	Symbol	Atomic mass
89	Actinium	Ac	(227)	60	Neodymium	Nd	144.24
13	Aluminum	Al	26.981539	10	Neon	Ne	20.1797
95	Americium	Am	(243)	93	Neptunium	Np	(237)
51	Antimony	Sb (L. *stibium*)	121.760	28	Nickel	Ni	58.6934
18	Argon	Ar	39.948	41	Niobium	Nb	92.90638
33	Arsenic	As	74.92159	7	Nitrogen	N	14.00674
85	Astatine	At	(210)	102	Nobelium	No	(259)
56	Barium	Ba	137.327	76	Osmium	Os	190.23
97	Berkelium	Bk	(247)	8	Oxygen	O	15.9994
4	Beryllium	Be	9.012182	46	Palladium	Pd	106.42
83	Bismuth	Bi	208.98037	15	Phosphorous	P	30.973762
5	Boron	B	10.811	78	Platinum	Pt	195.078
35	Bromine	Br	79.904	94	Plutonium	Pu	(244)
48	Cadmium	Cd	112.411	84	Polonium	Po	(209)
20	Calcium	Ca	40.078	19	Potassium	K (L. *kalium*)	39.0983
98	Californium	Cf	(251)	59	Praseodymium	Pr	140.90765
6	Carbon	C	12.0107	61	Promethium	Pm	(145)
58	Cerium	Ce	140.116	91	Protactinium	Pa	231.03588
55	Cesium	Cs	132.90543	88	Radium	Ra	(226)
17	Chlorine	Cl	35.4527	86	Radon	Rn	(222)
24	Chromium	Cr	51.9961	75	Rhenium	Re	186.207
27	Cobalt	Co	58.93320	45	Rhodium	Rh	102.90550
29	Copper	Cu (L. *cuprum*)	63.546	37	Rubidium	Rb	85.4678
96	Curium	Cm	(247)	44	Ruthenium	Ru	101.07
66	Dysprosium	Dy	162.50	62	Samarium	Sm	150.36
99	Einsteinium	Es	(252)	21	Scandium	Sc	44.955910
68	Erbium	Er	167.26	34	Selenium	Se	78.96
63	Europium	Eu	151.964	14	Silicon	Si	28.0855
100	Fermium	Fm	(257)	47	Silver	Ag (L. *argentum*)	107.8682
9	Fluorine	F	18.9984032	11	Sodium	Na (L. *natrium*)	22.989768
87	Francium	Fr	(223)	38	Strontium	Sr	87.62
64	Gadolinium	Gd	157.25	16	Sulfur	S	32.066
31	Gallium	Ga	69.723	73	Tantalum	Ta	180.9479
32	Germanium	Ge	72.61	43	Technetium	Tc	(98)
79	Gold	Au (L. *aurum*)	196.96654	52	Tellurium	Te	127.60
72	Hafnium	Hf	178.49	65	Terbium	Tb	158.92534
2	Helium	He	4.002602	81	Thallium	Tl	204.3833
67	Holmium	HO	164.93032	90	Thorium	Th	232.0381
1	Hydrogen	H	1.00794	69	Thulium	Tm	168.93421
49	Indium	In	114.818	50	Tin	Sn (L. *stannum*)	118.710
53	Iodine	I	126.90447	22	Titanium	Ti	47.867
77	Iridium	Ir	192.217	74	Tungsten	W (Ger. *Wolfram*)	183.84
26	Iron	Fe (L. *ferrum*)	55.845	106	Unnilhexium	Unh	(263)
36	Krypton	Kr	83.80	105	Unnilpentium	Unp	(262)
57	Lanthanum	La	138.9055	104	Unnilquadium	Unq	(261)
103	Lawrencium	Lr	(262)	107	Unnilseptium	Uns	(262)
82	Lead	Pb (L. *plumbum*)	207.2	92	Uranium	U	238.0289
3	Lithium	Li	6.941	23	Vanadium	V	50.9415
71	Lutetium	Lu	174.967	54	Xenon	Xe	131.29
12	Magnesium	Mg	24.3050	70	Ytterbium	Yb	173.04
25	Manganese	Mn	54.93805	39	Yttrium	Y	88.90585
101	Mendelevium	Md	(258)	30	Zinc	Zn	65.39
80	Mercury	Hg (L. *hydrargyrum*)	200.59	40	Zirconium	Zr	91.224
42	Molybdenum	Mo	95.94				

For radioactive elements that do not occur in nature, the mass number of the most stable isotope is given in parentheses.

By Symbol

Atomic no.	Name	Symbol	Atomic mass	Atomic no.	Name	Symbol	Atomic mass
89	Actinium	Ac	(227)	7	Nitrogen	N	14.00674
47	Silver	Ag (L. *argentum*)	107.8682	11	Sodium	Na (L. *natrium*)	22.989768
13	Aluminum	Al	26.981539	41	Niobium	Nb	92.90638
95	Americium	Am	(243)	60	Neodymium	Nd	144.24
18	Argon	Ar	39.948	10	Neon	Ne	20.1797
33	Arsenic	As	74.92159	28	Nickel	Ni	58.6934
85	Astatine	At	(210)	102	Nobelium	No	(259)
79	Gold	Au (L. *aurum*)	196.96654	93	Neptunium	Np	(237)
5	Boron	B	10.811	8	Oxygen	O	15.9994
56	Barium	Ba	137.327	76	Osmium	Os	190.23
4	Beryllium	Be	9.012182	15	Phosphorous	P	30.973762
83	Bismuth	Bi	208.98037	91	Protactinium	Pa	231.03588
97	Berkelium	Bk	(247)	82	Lead	Pb (L. *plumbum*)	207.2
35	Bromine	Br	79.904	46	Palladium	Pd	106.42
6	Carbon	C	12.0107	61	Promethium	Pm	(145)
20	Calcium	Ca	40.078	84	Polonium	Po	(209)
48	Cadmium	Cd	112.411	59	Praseodymium	Pr	140.90765
58	Cerium	Ce	140.116	78	Platinum	Pt	195.078
98	Californium	Cf	(251)	94	Plutonium	Pu	(244)
17	Chlorine	Cl	35.4527	88	Radium	Ra	(226)
96	Curium	Cm	(247)	37	Rubidium	Rb	85.4678
27	Cobalt	Co	58.93320	75	Rhenium	Re	186.207
24	Chromium	Cr	51.9961	45	Rhodium	Rh	102.90550
55	Cesium	Cs	132.90543	86	Radon	Rn	(222)
29	Copper	Cu (L. *cuprum*)	63.546	44	Ruthenium	Ru	101.07
66	Dysprosium	Dy	162.50	16	Sulfur	S	32.066
68	Erbium	Er	167.26	51	Antimony	Sb (L. *stibium*)	121.760
99	Einsteinium	Es	(252)	21	Scandium	Sc	44.955910
63	Europium	Eu	151.964	34	Selenium	Se	78.96
9	Fluorine	F	18.9984032	14	Silicon	Si	28.0855
26	Iron	Fe (L. *ferrum*)	55.845	62	Samarium	Sm	150.36
100	Fermium	Fm	(257)	50	Tin	Sn (L. *stannum*)	118.710
87	Francium	Fr	(223)	38	Strontium	Sr	87.62
31	Gallium	Ga	69.723	73	Tantalum	Ta	180.9479
64	Gadolinium	Gd	157.25	65	Terbium	Tb	158.92534
32	Germanium	Ge	72.61	43	Technetium	Tc	(98)
1	Hydrogen	H	1.00794	52	Tellurium	Te	127.60
2	Helium	He	4.002602	90	Thorium	Th	232.0381
72	Hafnium	Hf	178.49	22	Titanium	Ti	47.867
80	Mercury	Hg (L. *hydrargyrum*)	200.59	81	Thallium	Tl	204.3833
67	Holmium	Ho	164.93032	69	Thulium	Tm	168.93421
53	Iodine	I	126.90447	92	Uranium	U	238.0289
49	Indium	In	114.818	106	Unnilhexium	Unh	(263)
77	Iridium	Ir	192.217	105	Unnilpentium	Unp	(262)
19	Potassium	K (L. *kalium*)	39.0983	104	Unnilquadium	Unq	(261)
36	Krypton	Kr	83.80	107	Unnilseptium	Uns	(262)
57	Lanthanum	La	138.9055	23	Vanadium	V	50.9415
3	Lithium	Li	6.941	74	Tungsten	W (Ger. *Wolfram*)	183.84
103	Lawrencium	Lr	(262)	54	Xenon	Xe	131.29
71	Lutetium	Lu	174.967	39	Yttrium	Y	88.90585
101	Mendelevium	Md	(258)	70	Ytterbium	Yb	173.04
12	Magnesium	Mg	24.3050	30	Zinc	Zn	65.39
25	Manganese	Mn	54.93805	40	Zirconium	Zr	91.224
42	Molybdenum	Mo	95.94				

For radioactive elements that do not occur in nature, the mass number of the most stable isotope is given in parentheses.

By Atomic Mass

Atomic no.	Name	Symbol	Atomic mass	Atomic no.	Name	Symbol	Atomic mass
1	Hydrogen	H	1.00794	55	Cesium	Cs	132.90543
2	Helium	He	4.002602	56	Barium	Ba	137.327
3	Lithium	Li	6.941	57	Lanthanum	La	138.9055
4	Beryllium	Be	9.012182	58	Cerium	Ce	140.116
5	Boron	B	10.811	59	Praseodymium	Pr	140.90765
6	Carbon	C	12.0107	60	Neodymium	Nd	144.24
7	Nitrogen	N	14.00674	61	Promethium	Pm	(145)
8	Oxygen	O	15.9994	62	Samarium	Sm	150.36
9	Fluorine	F	18.9984032	63	Europium	Eu	151.964
10	Neon	Ne	20.1797	64	Gadolinium	Gd	157.25
11	Sodium	Na (L. *natrium*)	22.989768	65	Terbium	Tb	158.92534
12	Magnesium	Mg	24.3050	66	Dysprosium	Dy	162.50
13	Aluminum	Al	26.981539	67	Holmium	Ho	164.93032
14	Silicon	Si	28.0855	68	Erbium	Er	167.26
15	Phosphorous	P	30.973762	69	Thulium	Tm	168.93421
16	Sulfur	S	32.066	70	Ytterbium	Yb	173.04
17	Chlorine	Cl	35.4527	71	Lutetium	Lu	174.967
19	Potassium	K (L. *kalium*)	39.0983	72	Hafnium	Hf	178.49
18	Argon	Ar	39.948	73	Tantalum	Ta	180.9479
20	Calcium	Ca	40.078	74	Tungsten	W (Ger. *Wolfram*)	183.84
21	Scandium	Sc	44.955910	75	Rhenium	Re	186.207
22	Titanium	Ti	47.867	76	Osmium	Os	190.23
23	Vanadium	V	50.9415	77	Iridium	Ir	192.217
24	Chromium	Cr	51.9961	78	Platinum	Pt	195.078
25	Manganese	Mn	54.93805	79	Gold	Au (L. *aurum*)	196.96654
26	Iron	Fe (L. *ferrum*)	55.845	80	Mercury	Hg (L. *hydrargyrum*)	200.59
28	Nickel	Ni	58.6934	81	Thallium	Tl	204.3833
27	Cobalt	Co	58.93320	82	Lead	Pb (L. *plumbum*)	207.2
29	Copper	Cu (L. *cuprum*)	63.546	83	Bismuth	Bi	208.98037
30	Zinc	Zn	65.39	84	Polonium	Po	(209)
31	Gallium	Ga	69.723	85	Astatine	At	(210)
32	Germanium	Ge	72.61	86	Radon	Rn	(222)
33	Arsenic	As	74.92159	87	Francium	Fr	(223)
34	Selenium	Se	78.96	88	Radium	Ra	(226)
35	Bromine	Br	79.904	89	Actinium	Ac	(227)
36	Krypton	Kr	83.80	91	Protactinium	Pa	231.03588
37	Rubidium	Rb	85.4678	90	Thorium	Th	232.0381
38	Strontium	Sr	87.62	93	Neptunium	Np	(237)
39	Yttrium	Y	88.90585	92	Uranium	U	238.0289
40	Zirconium	Zr	91.224	95	Americium	Am	(243)
41	Niobium	Nb	92.90638	94	Plutonium	Pu	(244)
42	Molybdenum	Mo	95.94	96	Curium	Cm	(247)
43	Technetium	Tc	(98)	97	Berkelium	Bk	(247)
44	Ruthenium	Ru	101.07	98	Californium	Cf	(251)
45	Rhodium	Rh	102.90550	99	Einsteinium	Es	(252)
46	Palladium	Pd	106.42	100	Fermium	Fm	(257)
47	Silver	Ag (L. *argentum*)	107.8682	101	Mendelevium	Md	(258)
48	Cadmium	Cd	112.411	102	Nobelium	No	(259)
49	Indium	In	114.818	104	Unnilquadium	Unq	(261)
50	Tin	Sn (L. *stannum*)	118.710	103	Lawrencium	Lr	(262)
51	Antimony	Sb (L. *stibium*)	121.760	107	Unnilseptium	Uns	(262)
53	Iodine	I	126.90447	105	Unnilpentium	Unp	(262)
52	Tellurium	Te	127.60	106	Unnilhexium	Unh	(263)
54	Xenon	Xe	131.29				

For radioactive elements that do not occur in nature, the mass number of the most stable isotope is given in parentheses.

Appendix AA
DISSOCIATION CONSTANTS OF INORGANIC ACIDS AND BASES

The data in this table are presented as values of pK_a, defined as the negative logarithm of the acid dissociation constant K_a for the reaction

$$BH \rightleftharpoons B^- + H^+$$

Thus $pK_a = -\log K_a$, and the hydrogen ion concentration $[H^+]$ can be calculated from

$$K_a = \frac{[H^+][B^-]}{[BH]}$$

In the case of bases, the entry in the table is for the conjugate acid; e.g., ammonium ion for ammonia. The OH^- concentration in the system

$$NH_3 + H_2O \rightleftharpoons NH_4^+ + OH^-$$

can be calculated from the equation

$$K_b = K_{water}/K_a = \frac{[OH^-][NH_4^+]}{[NH_3]}$$

where $K_{water} = 1.01 \times 10^{-14}$ at 25 °C. Note that $pK_a + pK_b = pK_{water}$.

All values refer to dilute aqueous solutions at the temperature indicated. The table is arranged alphabetically by compound name.

Name	Formula	Step	$T/°C$	pK_a	Name	Formula	Step	$T/°C$	pK_a
Aluminum (III) ion	Al^{+3}		25	5.0	Hydrofluoric acid	HF		25	3.20
Ammonia	NH_3		25	9.25	Hydrogen peroxide	H_2O_2		25	11.62
Arsenic acid	H_3AsO_4	1	25	2.26	Hydrogen selenide	H_2Se	1	25	3.89
		2	25	6.76			2	25	11.0
		3	25	11.29	Hydrogen sulfide	H_2S	1	25	7.05
Arsenious acid	H_2AsO_3		25	9.29			2	25	19
Barium (II) ion	Ba^{+2}		25	13.4	Hydrogen telluride	H_2Te	1	18	2.6
Boric acid	H_3BO_3	1	20	9.27			2	25	11
		2	20	>14	Hydroxylamine	NH_2OH		25	5.94
Calcium (II) ion	Ca^{+2}		25	12.6	Hypobromous acid	HBrO		25	8.55
Carbonic acid	H_2CO_3	1	25	6.35	Hypochlorous acid	HClO		25	7.40
		2	25	10.33	Hypoiodous acid	HIO		25	10.5
Chlorous acid	$HClO_2$		25	1.94	Iodic acid	HIO_3		25	0.78
Chromic acid	H_2CrO_4	1	25	0.74	Lithium ion	Li^+		25	13.8
		2	25	6.49	Magnesium (II) ion	Mg^{+2}		25	11.4
Cyanic acid	HCNO		25	3.46	Nitrous acid	HNO_2		25	3.25
Germanic acid	H_2GeO_3	1	25	9.01	Perchloric acid	$HClO_4$		20	−1.6
		2	25	12.3	Periodic acid	HIO_4		25	1.64
Hydrazine	N_2H_4		25	8.1	Phosphoric acid	H_3PO_4	1	25	2.16
Hydrazoic acid	HN_3		25	4.6			2	25	7.21
Hydrocyanic acid	HCN		25	9.21			3	25	12.32

Modified from Lide DR, editor: *CRC handbook of chemistry and physics,* ed 76, New York, 1995, CRC Press.

Name	Formula	Step	$T/°C$	pK_a	Name	Formula	Step	$T/°C$	pK_a
Phosphorous acid	H_3PO_3	1	20	1.3	Sodium ion	Na^+		25	14.8
		2	20	6.70	Strontium (II) ion	Sr^{+2}		25	13.2
Pyrophosphoric acid	$H_4P_2O_7$	1	25	0.91	Sulfamic acid	NH_2SO_3H		25	1.05
		2	25	2.10	Sulfuric acid	H_2SO_4	2	25	1.98
		3	25	6.70	Sulfurous acid	H_2SO_3	1	25	1.85
		4	25	9.32			2	25	7.2
Selenic acid	H_2SeO_4	2	25	1.7	Telluric acid	H_2TeO_4	1	18	7.68
Selenious acid	H_2SeO_3	1	25	2.62			2	18	11.0
		2	25	8.32	Tellurous acid	H_2TeO_3	1	25	6.27
Silicic acid	H_4SiO_4	1	30	9.9			2	25	8.43
		2	30	11.8	Tetrafluoroboric acid	HBF_4		25	0.5
		3	30	12	Thiocyanic acid	$HSCN$		25	−1.8
		4	30	12	Water	H_2O		25	13.995

DISSOCIATION CONSTANTS OF ORGANIC ACIDS AND BASES

This table lists the acid-base dissociation constants of over 600 organic compounds, including many amino acids. All data apply to dilute aqueous solutions and are presented in the form of pK_a, which is the negative of the logarithm of the acid dissociation constant K_a. See the preceding table, "Dissociation Constants of Inorganic Acids and Bases", for further details on notation.

Compounds are listed by molecular formula in the Hill order.

Molecular formula	Name	Step	$T/°C$	pK_a	Molecular formula	Name	Step	$T/°C$	pK_a
CH_2O_2	Formic acid		20	3.75	$C_2H_3BrO_2$	Bromoacetic acid		25	2.69
CH_4N_2O	Urea		21	0.10	$C_2H_3ClO_2$	Chloroacetic acid		25	2.85
CH_5N	Methylamine		25	10.63	$C_2H_3IO_2$	Iodoacetic acid		25	3.12
$C_2HCl_3O_2$	Trichloracetic acid		25	0.70	C_2H_4OS	Thioacetic acid		25	3.33
$C_2H_2Cl_2O_2$	Dichloroacetic acid		25	1.48	$C_2H_4O_2$	Acetic acid		25	4.76
$C_2H_2O_3$	Glyoxylic acid		25	3.18	$C_2H_4O_3$	Glycolic acid		25	3.83
$C_2H_2O_4$	Oxalic acid	1	25	1.23	C_2H_5N	Ethyleneimine		25	8.01
		2	25	4.19	C_2H_5NO	Acetamide		25	0.63

Continued.

Molecular formula	Name	Step	$T/°C$	pK_a
$C_2H_5NO_2$	Glycine	1	25	2.35
		2	25	9.78
$C_2H_6O_2$	Ethylene glycol		25	14.22
$C_2H_7AsO_2$	Cacodylic acid	1	25	1.57
		2	25	6.27
C_2H_7N	Dimethylamine		25	10.68
C_2H_7N	Ethylamine		25	10.70
C_2H_7NO	Ethanolamine		25	9.50
$C_2H_7NO_3S$	Taurine	1	25	1.5
		2	25	9.061
C_2H_7NS	Cysteamine	1	25	8.35
		2	25	10.81
$C_2H_8N_2$	1,2-Ethanediamine	1	0	10.712
		2	0	7.564
$C_3H_3NO_2$	Cyanoacetic acid		25	2.45
C_3H_3NS	Thiazole		20	2.44
$C_3H_4N_2$	1H-Imidazole		25	6.953
$C_3H_4N_2S$	2-Thiazolamine		20	5.36
$C_3H_4O_2$	Acrylic acid		25	4.25
$C_3H_4O_3$	Pyruvic acid		25	2.39
$C_3H_4O_4$	Malonic acid	1	25	2.83
		2	25	5.69
$C_3H_5ClO_2$	2-Chloropropanoic acid		25	2.83
$C_3H_5ClO_2$	3-Chloropropanoic acid		25	3.98
$C_3H_6N_6$	Melamine		25	5.00
$C_3H_6O_2$	Propanoic acid		25	4.86
$C_3H_6O_3$	3-Hydroxypropanoic acid		25	4.51
$C_3H_6O_3$	Lactic acid		100	3.08
$C_3H_6O_4$	Glyceric acid		25	3.52
C_3H_7N	Azetidine		25	11.29
$C_3H_7NO_2$	L-Alanine	1	25	2.34
		2	25	9.87
$C_3H_7NO_2$	β-Alanine	1	25	3.55
		2	25	10.24
$C_3H_7NO_2$	Methylglycine	1	25	2.21
		2	25	10.12
$C_3H_7NO_2S$	Cysteine	1	25	1.92
		2	25	8.37
		3	25	10.70
$C_3H_7NO_3$	Serine	1	25	2.19
		2	25	9.21
$C_3H_7NO_5S$	l-Cysteic acid	1	25	1.3
		2	25	1.9
		3	25	8.70
$C_3H_7N_3O_2$	Glycocyamine		25	2.82
$C_3H_8O_3$	Glycerol		25	14.15
C_3H_9N	Propylamine		20	10.60
C_3H_9N	Trimethylamine		25	9.80
C_3H_9NO	1-Amino-2-methoxyethane		10	9.89
C_3H_9NO	Trimethylamine oxide		25	4.65
$C_3H_{10}N_2$	1,2-Propanediamine	1	25	9.82
		2	25	6.61
$C_3H_{10}N_2$	1,3-Propanediamine	1	10	10.94
		2	10	9.03
$C_3H_{11}N_3$	1,2,3-Triaminopropane	1	20	9.59
		2	20	7.95

Molecular formula	Name	Step	$T/°C$	pK_a
$C_4H_4N_2$	Pyrazine		27	0.65
$C_4H_4N_2$	Pyridazine		20	2.24
$C_4H_4N_2O_3$	Barbituric acid		25	4.01
$C_4H_4N_2O_5$	Alloxanic acid		25	6.64
$C_4H_4N_4O_2$	5-Nitropyrimidinamine		20	0.35
$C_4H_4O_4$	trans-Fumaric acid	1	18	3.03
		2	18	4.44
$C_4H_4O_4$	Maleic acid	1	25	1.83
		2	25	6.07
$C_4H_4O_5$	Oxaloacetic acid	1	25	2.22
		2	25	3.89
		3	25	13.03
$C_4H_5N_3$	2-Pyrimidinamine		20	3.45
$C_4H_6N_2$	1-Methylimidazol		25	6.95
$C_4H_6N_4O_3$	Allantoin		25	8.96
$C_4H_6O_2$	3-Butenoic acid		25	4.34
$C_4H_6O_2$	trans-Crotonic acid		25	4.69
$C_4H_6O_3$	Acetoacetic acid		18	3.58
$C_4H_6O_3$	2-Oxobutanoic acid		25	2.50
$C_4H_6O_4$	Methylmalonic acid	1	25	3.07
		2	25	5.76
$C_4H_6O_4$	Succinic acid	1	25	4.16
		2	25	5.61
$C_4H_6O_5$	Malic acid	1	25	3.40
		2	25	5.11
$C_4H_6O_6$	α-Tartaric acid	1	25	2.98
		2	25	4.34
$C_4H_6O_6$	meso-Tartaric acid	1	25	3.22
		2	25	4.82
$C_4H_6O_8$	Dihydroxytartaric acid		25	1.92
$C_4H_7ClO_2$	2-Chlorobutanoic acid		RT	2.86
$C_4H_7ClO_2$	3-Chlorobutanoic acid		RT	4.05
$C_4H_7ClO_2$	4-Chlorobutanoic acid		RT	4.52
$C_4H_7NO_2$	4-Cyanobutanoic acid		25	2.42
$C_4H_7NO_3$	N-Acetylglycine		25	3.669
$C_4H_7NO_4$	Aspartic acid	1	25	1.99
		2	25	3.90
		3	25	9.90
$C_4H_7N_3O$	Creatinine	1	25	4.83
		2		9.2
$C_4H_8N_2O_3$	Asparagine	1	20	2.17
		2	20	8.80
$C_4H_8N_2O_3$	N-Glycylglycine		25	3.139
$C_4H_8O_2$	Butanoic acid		25	4.83
$C_4H_8O_2$	2-Methylpropanoic acid		25	4.88
$C_4H_8O_3$	3-Hydroxybutanoic acid		25	4.70
$C_4H_8O_3$	4-Hydroxybutanoic acid		25	4.72
C_4H_9N	Pyrrolidine		25	11.27
C_4H_9NO	Morpholine		25	8.33
$C_4H_9NO_2$	2-Aminobutanoic acid	1	25	2.29
		2	25	9.83
$C_4H_9NO_2$	4-Aminobutanoic acid	1	25	4.031
		2	25	10.556
$C_4H_9NO_2$	N,N-Dimethylglycine		25	9.89
$C_4H_9NO_2$	2-Methylalanine	1	25	2.36
		2	25	10.21

Molecular formula	Name	Step	$T/°C$	pK_a	Molecular formula	Name	Step	$T/°C$	pK_a
$C_4H_9NO_2S$	Homocysteine	1	25	2.22	$C_5H_9NO_2$	Proline	1	25	1.952
		2	25	8.87			2	25	10.64
		3	25	10.86	$C_5H_9NO_3$	5-Aminolevulinic acid	1	25	4.05
$C_4H_9NO_3$	Homoserine	1	25	2.71			2	25	8.90
		2	25	9.62	$C_5H_9NO_3$	trans-4-Hydroxyproline	1	25	1.818
$C_4H_9NO_3$	DL-Methoxyalanine		25	2.037			2	25	9.662
$C_4H_9NO_3$	Threonine	1	25	2.09	$C_5H_9NO_3$	8-Hydroxypurine	1	20	2.56
		2	25	9.10			2	20	8.26
$C_4H_9N_3O_2$	Creatine	1	25	2.63	$C_5H_9NO_4$	L-Glutamic acid	1	25	2.13
		2	25	14.3			2	25	4.31
$C_4H_{10}N_2$	Piperazine	1	23	9.83	$C_5H_9N_3$	Histamine	1	25	6.04
		2	23	5.56			2	25	9.75
$C_4H_{10}N_2O$	2,4-Diaminobutanoic acid	1	25	1.85	$C_5H_{10}N_2O_2$	Diaminopimelic acid	1	25	1.8
		2	25	8.24			2	25	2.2
		3	25	10.44			3	25	8.8
$C_4H_{11}N$	Butylamine		20	10.77			4	25	9.9
$C_4H_{11}N$	sec-Butylamine		25	10.56	$C_5H_{10}N_2O_3$	L-Glutamine	1	25	2.17
$C_4H_{11}N$	tert-Butylamine		25	10.68			2	25	9.13
$C_4H_{11}N$	Diethylamine		40	11.02	$C_5H_{10}N_2O_3$	Glycylalanine		25	3.15
$C_4H_{12}N_2$	1,4-Butanediamine	1	20	10.80	$C_5H_{10}N_2O_4$	Glycylserine	1	25	2.98
		2	20	9.35			2	25	8.38
$C_4H_{12}O_2$	1,2-Dimethylaminoethane	1	25	10.40	$C_5H_{10}O_2$	2-Methylbutanoic acid		25	4.80
		2	25	8.26	$C_5H_{10}O_2$	3-Methylbutanoic acid		25	4.77
C_5H_4BrN	3-Bromopyridine		25	2.84	$C_5H_{10}O_2$	Pentanoic acid		25	4.84
C_5H_4ClN	3-Chloropyridine		25	2.84	$C_5H_{10}O_2$	Trimethylacetic acid		25	5.03
$C_5H_4N_4$	Purine	1	20	2.30	$C_5H_{11}N$	N-Methylpyrrolidine		25	10.32
		2	20	8.96	$C_5H_{11}N$	Piperidine		25	11.123
$C_5H_4N_4O_3$	Uric acid		12	3.89	$C_5H_{11}NO_2$	5-Aminopentanoic acid	1	25	4.27
C_5H_5N	Pyridine		25	5.25			2	25	10.766
C_5H_5NO	4-Pyridinol	1	20	3.20	$C_5H_{11}NO_2$	Betaine		0	1.83
		2	20	11.12	$C_5H_{11}NO_2$	Norvaline	1	25	2.32
C_5H_5NO	2(1H)-Pyridinone	1	20	0.75			2	25	9.81
		2	20	11.65	$C_5H_{11}NO_2$	N-Propylglycine	1	25	2.35
$C_5H_5N_5$	1H-Purin-6-amine	1	25	4.12			2	25	10.19
		2	25	9.83	$C_5H_{11}NO_2$	Valine	1	25	2.29
$C_5H_6N_2$	2-Methylpyrazine		27	1.45			2	25	9.74
$C_5H_6N_2$	2-Pyridinamine		20	6.82	$C_5H_{11}NO_2S$	Methionine	1	25	2.13
$C_5H_6N_2$	4-Pyridinamine		25	9.114			2	25	9.27
$C_5H_6O_4$	1,1-Cyclopropanedicarboxylic acid	1	25	1.82	$C_5H_{12}N_2O_2$	Ornithine	1	25	1.705
		2	25	7.43			2	25	8.69
$C_5H_6O_4$	Itaconic acid	1	25	3.85			3	25	10.76
		2	25	5.45	$C_5H_{13}N$	1-Amino-2,2-dimethylpropane		25	10.15
$C_5H_6O_4$	Mesaconic acid	1	25	3.09	$C_5H_{13}N$	Diethylmethylamine		25	10.35
		2	25	4.75	$C_5H_{13}N$	3-Methyl-1-butanamine		25	10.60
$C_5H_6O_5$	2-Oxoglutaric acid	1	25	2.47	$C_5H_{13}N$	2-Methyl-2-butanamine		19	10.85
		2	25	4.68	$C_5H_{13}N$	3-Pentanamine		17	10.59
$C_5H_7NO_3$	L-2-Pyrrolidone-5-carboxylic acid		25	3.32	$C_5H_{13}N$	Pentylamine		25	10.63
$C_5H_7N_3$	Methylaminopyrazine		25	3.39	$C_5H_{14}NO$	Choline		25	13.9
$C_5H_7N_3$	2,5-Pyridinediamine		20	6.48	$C_5H_{14}N_2$	Cadaverine	1	25	10.05
$C_5H_8N_2$	2,4-Dimethylimidazol		25	8.36			2	25	10.93
$C_5H_8O_4$	Dimethylmalonic acid		25	3.15	$C_6H_3ClN_4$	6-Chloropteridine		20	3.68
$C_5H_8O_4$	Glutaric acid	1	25	4.31	$C_6H_3N_3O_7$	Picric acid		25	0.38
		2	25	5.41	$C_6H_4Cl_2O$	2,3-Dichlorophenol		25	7.44
$C_5H_8O_4$	Methylsuccinic acid	1	25	4.13	$C_6H_4N_2O_3$	5-Hydroxylysine		25	2.13
		2	25	5.64	$C_6H_4N_2O_5$	2,4-Dinitrophenol		15	3.96

Continued.

Molecular formula	Name	Step	$T/°C$	pK_a	Molecular formula	Name	Step	$T/°C$	pK_a
$C_6H_4N_2O_5$	3,6-Dinitrophenol		15	5.15	$C_6H_8O_7$	Citric acid	1	20	3.14
$C_6H_4N_4$	Pteridine		20	4.05			2	20	4.77
$C_6H_5Br_2N$	3,5-Dibromoaniline		25	2.34			3	20	6.39
C_6H_5ClO	2-Chlorophenol		25	8.49	$C_6H_8O_7$	Isocitric acid	1	25	3.29
C_6H_5ClO	3-Chlorophenol		25	8.85			2	25	4.71
C_6H_5ClO	4-Chlorophenol		25	9.18			3	25	6.40
$C_6H_5Cl_2N$	2,4-Dichloroaniline		22	2.05	$C_6H_9NO_6$	γ-Carboxyglutamic acid	1	25	1.7
C_6H_5NO	2-Pyridinecarboxaldehyde		20	3.80			2	25	3.2
$C_6H_5NO_2$	Nitrobenzene		0	3.98			3	25	4.75
$C_6H_5NO_2$	Picolinic acid	1	25	1.07			4	25	9.9
		2	25	5.25	$C_6H_9N_3$	4,6-Dimethylpyrimidinamine		20	4.82
$C_6H_5NO_2$	3-Pyridinecarboxylic acid		25	4.85	$C_6H_9N_3O_2$	Histidine	1	25	1.80
$C_6H_5NO_2$	4-Pyridinecarboxylic acid		25	4.96			2	25	6.04
$C_6H_5NO_3$	2-Nitrophenol		25	7.17			3	25	9.33
$C_6H_5NO_3$	3-Nitrophenol		25	8.28	$C_6H_{10}O_3$	2-Oxo-3-methylpentanoic acid		25	2.3
$C_6H_5NO_3$	4-Nitrophenol		25	7.15	$C_6H_{10}O_4$	Adipic acid	1	25	4.43
$C_6H_5N_5O$	2-Amino-4-hydroxypteridine	1	20	2.27			2	25	5.41
		2	20	7.96	$C_6H_{10}O_4$	3-Methylglutaric acid		25	4.24
$C_6H_5N_5O_2$	Xanthopterin	2	20	6.59	$C_6H_{11}NO_2$	*l*-Pipecolic acid	1	25	2.28
		3	20	9.31			2	25	10.72
C_6H_6BrN	2-Bromoaniline		25	2.53				25	4.63
C_6H_6BrN	3-Bromoaniline		25	3.58	$C_6H_{11}NO_3$	Adipamic acid		25	4.63
C_6H_6BrN	4-Bromoaniline		25	3.86	$C_6H_{11}NO_4$	2-Aminoadipic acid	1	25	2.14
C_6H_6ClN	2-Chloroaniline		25	2.65			2	25	4.21
C_6H_6ClN	3-Chloroaniline		25	3.46			3	25	9.77
C_6H_6ClN	4-Chloroaniline		25	4.15	$C_6H_{11}N_3O_4$	Glycylasparagine	1	25	2.942
C_6H_6FN	2-Fluoroaniline		25	3.20			2	18	8.44
C_6H_6FN	3-Fluoroaniline		25	3.50	$C_6H_{11}N_3O_4$	*N*-(*N*-Glycylglycyl)glycine	1	25	3.225
C_6H_6FN	4-Fluoroaniline		25	4.65			2	25	8.09
C_6H_6IN	2-Iodoaniline		25	2.60	$C_6H_{12}N_2O_4S_2$	Cystine	1	35	2.1
$C_6H_6N_2O$	2-Pyridinecarboxaldehyde, oxime	1	20	3.59			2	35	8.0
		2	20	10.18	$C_6H_{12}O_2$	Hexanoic acid		25	4.85
$C_6H_6N_2O_2$	2-Nitroaniline		25	−0.26	$C_6H_{12}O_2$	4-Methylpentanoic acid		18	4.84
$C_6H_6N_2O_2$	3-Nitroaniline		25	2.466	$C_6H_{13}N$	Cyclohexylamine		24	10.66
$C_6H_6N_2O_2$	4-Nitroaniline		25	1.0	$C_6H_{13}N$	1,2-Dimethylpyrrolidine		26	10.20
C_6H_6O	Phenol		20	9.89	$C_6H_{13}N$	1-Methylpiperidine		25	10.08
$C_6H_6O_2$	Hydroquinone		20	10.35	$C_6H_{13}NO_2$	6-Aminohexanoic acid	1	25	4.373
$C_6H_6O_2$	Pyrocatechol		20	9.85			2	25	10.804
$C_6H_6O_2$	Resorcinol		25	9.81	$C_6H_{13}NO_2$	Isoleucine	1	25	2.32
$C_6H_6O_3S$	Benzenesulfonic acid		25	0.70			2	25	9.76
$C_6H_6O_6$	*cis*-Aconitic acid		25	1.95	$C_6H_{13}NO_2$	*L*-Leucine	1	25	2.328
$C_6H_6O_6$	*trans*-Aconitic acid	1	25	2.80			2	25	9.744
		2	25	4.46	$C_6H_{13}NO_2$	Norleucine	1	25	2.335
C_6H_7N	Aniline		25	4.63			2	25	9.83
C_6H_7N	2-Methylpyridine		20	5.97	$C_6H_{13}N_3O_3$	Citrulline	1	25	2.43
C_6H_7N	3-Methylpyridine		20	5.68			2	25	9.69
C_6H_7N	4-Methylpyridine		20	6.02	$C_6H_{14}N_2$	*cis*-1,2-Cyclohexanediamine	1	20	9.93
C_6H_7NO	Methoxypyridine		25	6.47			2	20	6.13
$C_6H_7NO_3S$	*o*-Aminobenzenesulfonic acid		25	2.48	$C_6H_{14}N_2$	*trans*-1,2-Cyclohexanediamine	1	20	9.94
$C_6H_7NO_3S$	*m*-Aminobenzenesulfonic acid		25	3.73			2	20	6.47
$C_6H_7NO_3S$	*p*-Aminobenzenesulfonic acid		25	3.24	$C_6H_{14}N_2$	2,5-Dimethylpiperazine	1	25	9.66
$C_6H_8N_2$	*N*-Methylpyridinamine		20	9.65			2	25	5.20
$C_6H_8O_6$	Ascorbic acid	1	24	4.10	$C_6H_{14}N_2O_2$	Lysine	1	25	2.16
		2	16	11.79			2	25	9.06
							3	25	10.54

Molecular formula	Name	Step	T/°C	pKₐ	Molecular formula	Name	Step	T/°C	pKₐ
$C_6H_{14}N_4O_2$	Arginine	1	25	1.82	C_7H_9N	2,4-Dimethylpyridine		25	6.99
		2	25	8.99	C_7H_9N	2,5-Dimethylpyridine		25	6.40
		3	25	12.48	C_7H_9N	2,6-Dimethylpyridine		25	6.65
$C_{10}H_{22}O_2$	3-Amino-3-methylpentane		16	11.01	C_7H_9N	3,4-Dimethylpyridine		25	6.46
$C_{10}H_{22}O_2$	Diisopropylamine		25	11.05	C_7H_9N	3,5-Dimethylpyridine		25	6.15
$C_{10}H_{22}O_2$	Hexylamine		25	10.56	C_7H_9N	2-Ethylpyridine		25	5.89
$C_{10}H_{22}O_2$	Triethylamine		25	10.75	C_7H_9N	N-Methylaniline		25	4.84
$C_6H_{16}N_2$	Hexamethylenediamine	1	0	11.857	C_7H_9N	o-Methylaniline		25	4.44
		2	0	10.762	C_7H_9N	m-Methylaniline		25	4.73
$C_7H_5BrO_2$	2-Bromobenzoic acid		25	2.84	C_7H_9N	p-Methylaniline		25	5.08
$C_7H_5BrO_2$	3-Bromobenzoic acid		25	3.86	C_7H_9NO	o-Anisidine		25	4.52
$C_7H_5ClO_2$	2-Chlorobenzoic acid		25	2.92	C_7H_9NO	m-Anisidine		25	4.23
$C_7H_5ClO_2$	3-Chlorobenzoic acid		25	3.82	C_7H_9NO	p-Anisidine		25	5.34
$C_7H_5ClO_2$	4-Chlorobenzoic acid		25	3.98	C_7H_9NS	4-Methylthioaniline		25	4.35
$C_7H_5IO_2$	2-Iodobenzoic acid		25	2.85	$C_7H_9N_5$	2-Dimethylaminopurine	1	20	4.00
$C_7H_5IO_2$	3-Iodobenzoic acid		25	3.80			2	20	10.24
$C_7H_5NO_3S$	Saccharin		18	11.68	$C_7H_{11}N_3O_2$	l-1-Methylhistidine	1	25	1.69
$C_7H_5NO_4$	Dinicotinic acid		25	2.80			2	25	6.48
$C_7H_5NO_4$	Dipicolinic acid	1	25	2.16			3	25	8.85
		2	25	4.76	$C_7H_{11}N_3O_2$	l-3-Methylhistidine	1	25	1.92
$C_7H_5NO_4$	Lutidinic acid		25	2.15			2	25	6.56
$C_7H_5NO_4$	2-Nitrobenzoic acid		18	2.16			3	25	8.73
$C_7H_5NO_4$	3-Nitrobenzoic acid		25	3.47	$C_7H_{12}O_2$	Cyclohexanecarboxylic acid		25	4.90
$C_7H_5NO_4$	4-Nitrobenzoic acid		25	3.41	$C_7H_{12}O_4$	Heptanedioic acid	1	25	4.71
$C_7H_5NO_4$	Quinolinic acid	1	25	2.43			2	25	5.58
		2	25	4.78	$C_7H_{13}NO$	3-Acetylpiperidine		25	3.18
$C_7H_6N_2$	Benzimidazole		25	5.532	$C_7H_{13}NO_4$	α-Ethylglutamic acid	1	25	3.846
$C_7H_6N_4O$	6-Hydroxy-4-methylpteridine	1	20	4.08			2	25	7.838
		2	20	6.41	$C_7H_{14}O_2$	Heptanoic acid		25	4.89
$C_7H_6O_2$	Benzoic acid		25	4.19	$C_7H_{15}N$	1,2-Dimethylpiperidine		25	10.22
$C_7H_6O_3$	o-Hydroxybenzoic acid	1	19	2.97	$C_7H_{15}N$	1-Ethylpiperidine		23	10.45
		2	18	13.40	$C_7H_{15}NO_3$	Carnitine		25	3.80
$C_7H_6O_3$	m-Hydroxybenzoic acid	1	19	4.06	$C_7H_{17}N$	2-Heptanamine		19	10.7
		2	19	9.92	$C_7H_{17}N$	Heptylamine		25	10.67
$C_7H_6O_3$	p-Hydroxybenzoic acid	1	19	4.48	$C_8H_6N_2$	Cinnoline		20	2.37
		2	19	9.32	$C_8H_6N_2$	Quinazoline		20	3.43
$C_7H_6O_4$	2,5-Dihydroxybenzoic acid	1	25	2.97	$C_8H_6N_2$	Quinoxaline		20	0.56
$C_7H_6O_4$	3,4-Dihydroxybenzoic acid	1	25	4.48	$C_8H_6N_2O$	5-Hydoxyquinazoline	1	20	3.62
		2	25	8.83			2	20	7.41
		3	25	12.6	$C_8H_6O_4$	o-Phthalic acid	1	25	2.89
$C_7H_6O_4$	3,5-Dihydroxybenzoic acid	1	25	4.04			2	25	5.51
$C_7H_6O_4$	Dihydroxymalic acid		25	1.92	$C_8H_6O_4$	m-Phthalic acid	1	25	3.54
$C_7H_6O_5$	Gallic acid		25	4.41			2	18	4.60
$C_7H_6O_5$	2,4,6-Trihydroxybenzoic acid		25	1.68	$C_8H_6O_4$	p-Phthalic acid	1	25	3.51
$C_7H_7NO_2$	2-Aminobenzoic acid	1	25	2.108			2	16	4.82
		2	25	4.946	$C_8H_6O_4$	Terephthalic acid		25	3.51
$C_7H_7NO_2$	3-Aminobenzoic acid	2	25	4.78	$C_8H_7ClO_2$	2-Chlorophenylacetic acid		25	4.07
$C_7H_7NO_2$	4-Aminobenzoic acid	1	25	2.501	$C_8H_7ClO_2$	3-Chlorophenylacetic acid		25	4.14
		2	25	4.874	$C_8H_7ClO_2$	4-Chlorophenylacetic acid		25	4.19
$C_7H_8N_4O_2$	Theobromine		18	7.89	$C_8H_7ClO_3$	2-Chlorophenoxyacetic acid		25	3.05
C_7H_8O	o-Cresol		25	10.20	$C_8H_7ClO_3$	3-Chlorophenoxyacetic acid		25	3.10
C_7H_8O	m-Cresol		25	10.01	$C_8H_7NO_4$	2-Nitrophenylacetic acid		25	4.00
C_7H_8O	p-Cresol		25	10.17	$C_8H_7NO_4$	3-Nitrophenylacetic acid		25	3.97
C_7H_9N	Benzylamine		25	9.33	$C_8H_7NO_4$	4-Nitrophenylacetic acid		25	3.85
C_7H_9N	2,3-Dimethylpyridine		25	6.57	$C_8H_8N_2$	2-Methylbenzimidazole		25	6.19

Continued.

Molecular formula	Name	Step	T/°C	pKa	Molecular formula	Name	Step	T/°C	pKa
C8H8O2	Phenylacetic acid		18	4.28	C9H7NO3	m-Cyanophenoxyacetic acid		25	3.03
C8H8O2	o-Toluic acid		25	3.91	C9H7NO3	p-Cyanophenoxyacetic acid		25	2.93
C8H8O2	m-Toluic acid		25	4.27	C9H8N2	1-Isoquinolinamine		20	7.59
C8H8O2	p-Toluic acid		25	4.36	C9H8N2	3-Quinolinamine		20	4.91
C8H8O3	DL-Mandelic acid		25	3.85	C9H8O2	cis-Cinnamic acid		25	3.89
C8H8O4	Homogentisic acid		25	4.40	C9H8O2	trans-Cinnamic acid		25	4.44
C8H9NO2	2-(Methylamino)benzoic acid		25	5.34	C9H9ClO2	3-(2-Chlorophenyl)propanoic acid		25	4.58
C8H9NO2	3-(Methylamino)benzoic acid		25	5.10	C9H9ClO2	3-(3-Chlorophenyl)propanoic acid		25	4.59
C8H9NO2	4-(Methylamino)benzoic acid		25	5.04	C9H9ClO2	3-(4-Chlorophenyl)propanoic acid		25	4.61
C8H9NO2	Phenylglycine	1	25	1.83	C9H9I2NO3	3,5-Diiodotyrosine	1	25	2.12
		2	25	4.39			2	25	5.32
C8H10BrN	4-Bromo-N,N-dimethylaniline		25	4.23			3	25	9.48
C8H10ClN	3-Chloro-N,N-dimethylaniline		20	3.83	C9H9NO3	Hippuric acid		25	3.62
C8H10ClN	4-Chloro-N,N-dimethylaniline		20	4.39	C9H9NO4	3-(2-Nitrophenyl)propanoic acid		25	4.50
C8H10N2O2	N,N-Dimethyl-3-nitroaniline		25	2.62	C9H9NO4	3-(4-Nitrophenyl)propanoic acid		25	4.47
C8H11N	N,N-Dimethylaniline		25	5.15	C9H10INO3	3-Iodotyrosine	1	25	2.2
C8H11N	N-Ethylaniline		24	5.12			2	25	8.7
C8H11N	Phenylethylamine		25	9.84			3	25	9.1
C8H11N	2,4,6-Trimethylpyridine		25	7.43	C9H10N2	2-Ethylbenzimidazole		25	6.18
C8H11NO	o-Phenetidine		28	4.43	C9H10O2	Mesitylenic acid		25	4.32
C8H11NO	m-Phenetidine		25	4.18	C9H10O2	α-Phenylpropanoic acid		25	4.64
C8H11NO	p-Phenetidine		28	5.20	C9H10O2	β-Phenylpropanoic acid		25	4.37
C8H11NO	Tyramine	1	25	9.74	C9H11N	N-Allylaniline		25	4.17
		2	25	10.52	C9H11N	1-Aminoindane		22	9.21
C8H11NO2	Dopamine	1	25	8.9	C9H11NO2	Phenylalanine	1	25	2.20
		2	25	10.6			2	25	9.31
C8H11NO3	Noradrenaline	1	25	8.64	C9H11NO3	Tyrosine	1	25	2.20
		2	25	9.70			2	25	9.21
C8H12N2O3	Veronal		25	7.43			3	25	10.46
C8H14O4	Octanedioic acid		25	4.52	C9H11NO4	L-3,4-Dihydroxyphenylalanine	1	25	2.32
C8H16N2O3	N-Glycylleucine		25	3.18			2	25	8.72
C8H16N2O3	N-Leucylglycine	1	25	3.25			3	25	9.96
		2	25	8.2			4	25	11.79
C8H16N2O4S2	Homocystine	1	25	1.59	C9H12N2O2	Tyrosineamide		25	7.33
		2	25	2.54	C9H13NO3	D-Adrenaline	1	25	8.66
		3	25	8.52			2	25	9.95
		4	25	9.44	C9H14N4O3	N-β-Alanylhistidine	1	20	2.73
C8H16O2	Octanoic acid		25	4.89			2	20	6.87
C8H17N	2,2,4-Trimethylpiperidine		30	11.04			3	20	9.73
C8H19N	Dibutylamine		21	11.25	C9H14N4O3	L-Carnosine	1	25	2.62
C8H19N	N-Methyl-2-heptanamine		17	10.99			2	25	6.66
C8H19N	Octylamine		25	10.65			3	25	9.24
C9H6BrN	3-Bromoquinoline		25	2.69	C9H18O2	Nonanic acid		25	4.96
C9H7ClO2	o-Chlorocinnamic acid		25	4.23	C9H19N	1-Butylpiperidine		23	10.47
C9H7ClO2	m-Chlorocinnamic acid		25	4.29	C9H19N	2,2,6,6-Tetramethylpiperidine		25	11.07
C9H7ClO2	p-Chlorocinnamic acid		25	4.41	C9H21N	Nonylamine		25	10.64
C9H7N	Isoquinoline		20	5.42	C10H7NO2	8-Quinolinecarboxylic acid		25	1.82
C9H7N	Quinoline		20	4.90	C10H8O	1-Naphthol		25	9.34
C9H7NO	7-Isoquinolinol	1	20	5.68	C10H8O	2-Naphthol		25	9.51
		2	20	8.90	C10H9N	2-Methylquinoline		20	5.83
C9H7NO	3-Quinolinol	1	20	4.28	C10H9N	4-Methylquinoline		20	5.67
		2	20	8.08	C10H9N	5-Methylquinoline		20	5.20
C9H7NO	8-Quinolinol	1	20	5.017	C10H9N	α-Naphthylamine		25	3.92
		2	25	9.812	C10H9N	β-Naphthylamine		25	4.16
C9H7NO3	o-Cyanophenoxyacetic acid		25	2.98	C10H9NO	1-Amino-6-hydroxynaphthalene		25	3.97

Continued.

Molecular formula	Name	Step	T/°C	pKa	Molecular formula	Name	Step	T/°C	pKa
C₁₀H₉NO	6-Methoxyquinoline		20	5.03	C₁₁H₁₆N₂O₂	Pilocarpine		30	6.87
C₁₀H₁₀O₂	o-Methylcinnamic acid		25	4.50	C₁₁H₂₅N	Undecylamine		25	10.63
C₁₀H₁₀O₂	m-Methylcinnamic acid		25	4.44	C₁₂H₈N₂	1,10-Phenanthroline		25	4.84
C₁₀H₁₀O₂	p-Methylcinnamic acid		25	4.56	C₁₂H₁₁N	2-Aminobiphenyl		22	3.82
C₁₀H₁₂N₂	Tryptamine		25	10.2	C₁₂H₁₁N	2-Benzylpyridine		25	5.13
C₁₀H₁₂N₂O	5-Hydroxytryptamine	1	25	9.8	C₁₂H₁₁N	Diphenylamine		25	0.79
		2	25	11.1	C₁₂H₁₁N₃	4-Aminoazobenzene		25	2.82
C₁₀H₁₂O₂	4-Phenylbutanoic acid		25	4.76	C₁₂H₁₂N₂	p-Benzidine	1	30	4.66
C₁₀H₁₂O₃	2-(m-Anisyl)propanoic acid		25	4.65			2	30	3.57
C₁₀H₁₂O₃	2-(p-Anisyl)propanoic acid		25	4.69	C₁₂H₁₃N	N,N-Dimethyl-1-naphthylamine		25	4.83
C₁₀H₁₂O₃	2-(o-Anisyl)propanoic acid		25	4.80	C₁₂H₁₃N	N,N-Dimethyl-2-naphthylamine		25	4.566
C₁₀H₁₄N₂	Nicotine	1	25	8.02	C₁₂H₂₇N	Dodecylamine		25	10.63
		2	25	3.12	C₁₃H₉N	Acridine		20	5.58
C₁₀H₁₅N	N,N-Diethylaniline		22		C₁₃H₉N	Phenanthridine		20	5.58
C₁₀H₁₅NO	d-Ephedrine		10	10.139	C₁₃H₁₀N₂	2-Phenylbenzimidazole	1	25	5.23
C₁₀H₁₅NO	l-Ephedrine		10	9.958			2	25	11.91
C₁₀H₁₇N₃O₆S	l-Glutathione	1	25	2.12	C₁₃H₁₀O₂	2-Phenylbenzoic acid		25	3.46
		2	25	3.59	C₁₃H₁₂N₂O	4-(p-Aminobenzoyl)aniline	1	25	2.93
		3	25	8.75	C₁₃H₁₃N	4-Benzylaniline		25	2.17
		4	25	9.65	C₁₃H₂₉N	Tridecylamine		25	10.63
C₁₀H₁₇N₅O₆	Tetraglycylglycine	1	20	3.10	C₁₄H₁₂O₂	Diphenylacetic acid		25	3.94
		2	20	8.02	C₁₄H₁₅N₃	4-Dimethylaminoazobenzene		25	3.226
C₁₀H₁₈N₄O₅	L-Argininosuccinic acid	1	25	1.62	C₁₄H₃₁N	Tetradecylamine		25	10.62
		2	25	2.70	C₁₅H₁₁I₄NO₄	L-Thyroxine	1	25	2.2
		3	25	4.26			2	25	6.45
		4	25	9.58			3	25	10.1
C₁₀H₁₉N	Bornylamine		25	10.17	C₁₅H₃₃N	Pentadecylamine		25	10.61
C₁₀H₁₉N	Neobornylamine		25	10.01	C₁₆H₃₅N	Hexadecylamine		25	10.63
C₁₀H₂₁N	Butylcyclohexylamine		25	11.23	C₁₇H₁₉NO₃	Morphine		25	8.21
C₁₀H₂₃N	Decylamine		25	10.64	C₁₈H₂₁NO₃	Codeine		25	8.21
C₁₁H₈N₂	Perimidine		20	6.35	C₁₈H₃₉N	Octadecylamine		25	10.60
C₁₁H₈O₂	1-Naphthoic acid		25	3.70	C₂₀H₂₁NO₄	Papaverine		25	6.40
C₁₁H₈O₂	2-Naphthoic acid		25	4.17	C₂₀H₂₄N₂O₂	Quinine	1	25	8.52
C₁₁H₁₁N	Methyl-1-naphthylamine		27	3.67			2	25	4.13
C₁₁H₁₂N₂O₂	Tryptophan	1	25	2.46	C₂₁H₂₂N₂O₂	Strychnine		25	8.26
		2	25	9.41	C₂₃H₂₆N₂O₄	Brucine	1	25	8.28

Appendix BB
CONCENTRATION OF ACIDS AND BASES—COMMON COMMERCIAL STRENGTHS

	Molecular weight	Moles per liter	Grams per liter	Percent by weight	Specific gravity
Acetic acid	60.05	6.27	376	36	1.045
Acetic acid, glacial	60.05	17.4	1,045	99.5	1.05
Butyric acid	88.1	10.3	912	95	0.96
Formic acid	46.02	23.4	1,080	90	1.20
		5.75	264	25	1.06
Hydriodic acid	127.9	7.57	969	57	1.70
		5.51	705	47	1.50
		0.86	110	10	1.1
Hydrobromic acid	80.92	8.89	720	48	1.50
		6.82	552	40	1.38
Hydrochloric acid	36.5	11.6	424	36	1.18
		2.9	105	10	1.05
Hydrocyanic acid	27.03	25.0	676	97	0.697
		0.74	19.9	2	0.996
Hydrofluoric acid	20.01	32.1	642	55	1.167
		28.8	578	50	1.155
Hydrofluosilicic acid	144.1	2.65	382	30	1.27
Hypophosphorous acid	66.0	9.47	625	50	1.25
		5.14	339	30	1.13
		1.57	104	10	1.04
Lactic acid	90.1	11.3	1,020	85	1.2
Nitric acid	63.02	15.99	1,008	71	1.42
		14.9	938	67	1.40
		13.3	837	61	1.37
Perchloric acid	100.5	11.65	1,172	70	1.67
		9.2	923	60	1.54
Phosphoric acid	98.0	14.7	1,445	85	1.70
Sulfuric acid	98.1	18.0	1,766	96	1.84
Sulfurous acid	82.1	0.74	61.2	6	1.02
Ammonia water	17.0	14.8	252	28	0.898
Potassium hydroxide	56.1	13.5	757	50	1.52
		1.94	109	10	1.09
Sodium carbonate	106.0	1.04	110	10	1.10
Sodium hydroxide	40.0	19.1	763	50	1.53
		2.75	111	10	1.11

Appendix CC
MOLECULAR WEIGHT TO MOLAR AMOUNTS: CONVERSION FACTORS

This table is used to convert gram amounts of subtances to molar amounts. To convert a number of grams of a substance to an equivalent number of moles, multiply the number of grams by the factor given for the substance. These factors can also be used to convert milligrams to millimoles, micrograms to micromoles, kilograms to kilomoles, etc.

Substance	Molecular weight	Factor
Acetaldehyde	44.05	0.0227
Acetoacetic acid	102.09	0.009795
Acetoin	88.10	0.01135
Acetone	58.08	0.01722
Acetonitrile	41.05	0.02436
Acetylcholine	163.22	0.006127
Acetyldigitoxin	809.96	0.001235
Acetylneuraminic acid	309.28	0.003233
ACTH (adrenocorticotropic hormone)	4,500	0.0002222
Adenine	135.14	0.007400
Adenosine diphosphate (ADP)	427.22	0.002341
Adenosine monophosphate (AMP)	347.23	0.002880
Adenosine triphosphate (ATP)	507.21	0.001972
Adipic acid	146.14	0.006843
Alanine	89.09	0.01122
Albumin	69,000	0.00001449
Aldosterone	360.44	0.002774
Allantoin	158.12	0.006324
Allotetrahydrocortisone	364.47	0.002744
Aluminum	26.98	0.03706
p-Aminobenzoic acid	137.13	0.007292
Aminobutyric acid (aminoisobutyric acid)	103.12	0.009697
p-Aminohippuric acid	194.19	0.005150
δ-Aminolevulinic acid (ALA)	131.13	0.007626
Ammonia	17.03	0.05872
Androstenediol	290.43	0.003443
Androstenedione	286.40	0.003492
Androsterone	290.43	0.003443
Anserine	240.26	0.004162
α-1-Antitrypsin	45,000	0.00002222
Arabinose	150.13	0.006661
Arachidonic acid	304.46	0.003285
Arginine	174.20	0.005741
Arsenic	74.92	0.01335
Asparagine	132.12	0.007569
Aspartic acid	133.10	0.007513

Continued.

Substance	Molecular weight	Factor
Bicarbonate	61.02	0.01639
Bilirubin	584.65	0.001710
Biotin	244.31	0.004093
Boron	10.81	0.09251
Bromine (bromide)	79.90	0.01252
Bromsulphalein sodium (BSP)	838.0	0.001193
Bufotenine	204.26	0.004896
Butylene glycol	90.12	0.01110
Calcium	40.08	0.2495
Carbon dioxide (CO_2)	440.1	0.02272
Carbon monoxide (CO)	28.01	0.03570
Carnitine	161.20	0.006203
Carnosine	226.23	0.004420
Carotene (β-carotene)	536.85	0.001863
Ceruloplasmin	160,000	0.00000625
Chenodeoxycholic acid	392.56	0.002547
Chlorine (chloride)	35.45	0.02821
Cholesterol (total)	386.64	0.002586
Cholic acid	408.56	0.002448
Choline	121.18	0.008252
Citric acid	192.12	0.005205
Citrulline	175.19	0.005708
Cobalt	58.93	0.01697
Copper	63.55	0.01574
Coproporphyrin	654.73	0.001527
Corticosteroids; use Cortisol		
Corticosterone	346.45	0.002886
Cortisol	362.47	0.002759
Cortisone	360.46	0.002774
Creatine	131.14	0.007625
Creatinine	113.12	0.008840
Cresol	108.13	0.009248
Cyanide	26.02	0.03843
Cystamine	152.29	0.006566
Cystathionine	222.28	0.004499
Cystine	240.30	0.004161
Dehydroepiandrosterone	288.41	0.003467
Deoxycholic acid	392.56	0.002547
Diethylbarbituric acid (barbital)	184.19	0.005429
Digitoxin	764.92	0.001307
Digoxin	780.92	0.001281
Dihydroxyacetone	90.08	0.01110
Dihydroxyphenylacetic acid (homogentisic acid)	168.14	0.005947
Dimethylamine	45.08	0.02218
Dimethyltryptamine	188.26	0.005312

Substance	Molecular weight	Factor
Dopa	197.19	0.005071
Dopamine	153.18	0.006528
Epinephrine (Adrenalin)	183.20	0.005459
Epitestosterone	288.43	0.003467
Ergothioneine	229.29	0.004361
Estradiol	272.37	0.003671
Estriol	288.37	0.003468
Estrone	270.36	0.003699
Ethanolamine	61.08	0.01637
Ethyl alcohol	47.07	0.2171
Etiocholanolone	290.45	0.003443
Fibrinogen	340,000	0.000002941
Fluorine (fluoride)	19.00	0.05263
Folic acid	441.40	0.002266
Fructose	180.16	0.005551
Fucose	164.16	0.006092
Galactose	180.16	0.005551
Glucose	180.16	0.005551
Glucuronic acid	194.14	0.005151
Glutamic acid	147.13	0.006797
Glutamine	146.15	0.006842
Glutaric acid	132.11	0.007569
Glutathione	307.33	0.003254
Glycerol	92.09	0.01086
Glycine	75.07	0.01332
Glyoxylic acid	74.04	0.01351
Gold	196.97	0.005077
Growth hormone (human)	22,124	0.00004520
Guanidine	59.07	0.01693
Guanidoacetic acid (glycocyamine)	117.11	0.008539
Guanosine triphosphate	523.19	0.001911
Haptoglobin	85,000	0.00001176
Hemoglobin (tetramer)	64,500	0.00001550
Hemoglobin/4 (monomer)	16,125	0.00006202
Hexosamines (glucosamine, etc.)	179.17	0.005581
Hippuric acid	179.17	0.005581
Histamine	111.15	0.008997
Histidine	155.16	0.006445
Homogentisic acid	168.14	0.005947
Homovanillic acid	182.18	0.005489
β-Hydroxybutyric acid	104.10	0.009606
11-Hydroxycorticosteroids; use Cortisol		
17-Hydroxycorticosteroids; use Cortisol		
5-Hydroxyindoleacetic acid (5-HIAA)	191.19	0.005230
Hydroxyphenylacetic acid (mandelic acid)	152.14	0.006573

Continued.

Substance	Molecular weight	Factor
Hydroxyprogesterone	330.45	0.003026
Hydroxyproline	131.13	0.007626
Hypoxanthine	136.11	0.007347
IgA	180,000	0.000005556
IgD	180,000	0.000005556
IgE	200,000	0.000005000
IgG	150,000	0.000006667
IgM	900,000	0.000001111
Indican (potassium indoxyl sulfate)	251.32	0.003979
Indoleacetic acid	175.18	0.005708
Inosine	268.23	0.003728
Inositol	180.16	0.005551
Insulin (bovine)	5,733	0.0001744
Insulin (bovine, 52%; porcine, 48%)	5,754	0.0001738
Insulin (human)	5,807	0.0001722
Insulin (porcine)	5,777	0.0001731
Iodine	126.90	0.007880
Iron	55.85	0.01791
Isoleucine	131.17	0.007624
17-Ketogenic steroids; use Cortisol		
Ketoglutaric acid	146.10	0.006845
Ketoisovaleric acid	116.13	0.008611
17-Ketosteroids; use Androsterone		
Kynurenic acid	189.16	0.005287
Kynurenine	208.21	0.004803
Lactic acid	90.08	0.01110
Lactose	342.30	0.002921
Lead	207.20	0.004826
Lecithin	677.92	0.001475
Leucine	131.17	0.007624
Linoleic acid	280.44	0.003566
Linolenic acid	278.42	0.003592
Lipoic acid	206.33	0.004847
Lithium	6.94	0.1441
Lithocholic acid	376.56	0.002656
Lysine	146.19	0.006840
Magnesium	24.31	0.04114
Malic acid	134.09	0.007458
Mandelic acid	152.14	0.006573
Manganese	54.94	0.01820
Mercury	200.59	0.004985
Metanephrine, metadrenaline	197.23	0.005070
Methanol	32.04	0.03121
Methionine	149.21	0.006702
5-Methoxytryptamine	190.24	0.005257
Methyl digitoxin	779.92	0.001282

Substance	Molecular weight	Factor
Methylamine	31.06	0.03220
Methylhistidine	169.18	0.005911
Methylmalonic acid	118.09	0.008468
Methylnicotinamide	137.16	0.007291
Molybdenum	95.94	0.01042
Nicotinamide adenine dinucleotide (NAD, nadide)	663.44	0.001507
Nicotinamide adenine dinucleotide phosphate (NADP)	743.44	0.001345
Nicotinic acid	123.11	0.008123
Nitrate	62.01	0.01613
Nitrite	46.01	0.02173
Nitrogen	14.01	0.07138
Norepinephrine (noradrenaline)	169.18	0.005911
Normetanephrine (normetadrenaline)	183.20	0.005459
Oleic acid	282.45	0.003540
Ornithine	132.16	0.007567
Orotic acid	156.10	0.006406
Oxalacetic acid	132.07	0.007572
Oxalic acid	90.04	0.01111
Pantothenic acid	219.23	0.004561
Phenacetin (acetophenetidin)	179.21	0.005580
Phenol	94.11	0.01063
Phenolsulfonphthalein (PSP)	354.37	0.002822
Phenylalanine	165.19	0.006054
Phenylpyruvic acid	164.17	0.006091
Phospholipids	774	0.001292
Phosphorus	30.97	0.03229
Piperidine	85.15	0.01174
Porphobilinogen	226.23	0.004420
Porter-Silber chromogens; use Cortisol		
Potassium	39.10	0.02558
Prednisolone	360.44	0.002774
Prednisone	358.44	0.002790
Pregnanediol	320.50	0.003120
Pregnanetriol	336.50	0.002972
Pregnanolone	318.48	0.003140
Progeterone	314.45	0.003180
Proline	115.13	0.008686
Propoxyphene	339.48	0.002946
Prostaglandin E_1	354.49	0.002821
Prostaglandin E_2	352.48	0.002837
Prostaglandin E_3	350.46	0.002853
Prostaglandin $F_{1\alpha}$	355.50	0.002813
Prostaglandin $F_{2\alpha}$	354.49	0.002821
Prostaglandin $F_{3\alpha}$	351.47	0.002845
Prothrombin	68,900	0.00001451

Continued.

Substance	Molecular weight	Factor
Protoporphyrin IX	562.64	0.001777
Pyridoxal-5-phosphate	247.15	0.004046
Pyridoxic acid	183.16	0.005460
Pyrocatechol	110.11	0.009082
Pyrophosphate	173.94	0.005749
Pyruvic acid (pyruvate)	88.06	0.01136
Ribose	150.13	0.006661
Ribosyluracil (uridine)	244.20	0.004095
Ribulose	150.13	0.006661
Rubidium	85.47	0.01170
Salicylic acid	138.12	0.007240
Selenium	78.96	0.01266
Serine	105.09	0.009516
Serotonin	176.21	0.005675
Silicon dioxide	60.09	0.01664
Sodium	22.99	0.04350
Sorbitol	182.17	0.005489
Spermidine	145.25	0.006885
Spermine	202.34	0.004942
Stercobilinogen	596.77	0.001676
Succinic acid	118.09	0.008468
Sucrose	342.30	0.002921
Sulfate	96.06	0.01041
Sulfur	32.06	0.03119
Taurine	125.14	0.007991
Testosterone	288.41	0.003467
Tetrahydrocortisol	366.48	0.002729
Tetrahydrocortisone	364.47	0.002744
Thallium	204.37	0.004893
Thiocyanate	58.08	0.01722
Threonine	119.12	0.008395
Thyroid-stimulating hormone (TSH)	25,000	0.00004
Thyroxin	776.93	0.001287
Transferrin	80,000	0.00001250
Triglycerinde	875	0.001143
Triiodothyronine	651.01	0.001536
Trypsin	24,000	0.00004167
Tryptamine	160.21	0.006242
L-Tryptophane	204.22	0.004897
Tyrosine	181.19	0.005519
Urea	60.06	0.01665
Urea nitrogen	28.02	0.03569
Uric acid	168.11	0.005948
Uridine	244.20	0.004095
Uridine-5-monophosphate	324.19	0.003085

Substance	Molecular weight	Factor
Urobilinogen	590.73	0.001693
Urocanic acid	138.12	0.007240
Uroporphyrin	830.77	0.001204
Valine	117.15	0.008536
Vanillic acid	168.14	0.005947
Vanillymandelic acid (VMA, 4-hydroxy-3-methoxy mandelic acid)	198.17	0.005046
Vitamin A (retinol)	286.44	0.003491
Vitamin B_1 (thiamine, aneurine)	337.27	0.002965
Vitamin B_2 (riboflavin, lactoflavin)	376.36	0.002657
Vitamin B_6 (pyridoxine, adermine)	169.18	0.005911
Vitamin B_{12} (cyanocabalamin)	1,357.44	0.007367
Vitamin C (ascorbic acid)	176.12	0.005678
Vitamin D_2 (ergocalciferol)	396.63	0.002521
Vitamin D_3 (cholecalciferol)	384.62	0.002600
Vitamin E (α-tocopherol)	430.69	0.002322
Vitamin K	450.68	0.002219
Xanthine	152.11	0.006574
Xanthurenic acid	205.16	0.004874
Xylose	150.13	0.006661
Xylulose	150.13	0.006661
Zinc	65.38	0.01530

Appendix DD
CLINICAL TESTS WITH UNITS, NORMAL VALUES, AND CONVERSION FACTORS

Test	Sample type	Kind of quantity	Synonyms	Atomic or molecular mass	Current units (A)
Acid phosphatase	Serum	Enzyme concentration (Jacobsson, 1960)			
Acids (H)	24-hour urine	Amount of substance (Jørgensen, 1957)	Net acid		mEq/24 h (mEq/d)
Alanine aminotransferase	Serum	Enzyme concentration (Laursen et al., 1958)	Glutamic-alanine transaminase, glutamic-pyruvic transaminase, GPT, SGPT		
Albumin	Serum	Mass concentration	Albumin percent		g/100 ml
					Percent
Albumin	Spinal fluid	Mass concentration			mg/100 ml
Albumin	Serum protein	Mass fraction	Albumin percent		Percent
Alkaline phosphatase	Serum	Enzyme concentration (Bessey et al., 1946)			
Amino acid nitrogen (N)	Fasting serum	Molar concentration		A = 14.01 for N	mg/100 ml
Ammonia	Plasma	Molar concentration		M = 17.03 for NH_3	μg/100 ml (as NH_3)

*Numbers without parentheses are in scientific notation; numbers in parentheses are in real numbers.

Conversion factors*		Recommended units (B)	Normal values		Comments
A to B	B to A		Conventional	Recommended SI	
				At 30 °C: prostatic, 0-3 U/L; total, 0-9 U/L	Measured in international units. Conversion between values generated by two methods requires an empirically constructed function.
1	1	mmol/d	50 mEq/24 h (mEq/d)	50 mmol/d	Alternative quantity (Jørgensen, 1957) Patient (urine) acids (H, excreted), mole rate (24 h). $1 \text{ mmol/d} = 1.16 \times 10^{-2} \ \mu\text{mol/s}$.
				At 30°C: M, 6-21 U/L; F, 4-17 U/L	Measured in international units. Conversion between values generated by two methods requires an empirically constructed function.
10^1 (10)	10^{-1} (0.1)	g/L	3.8-5.0 g/100 ml	38-50 g/L	It is presumed that percent is incorrectly used for g/100 ml.
10^1 (10)	10^{-1} (0.1)	g/L	3.8%-5.0%		
10^{-2} (0.01)	10^2 (100)	g/L	10-30 mg/100 ml	0.1-0.3 g/L	
10^{-2} (0.01)	10^2 (100)	kg/kg	Approx 6.9%	Approx 0.69 kg/kg	
				Approx. 26 U/L	Measured in international units. Conversion between values generated by two methods requires an empirically constructed function.
7.138×10^{-1} (0.7138)	1.401	mmol/L	2.9-5.8 mg/100 ml	2.1-4.2 mmol/L	
5.872×10^{-1} (0.5872)	1.703	μmol/L	40-80 μg/100 ml	23.5-47.0 μmol/L (enzymatic method)	The values for plasma ammonia, molar concentration; plasma ammonia nitrogen (N), molar concentration; and plasma nitrogen (N, ammonia), molar concentration are equal.

Continued.

CLINICAL TESTS WITH UNITS, NORMAL VALUES, AND CONVERSION FACTORS—cont'd

Test	Sample type	Kind of quantity	Synonyms	Atomic or molecular mass	Current units (A)
Ammonia	24-hour urine	Amount of substance	Ammonia excretion	$M = 17.03$ for NH_3	mg/d (as NH_3)
Ascorbic acid	Fasting serum	Molar concentration	Vitamin C	$M = 176.12$ for ascorbic acid	mg/100 ml (as ascorbic acid)
Asparate amino-transferase	Serum	Enzyme concentration (Laursen et al., 1959)	Glutamic-aspartic trans-aminase, glutamic-oxaloacetic transami-nase, GOT, SGOT		
Bilirubin (total)	Fasting serum	Molar concentration		$M = 584.65$ for unconjugated bilirubin as un-dissociated acid	mg/100 ml
Bilirubin	Urine	Arbitrary molar con-centration (Rosen-bach, 1876; 0-1)	Gemlin's reaction		
Blood	Feces	Arbitrary specific vol3ume content (Gregersen, 1916; 0-1)	Benzidine reaction		
Blood	Patient	Specific volume con-tent	Blood content		ml/100 g
Calcium ion (Ca, total)	Fasting serum	Molar concentration	Calcium	$A = 40.08$ for Ca	mg/100 ml _____ mEq/L

*Numbers without parentheses are in scientific notation; numbers in parentheses are in real numbers.

Conversion factors*		Recommended units (B)	Normal values		Comments
A to B	**B to A**		**Conventional**	**Recommended SI**	
5.872×10^{-2} (0.05872)	1.703×10^{1} (17.03)	mmol/d	500-1,200 mg/d	29-70 mmol/d	Alternative quantity: patient (urine) ammonia (excreted), mole rate. 1 mmol/d = 1.16×10^{-2} μmol/s. The values of 24-hour urine ammonia, mole rate; 24 hr urine ammonia nitrogen (N), mole rate; and 24-hr urine nitrogen (N, ammonia), mole rate are equal.
5.678×10^{1} (56.78)	1.761×10^{-2} (0.01761)	μmol/L	0.5-1.5 mg/100 ml	28.4-85.2 μmol/L	
				At 30°C: without P-5-P: M, 7-21 U/L; F, 6-18 U/L. with P-5-P: 12-29 U/L (females slightly lower)	Measured in international units. Conversion between values generated by two methods requires an empirically constructed function.
1.710×10^{1} (17.1)	5.847×10^{-2} (0.05847)	μmol/L	0.2-1.0 mg/100 ml	3.4-17.1 μmol/L	If the method of determination does not yield identical photometric readings for the same molar concentrations of conjugated bilirubin, add the name of the method.
				0 arbitrary units	Use 0 arbitrary units instead of −; use 0 or 1 for ±.
				0 arbitrary units	Use 0 arbitrary units instead of −; use 0 or 1 for ±.
10^{1} (10)	10^{-1} (0.1)	ml/kg	Approx. 7.0 ml/100 g	Approx. 70 ml/kg	
2.495×10^{-1} (0.2495)	4.008	mmol/L	8.5-10.8 mg/100 ml	2.1-2.7 mmol/L	The calcium ion is found in serum as free ion, chelated to citrate, and bound to proteins. Free ions and chelted form are dialyzable; the protein-bound form is nondialyzable.
5.000×10^{-1} (0.5)	2.0	mmol/L	4.2-5.4 mEq/L		To convert mg/100 ml to mEq/L, multiply by 0.499; to convert mEq/L to mg/100 ml, multiply by 2.004.

Continued.

CLINICAL TESTS WITH UNITS, NORMAL VALUES, AND CONVERSION FACTORS—cont'd

Test	Sample type	Kind of quantity	Synonyms	Atomic or molecular mass	Current units (A)
Calcium ion (Ca)	24-hour urine	Amount of substance	Calcium excretion	A = 40.08 for Ca	mg/d
					mEq/d
Capillary bleeding time	Patient	Time difference (Duke, 1910)	Bleeding time		min
					min
Carbon dioxide	Alveolar gas	Partial pressure	Alveolar carbon dioxide tension		mm Hg
					mm Hg
Carbon dioxide	Gas	Partial pressure (arterial blood equilibration)	Carbon dioxide pressure, P_{CO_2}		mm Hg
					mm Hg
Carbonate (total + CO_2)	Plasma	Molar concentration	Alkali reserve, bicarbonate, total carbon dioxide		Volume percent (as carbon dioxide at 0°C, 1013 mbar, dry, having a molar volume of 22.26 L/mol.
Cells	Spinal fluid	Particle concentration	Cell content, cells		Per μl (cumm, mm^3)
					Thirds

*Numbers without parentheses are in scientific notation; numbers in parentheses are in real numbers.

Conversion factors*		Recommended units (B)	Normal values		Comments
A to B	B to A		Conventional	Recommended SI	
2.495×10^{-2} (0.02495)	4.008×10^{1} (40.08)	mmol/d	50-150 mg/d	1.25-3.74 mmol/d (Varies with intake)	Alternative quantity: patient (urine), calcium ion (Ca, excreted), mole rate. 1 mmol/d = 11.57 nmol/s. To convert mg/d to mEq/d, multiply by 0.0499; to convert mEq/d to mg/d, multiply by 20.04.
5.000×10^{-1} (0.5)	2.0	mmol/d	2.5-7.48 mEq/d		
6.00×10^{-2} (0.06)	1.667×10^{1} (16.67)	ks	Approx. 3.83 min.	Approx. 0.23 ks	Some prefer the unit *second* even if reproducibility does not permit three significant figures, i.e., the value 230 s instead of 0.23 ks.
6.000×10^{1} (60)	1.667×10^{-2} (0.01667)	s	Approx. 3.83 min.	Approx. 230 s	
1.333	7.502×10^{-1} (0.7502)	mbar	Approx. 40.5 mm Hg	Approx. 54 mbar	A measured liquid height of water or mercury must be corrected for the temperature of the liquid and for the local acceleration of free fall whether the conversion is to conventional millimeters of mercury or to millibars or to kilonewtons per square meter (kPa). Exact measurements refer to a relative error of less than 10^{-2}.
1.333×10^{-1} (0.1333)	7.502	kN/m^2 (kPa)		Approx. 5.4 kN/m^2 (kPa)	
1.333	7.502×10^{-1} (0.7502)	mbar	35-45 mm Hg	46-60 mbar	A measured liquid height of water or mercury must be corrected for the temperature of the liquid and for the local acceleration of free fall whether the conversion is to conventional millimeters of mercury or to millibars or kilonewtons per square meter (kPa). Exact measurements refer to a relative error of less than 10^{-2}.
1.333×10^{-1} (0.1333)	7.502	kN/m^2 (kPa)	35-45 mm Hg	4.6-6.0 kN/m^2 (kPa)	
4.492×10^{-1} (0.4492)	2.226	mmol/L	51-67 volume percent	23-30 mmol/L	The "concentration" of hydrogen carbonate (HCO$_3^-$) has been called the "combined carbon dioxide capacity."
1	1	$\times 10^6$/L	<10/μl (cumm, mm^3)	<10 $\times 10^6$/L	The term *thirds* refers to approximately one third the volume of a counting chamber having a volume of 3.2 μl.
3.125×10^{-1} (0.315)	3.2	$\times 10^6$/L			

Continued.

CLINICAL TESTS WITH UNITS, NORMAL VALUES, AND CONVERSION FACTORS—cont'd

Test	Sample type	Kind of quantity	Synonyms	Atomic or molecular mass	Current units (A)
Chloride	Serum	Molar concentration		A = 35.46 for Cl	mg/100 ml
					mEq/L
Chloride	Urine	Molar concentration		A = 35.46 for Cl	mg/100 ml
					mEq/L
Chloride	24-hour urine	Amount of substance	Chloride excretion	A = 35.46 for Cl	mg/24 h (mg/d)
					mEq/24 h (mEq/d)
Chloride	Feces	Specific mole content		A = 35.46 for Cl	mg/100 g
					mEq/kg
Cholesterol (total)	Fasting serum	Molar concentration	Total cholesterol	M = 386.64 for cholesterol	mg/100 ml
Citrate	Serum	Molar concentration	Citric acid	M = 192.12 for citric acid	mg/100 ml (as citric acid)
Coagulation	Blood	Time difference (Biggs, et al., 1957)	Coagulation time		min
					min
Copper ion (Cu, total)	Serum	Molar concentration		A = 63.54 for Cu	μg/100 ml

*Numbers without parentheses are in scientific notation; numbers in parentheses are in real numbers.

Conversion factors*		Recommended units (B)	Normal values		Comments
A to B	B to A		Conventional	Recommended SI	
2.820×10^{-1} (0.282)	3.546	mmol/L	347-375 mg/ 100 ml	98-106 mmol/L	To convert mg/100 ml to mEq/L, multiply by 0.282; to convert mEq/L to mg/100 ml, multiply by 3.546.
1	1	mmol/L	98-106 mEq/L		
2.820×10^{-1} (0.282)	3.546	mmol/L	See Chloride, 24-hour urine	See Chloride, 24-hour urine	To convert mg/100 ml to mEq/L, multiply by 0.282; to convert mEq/L to mg/100 ml, multiply by 3.546.
1	1	mmol/L	See Chloride, 24-hour urine		
2.820×10^{-2} (0.0282)	3.546×10^{1} (35.46)	mmol/d	3,900-8,890 mg/d	110-250 mmol/d (varies with intake)	Alternative quantity: patient (urine), chloride (excreted), mole rate. 1 mmol/d = 1.16×10^{-2} μmol/s. To convert mg/24 h to mEq/24 h, multiply by 0.028; to convert mEq/24 h to mg/24 h, multiply by 35.46.
1	1	mmol/d	110-250 mEq/d		
2.820×10^{-1} (0.282)	3.546	mmol/kg	Approx. 2.0 mg/100 g	Approx. 0.6 mmol/kg	To convert mg/100 g to mEq/kg, multiply by 0.282; to convert mEq/kg to mg/100 g, multiply by 3.546.
1	1	mmol/kg	Approx. 0.6 mEq/kg		
2.586×10^{-2} (0.02586)	3.866×10^{1} (38.66)	mmol/L	140-250 mg/ 100 ml (varies with diet, age, and season)	3.62-6.46 mmol/L (varies with diet, age, and season)	The designation *total* signifies that free and several kinds of esterified cholesterol are represented by the same formula unit.
5.205×10^{1} (52.05)	1.921×10^{-2} (0.01921)	μmol/L	Approx. 2.2 mg/100 ml	Approx. 115 μmol/L	
6.000×10^{-2} (0.06)	1.667×10^{1} (16.67)	ks	Approx. 21.6 min	Approx. 1.3 ks	Some will prefer the unit *second* even if the reproducibility does not permit three significant figures, i.e., the value 1,300 s instead of 1.30 ks.
6.000×10^{1} (60)	1.667×10^{-2} (0.01667)	s	Approx. 21.6 min	Approx. 1,300 s	
1.574×10^{-1} (0.1574)	6.354	μmol/L	M, 70-140 μg/ 100 ml; F, 80-155 μg/ 100 ml	M, 11.0-22.0 μmol/L; F, 12.6-24.4 μmol/L	

Continued.

CLINICAL TESTS WITH UNITS, NORMAL VALUES, AND CONVERSION FACTORS—cont'd

Test	Sample type	Kind of quantity	Synonyms	Atomic or molecular mass	Current units (A)
Coproporphyrins (I + III)	24-hour urine	Amount of substance	Coproporphyrin excretion	M = 654.73 for coproporphyrin	μg/24 h (μ/d)
Creatinine	Fasting serum	Molar concentration		M = 113.12 for creatinine	mg/100 ml (as creatinine)
Creatinine	24-hour urine	Amount of substance	Creatinine excretion	M = 113.12 for creatinine	g/24 h (g/d) (as creatinine)
Creatinine clearance (endogenous)	Kidneys	Clearance (in, plasma; out, urine; output volume rate > 33 μl/s or > 2.0 ml/min.)	Creatinine clearance	M = 113.12 for creatinine	ml/min
Cyanocobalamin	Serum	Molar concentration	B$_{12}$, Vitamin B$_{12}$	M = 1,357.4 for the cyano compound	$\mu\mu$g/ml
Eosinophil granulocytes	Blood	Particle concentration	Eosinophil count		per μl (cumm, mm^3)
Erythrocytes	Blood	Particle concentration	Erythrocyte count		Millions per μl (millions per cumm or mm^3)

*Numbers without parentheses are in scientific notation; numbers in parentheses are in real numbers.

Conversion factors*		Recommended units (B)	Normal values		Comments
A to B	B to A		Conventional	Recommended SI	
1.527	6.548×10^{-1} (0.6548)	nmol/d	<200 μg/d	91.6-274.8 nmol/d	Alternative quantity: Patient (urine), coproporphyrins (I + III, excreted), mole rate. 1 mmol/d = 1.16×10^{-2} pmol/s.
8.840×10^{-2} (0.0884)	1.131×10^{1} (11.31)	mmol/L	Nonspecific method: M, 0.9-1.5 mg/100 ml; F, 0.8-1.2 mg/100 ml Specific method: M, 0.6-1.2 mg/100 ml; F, 0.5-1.0 mg/100 ml	Nonspecific method: M, 0.08-0.12 mmol/L; F, 0.07-0.11 mmol/L Specific method: M, 0.05-0.11 mmol/L; F, 0.04-0.09 mmol/L	
8.840	1.131×10^{-1} (0.1131)	mmol/d	M, 1.0-2.0 g/24 h; F, 0.8-1.8 g/24 h	M, 8.8-17.7 mmol/d; F, 7.1-15.9 mmol/d	Alternative quantity: patient (urine), creatinine (excreted), mole rate. 1 mmol/d = 1.16×10^{-2} μmol/s. The quantity "24-hour urine creatinine (N), mole rate" yields results having numerical values exactly 3 times as high.
1.667×10^{-2} (0.01667)	60	ml/s	97.2-136.8 ml/min	1.62-2.28 ml/s	
7.367×10^{-1} (0.7367)	1.357	pmol/L	Approx. 488 μμg/ml	Approx. 360 pmol/L	Results vary with the different microbiological methods of determination.
10^{-3} (0.001)	10^{3} (1,000)	$\times 10^{9}$/L	50-250/μl	$0.05\text{-}0.25 \times 10^{9}$/L	The unit "$\times 10^{9}$/L" has been chosen because the quantity "Blood leukocytes (total), particle concentration" is given in the same unit. Furthermore, the precision usually does not lend validity to a result such as 204×10^{6}/L.
1	1	$\times 10^{12}$/L	Approx. 5.1 million/μl	Approx. 5.1×10^{12}/L	

Continued.

CLINICAL TESTS WITH UNITS, NORMAL VALUES, AND CONVERSION FACTORS—cont'd

Test	Sample type	Kind of quantity	Synonyms	Atomic or molecular mass	Current units (A)
Erythrocytes	Blood	Volume fraction	Hematocrit, packed cell volume, PCV		Percent
Erythrocytes	Blood	Diameter (mean)	Halometry		
Erythrocytes	Blood	Volume (mean)	Index volumetricus, mean cell volume, MCV		μ^3 (cubic microns)
					mpl (millipicoliter)
Erythrocytes	Urine	Number (Addis, 1949)	Sediment count		Millions
Fatty acids (carboxyl, total)	24-hour feces	Amount of substance			mEq/d
Fetal hemoglobin (Fe)	Blood hemoglobin	Mole fraction (of Hb (Fe, total)	Alkali-stable hemoglobin, Hemoglobin F		Percent
Fibrinogen	Plasma	Mass concentration			mg/100 ml
Fluid (filtrated)	Glomeruli	Volume rate	Glomerular filtration rate, GFR		ml/min
Freezing point depression	Serum	Temperature difference			

*Numbers without parentheses are in scientific notation; numbers in parentheses are in real numbers.

Conversion factors*		Recommended units (B)	Normal values		Comments
A to B	B to A		Conventional	Recommended SI	
10^{-2} (0.01)	10^2 (100)	L/L	Approx. 43%	Approx. 0.43 L/L	The quantity is dimensionless and the unit symbol "L/L" equals unity (1) and may be omitted.
				7.4 μm	
1	1	fl	80-100 μ^3	80-100 fl	
1	1	fl			
1	1	$\times 10^6$	Approx. 1.1 million	Approx. 1.1×10^6	The reference "Addis" implies that the number is counted in the urine collected during 12 hours overnight.
1	1	mmol/d		Approx. 12 mmol/d	Only the *amount of substance* can be measured by titration methods. Only *mass* can be measured by extraction and weighing.
10^{-2} (0.01)	10^2 (100)	mol/mol		Approx. 0.01 mol/mol	The quantity is dimensionless; the unit symbol "mol/mol" equals unity (1) and may be omitted.
10^{-2} (0.01)	10^2 (100)	g/L	200-400 mg/100 ml	2.0-4.0 g/L	
1.667×10^{-2} (0.01667)	6.000×10^1 (60)	ml/s	Approx. 126 ml/min	Approx. 2.1 ml/s	This designation requires an acceptable method of determination, e.g., inulin clearance. If creatinine clearance is used it may be advisable, after the kind of quantity, to add "creatinine, clear (endog.)" In some instances the interest centers on the substances cleared, in which case a proper name would be "kidneys, creatinine, clear (endog.)."
				545 mdeg., 0.545°C	

Continued.

CLINICAL TESTS WITH UNITS, NORMAL VALUES, AND CONVERSION FACTORS—cont'd

Test	Sample type	Kind of quantity	Synonyms	Atomic or molecular mass	Current units (A)
Gas	Alveolus	Pressure			mm Hg
					mm Hg
Glucose	Fasting plasma	Molar concentration	Fasting blood sugar	M = 180.16 for glucose	mg/100 ml
Glucose	Urine	Arbitrary molar concentration (Clinistix, 0-1)	Glucose, qualitative; Sugar		
Glucose	Urine	Molar concentration		M = 180.16 for glucose	mg/100 ml
					Percent
Glucose	24-hour urine	Amount of substance	Glucose excretion	M = 180.16 for glucose	g/24 h (g/d)
Haptoglobin (Hb [Fe])	Serum	Molar concentration (hemoglobin saturation)		One fourth of a whole hemoglobin molecule (HB$_4$) contains one iron atom and has an average M = 16,115.	mg/100 ml (of hemoglobin bound)
Hemoglobin (Fe)	Blood	Molar concentration	Blood percent, hemoglobin percent	One fourth of a whole hemoglobin molecule (HB$_4$) contains one iron atom and has an average M = 16,115.	g/100 ml
					Percent

*Numbers without parentheses are in scientific notation; numbers in parentheses are in real numbers.

Conversion factors*		Recommended units (B)	Normal values		Comments
A to B	B to A		Conventional	Recommended SI	
1.333	7.502×10^{-1} (0.7502)	mbar		1,013 mbar	A measured liquid height of water or mercury must be corrected for the temperature of the liquid and for the local acceleration of free fall whether the conversion is to conventional millimeters of mercury or to millibars or kilonewtons per square meter (kPa). Exact measurements refer to a relative error of less than 10^{-2}.
1.333×10^{-1} (0.1333)	7.502	kN/m² (kPa)		101.3 kN/m² (kPa)	
5.551×10^{-2} (0.0551)	1.802×10^{1} (18.02)	mmol/L	70-105 mg/100 ml	3.89-5.83 mmol/L	
				0 arbitrary units	Use 0 arbitrary units instead of −; use 0 or 1 for ±.
5.551×10^{-2} (0.0551)	1.802×10^{1} (18.02)	mmol/L	<30 mg/100 ml	<1.67 mmol/L	It is presumed that percent is incorrectly used for g/100 ml.
5.551×10^{1} (55.51)	1.802×10^{-2} (0.01802)	mmol/L	<0.03%		
5.551	1.802×10^{-1} (0.1802)	mmol/d	0.5-1.5 g/d	2.78-8.34 mmol/d	Alternative quantity: patient (urine), glucose (excreted), mole rate. 1 mmol/d = 11.57 nmol/s. The methodology may be appended by nonspecific methods.
6.205×10^{-1} (0.6205)	1.612	μmol/L	70-140 mg/100 ml	43.4-86.8 μmol/L	Alternative quantity: serum hemoglobin (Fe, haptoglobin bound), molar concentration (hemoglobin saturation) = μmol/L.
6.205×10^{-1} (0.6205)	1.612	mmol/L	M, 14-17 g/100 ml; F, 12-15 g/100 ml	M, 8.7-10.5 mmol/L; F, 7.4-9.3 mmol/L	A value of 100% is assumed to correspond to 148 g/L or 14.8 g/100 ml.
9.183×10^{-2} (0.09183)	1.089×10^{1} (10.89)	mmol/L			

Continued.

CLINICAL TESTS WITH UNITS, NORMAL VALUES, AND CONVERSION FACTORS—cont'd

Test	Sample type	Kind of quantity	Synonyms	Atomic or molecular mass	Current units (A)
Hemoglobin (Fe)	Blood (erythrocyte)	Mole rate (mean)	Colorimetric index, index colorimetricus, mean cell hemoglobin, MCH	One fourth of a whole hemoglobin molecule (HB_4) contains one iron atom and has an average $M = 16,115$.	$\mu\mu g$
Hemoglobin (Fe)	Blood (erythrocyte)	Molar concentration (mean)	Mean cell hemoglobin concentration, MCHC, saturation index	One fourth of a whole hemoglobin molecule (HB_4) contains one iron atom and has an average $M = 16,115$.	g/100 ml (%)
Homogentisate	Urine	Arbitrary molar concentration (method; 0-1)	Alkapton		
Hydrogen carbonate	Plasma	Molar concentration (blood, $Pco_2 = 53$ mbar, 38°C)	Saturated bicarbonate		mEq/L
17-Hydroxycorticosteroids	24-hour urine	Mole rate	17-ketogenic steroids	$M = 361.5$ for cortisol	mg/d
Iodine (I, protein bound)	Fasting serum	Molar concentration	Protein bound iodine, PBI	$A = 126.9$ for I	$\mu g/100$ ml
Iron ion (Fe, transferrin bound)	Fasting serum	Molar concentration	Iron	$A = 55.85$ for Fe	$\mu g/100$ ml
17-Ketosteroids (as androsterone)	24-hour urine	Mole rate		$M = 290.43$ for androsterone	mg/d
Lead (Pb)	Blood	Molar concentration		$A = 207.2$ for Pb	$\mu g/100$ ml
Leukocytes (total)	Blood	Particle concentration	Leukocyte count		Per μl (cumm, mm^3)
Lipids (total)	Fasting serum	Mass concentration	Fat		mg/100 ml

*Numbers without parentheses are in scientific notation; numbers in parentheses are in real numbers.

Conversion factors*		Recommended units (B)	Normal values		Comments
A to B	B to A		Conventional	Recommended SI	
6.205×10^{-2} (0.06205)	1.612×10^{1} (16.12)	fmol	26-34 $\mu\mu$g	1.6-2.1 fmol	
6.205×10^{-1} (0.6205)	1.612	mmol/L	31-37 g/100 ml (%)	19-23 mmol/L	
				0 arbitrary units	Use 0 arbitrary units instead of $-$; use 0 or 1 for $\pm$.
1	1	mmol/L	Approx. 23.6 mEq/L	Approx. 23.6 mmol/L	
2.766	3.615×10^{-1} (0.3615)	μmol/d	3.0-10.0 mg/d	8.3-27.7 μmol/d	
7.880×10^{-2} (0.0788)	1.269×10^{1} (12.69)	μmol/L	4.0-8.0 μg/100 ml	0.32-0.63 μmol/L	
1.791×10^{-1} (0.1791)	5.585	μmol/L	60-150 μg/100 ml	10.7-26.9 μmol/L	
3.443	2.904×10^{-1} (0.2904)	μmol/d	M, 8-20 mg/d; F, 6-15 mg/d (declines after age 60)	M, 27.5-68.8 μmol/d; F, 20.7-51.6 μmol/d	
4.826×10^{-2} (0.04826)	2.072×10^{1} (20.72)	μmol/L	<50.3 μg/100 ml	<2.43 μmol/L	
10^{-3} (0.001)	10^{3} (1,000)	$\times 10^{9}$/L	Approx. 7,500/μl	Approx. 7.5 $\times$ 10^{9}/L	
10^{-2} (0.01)	10^{2} (100)	g/L	400-700 mg/100 ml	4.0-7.0 g/L	Only the *amount of substance* can be measured by titration methods. Only the *mass* can be measured by extraction and weighing.

Continued.

CLINICAL TESTS WITH UNITS, NORMAL VALUES, AND CONVERSION FACTORS—cont'd

Test	Sample type	Kind of quantity	Synonyms	Atomic or molecular mass	Current units (A)
Lipids (total)	Dry feces	Mass fraction (method)	Lipid percent, fat		Percent
Lymphocytes	Blood (leuko-cytes)	Particle fraction	Differential count, lymphocytes		Percent
Magnesium ion (Mg)	Serum	Molar concentration	Magnesium	A = 24.32 for Mg	mg/100 ml
					mEq/L
Methylketones	Urine	Arbitrary molar concentration (Acetest, 0-1)	Acetone bodies, Ketone bodies, Legal's reaction		
Nitrogen (N, nonprotein)	Serum	Molar concentration	Nonprotein nitrogen, NPN	A = 14.01 for N	mg/100 ml
Nitrogen (N)	24-hour urine	Amount of substance	Nitrogen excretion	A = 14.01 for N	g/24 h (g/d)
Osmotic pressure reaction	Blood (erythro-cyte)	Arbitrary pressure (Parpart et al., 1947)	Osmotic fragility test, osmotic resistance		mEq/L
					Percent NaCl
Oxyhemo-globin (Fe)	Arterial blood (Hemoglo-bin)	Mole fraction (of hemoglobin [Fe, total])	Oxygen saturation		Percent
Phenylpyruvate	Urine	Arbitrary molar concentration (method; 0-1)	Phenylpyruvic acid		

*Numbers without parentheses are in scientific notation; numbers in parentheses are in real numbers.

Conversion factors*		Recommended units (B)	Normal values		Comments
A to B	**B to A**		**Conventional**	**Recommended SI**	
10^1 (10)	10^{-1} (0.1)	g/kg	15%-25% of dry weight	<250 g/kg	Only the *amount of substance* can be measured by titration methods. Only the *mass* can be measured by extraction and weighing.
10^{-2} (0.01)	10^2 (100)	1 (unity)	Approx. 30%	Approx. 0.30	Another possibility is to calculate the quantity: blood lymphocytes, particle concentration, given in the unit "$\times 10^9$/L" (absolute count).
4.112×10^{-1} (0.4112)	2.432	mmol/L	1.7-3.16 mg/ 100 ml	0.7-1.3 mmol/L	The concentration of electrovalencies is given by the quantity "serum magnesium ion $(Mg^{2+})_{0.5}$, molar concentration." To convert mg/100 ml to m/Eq/L, multiply by 0.822; to convert mEq/L to mg/100 ml, multiply by 1.216.
5.000×10^{-1} (0.5)	2.0	mmol/L	1.4-2.6 mEq/L		
				0 arbitrary units	Use 0 arbitrary units instead of −; use 0 or 1 for ±.
7.138×10^{-1} (0.7138)	1.401	mmol/L	20-35 mg/100 ml	14.3-25.0 mmol/L	
7.138×10^{-2} (0.07138)	1.401×10^1 (14.01)	mol/d	Approx. 14.8 g/24 h (g/d)	Approx. 1.06 mol/d	Alternative quantity: patient (urine); nitrogen (N, eliminated), mole rate. 1 mol/d = 11.57 μmol/s.
1	1	Arbitrary unit	Approx. 140 mEq/L	Approx. 140 arbitrary units	The arbitrary pressure by the example yields results numerically equal to the molar concentration of ions in an aqueous solution of sodium chloride surrounding the erythrocytes when half of their total content of hemoglobin becomes free.
3.422×10^2 (342.2)	2.923×10^{-3} (0.002923)	Arbitrary unit	Approx. 0.41%		
10^{-2} (0.01)	10^2 (100)	mol/mol	90%-96%	0.90-0.96 mol/mol	The quantity is demensionless; the unit symbol "mol/mol" equals unity (1) and may be omitted.
				0 arbitrary units	Use 0 arbitrary units instead of −; Use 0 or 1 for ±.

Continued.

CLINICAL TESTS WITH UNITS, NORMAL VALUES, AND CONVERSION FACTORS—cont'd

Test	Sample type	Kind of quantity	Synonyms	Atomic or molecular mass	Current units (A)
Phosphorus (P, inorganic)	Serum	Molar concentration	Phosphorus	A = 30.97 for P	mg/100 ml (as P)
Phosphate (P, total)	24-hour urine	Amount of substance	Phosphorus excretion	A = 30.97 for P	g/d (as P)
Plasma	Arterial blood	pH (37°C)			pH
Porphobilin-ogen	24-hour urine	Amount of substance	Porphobilinogen excretion	M = 226.24 for porphobilino-gen	μg/24 h (μg/d)
Potassium ion	Serum	Molar concentration	Potassium	A = 39.10 for K	mg/100 ml
					mEq/L
Potassium	24-hour urine	Amount of substance	Potassium excretion	A = 39.10 for K	mg/d
					mEq/d
Protein	Fasting serum	Mass concentration	Protein		g/100 ml
					Percent
Protein	Urine	Arbitrary mass concentration (Albustix, 0-1)	Protein, qualitative; protein reaction		
Protein	24-hour urine	Amount of substance	Protein excretion		mg/24 h (mg/d)

*Numbers without parentheses are in scientific notation; numbers in parentheses are in real numbers.

Conversion factors*		Recommended units (B)	Normal values		Comments
A to B	B to A		Conventional	Recommended SI	
3.229×10^{-1} (0.3229)	3.097	mmol/L	3.0-4.5 mg/100 ml	0.97-1.45 mmol/L	The conversion from equivalent concentration of phosphate to other concentration concepts requires measurement of the pH.
3.229×10^{1} (32.29)	3.097×10^{-2} (0.03097)	mmol/d	0.9-1.3 g/d	29-42 mmol/d	Alternative quantity: patient (urine), phosphate (plasma, total, excreted), mole rate. 1 mmol/d = 1.6×10^{-2} μmol/s.
Antilog of (9 − pH)		cH (in nmol/L)	7.35-7.45	35.5-45 cH (in nmol/L)	With its present definition pH is a dimensionless kind of quantity. cH in nmol/L = antilog of (9 minus the pH).
4.420×10^{-3} (0.00442)	2.262×10^{2} (226.2)	μmol/d	0-1990 μg/24 h (μg/d)	0-8.8 μmol/d	Alternative quantity: patient (urine), porphobilinogen (excreted), mole rate. 1 μmol/d = 11.57 pmol/s.
2.558×10^{-1} (0.2558)	3.910	mmol/L	13.7-20.7 mg/100 ml	3.5-5.3 mmol/L	To convert mg/100 ml to mEq/L, multiply by 0.256; to convert mEq/L to mg/100 ml, multiply by 3.910.
1	1	mmol/L	3.5-5.3 mEq/L		
2.558×10^{-2} (0.02558)	3.910×10^{1} (39.1)	mmol/d	1,173-3,519 mg/d	30-90 mmol/d	To convert mg/d to mEq/d, multiply by 0.0256; to convert mEq/d to mg/d, multiply by 39.1.
1	1	mmol/d	30-90 mEq/d		
10^{1} (10)	10^{-1} (0.1)	g/L	6.0-8.2 g/100 ml	60-82 g/L	It is presumed that percent is incorrectly used for g/100 ml.
10^{1} (10)	10^{-1} (0.1)	g/L	6.0%-8.2%		
				0 arbitrary units	Use 0 arbitrary units instead of −; Use 0 or 1 for ±.
1	1	mg/d	50-100 mg/d	50-100 mg/d	Alternative quantity: patient (urine), protein (excreted), mass rate. 1 mg/d = 1.16×10^{-2} μg/s. It may be advantageous to state the method used, e.g., 24-hour urine protein, mass rate (Kjeldahl).

Continued.

CLINICAL TESTS WITH UNITS, NORMAL VALUES, AND CONVERSION FACTORS—cont'd

Test	Sample type	Kind of quantity	Synonyms	Atomic or molecular mass	Current units (A)
Prothrombin (Factors II, VII, and X)	Plasma	Relative arbitrary molar concentration (actual/normal)	Prothrombin, P-P		Percent
Reticulocytes	Blood (erythrocytes)	Particle fraction	Reticulocyte count		Per mille (‰) (per 1,000 RBC)
					Percent (%) (per 100 RBC)
Sedimentation reaction	Blood	Arbitrary length (Westergren, 1926; 1 h)	Erythrocyte sedimentation rate, ESR, Sedimentation rate		mm/h (velocity)
Serum	Blood	Relative density, $\left(\dfrac{\text{S, 20°C}}{\text{H}_2\text{O, 20°C}}\right) = 1.026$	Specific gravity		
Sodium ion	Serum	Molar concentration	Sodium	A = 22.99 for Na	mg/100 ml
					mEq/L
Sodium	24-hour urine	Amount of substance	Sodium excretion	A = 22.99 for Na	mg/d
					mEq/d
Surface	Blood (erythrocyte)	Area (mean)			
Thrombocytes	Plasma	Particle concentration	Platelets, thrombocyte count, platelet count		per μl (cumm, mm^3)

*Numbers without parentheses are in scientific notation; numbers in parentheses are in real numbers.

Conversion factors*		Recommended units (B)	Normal values		Comments
A to B	B to A		Conventional	Recommended SI	
10^{-2} (0.01)	10^2 (100)	1 (unity)		1.00	Alternative designation: plasma prothrombin, relative arbitrary molar concentration (actual/normal), (Owren and As, 1951). The quantity is not to be confused with "plasma prothrombin, relative molar concentration (actual/normal)," which refers to the concentration of factor II alone. The designation "prothrombin time" denotes another kind of measurement altogether.
10^{-3} (0.001)	10^3 (1000)	1 (unity)	Approx. 6 ‰	Approx. 0.006	The quantity "blood reticulocytes, particle concentration" may be preferred. The unit "$\times 10^{-3}$" may be preferred, giving the value of 6×10^{-3}.
10^{-2} (0.01)	10^2 (100)	1 (unity)	Approx. 0.6%		
1	1	Arbitrary unit	5 mm/h	5 Arbitrary units	The result depends totally on the specific method.
				Approx. 1.026	Alternative quantity: serum, relative density $\left(\dfrac{S, 20°C}{H_2O, 20°C}\right) = 1.026$
4.350×10^{-1} (0.435)	2.299	mmol/L	310-340 mg/ 100 ml	135-148 mmol/L	To convert mg/100 ml to mEq/L, multiply by 0.435; to convert mEq/L to mg/100 ml, multiply by 2.299.
1	1	mmol/L	135-148 mEq/L		
4.350×10^{-2} (0.0435)	2.299×10^1 (22.99)	mmol/d	920-5058 mg/d	40-220 mmol/d	To convert mg/d to mEq/d, multiply by 0.043; to convert mEq/d to mg/d, multiply by 22.99.
1	1	mmol/d	40-220 mEq/d		
				Approx. 138 μm^2	
10^{-3} (0.001)	10^3 (1,000)	$\times 10^9$/L	Approx. 300,000/μl	Approx. 300 $\times$ 10^9/L	

Continued.

CLINICAL TESTS WITH UNITS, NORMAL VALUES, AND CONVERSION FACTORS—cont'd

Test	Sample type	Kind of quantity	Synonyms	Atomic or molecular mass	Current units (A)
Transferrin (Fe)	Fasting serum	Molar concentration (Fe saturation)	Total iron binding capacity, TIBC	A = 55.85 for Fe	μg/100 ml
Urate	Fasting serum	Molar concentration	Uric acid	M = 168.11 for uric acid	mg/100 ml
Urate (total)	24-hour urine	Amount of substance	Uric acid excretion	M = 168.11 for uric acid	mg/24 h (mg/d)
Urea	Fasting serum	Molar concentration	Blood urea	M = 60.06 for urea	mg/100 ml
Urea	24-hour urine	Amount of substance	Urea excretion	M = 60.06 for urea	g/24 h (g/d)
Urea clearance	Kidneys	Clearance (in, plasma; out, urine; output volume rate > 33 μl/s or > 2 ml/min)	Maximum clearance		ml/min
Urea nitrogen (N)	Fasting serum	Molar concentration	Serum urea nitrogen	M = 28.02 for N in urea	mg/100 ml
Urea nitrogen (N)	24-hour urine	Mole rate	Urea nitrogen excretion	M = 28.02 for N in urea	g/d

*Numbers without parentheses are in scientific notation; numbers in parentheses are in real numbers.

Conversion factors*		Recommended units (B)	Normal values		Comments
A to B	B to A		Conventional	Recommended SI	
1.791×10^{-1} (0.1791)	5.583	μmol/L	270-380 μg/ 100 ml	48.4-68.1 μmol/L	Probably *Serum transferrin (Fe), molar concentration (Fe saturation) $\times$ 0.5 = Serum transferrin, molar concentration,* as one transferrin molecule seems to bind two iron atoms. By immunological methods the quantity "serum transferrin, mass concentration" is determined. The problem is compounded by the existence of several kinds of transferrin having different relative molecular masses. Their individual antigenic properties are not known.
5.948×10^{-2} (0.05948)	1.681×10^{1} (16.81)	mmol/L	2.5-7.1 mg/100 ml	0.15-0.42 mmol/L	
5.948×10^{-3} (0.005948)	1.681×10^{2} (168.1)	mmol/d	250-750 mg/24 h (mg/d)	1.49-4.46 mmol/d	Alternative quantity: patient (urine), urate (total excreted), mole rate. 1 mmol/d = 11.57 nmol/s.
1.665×10^{-1} (0.1665)	6.006	mmol/L	15-39 mg/100 ml	2.50-6.41 mmol/L	
1.665×10^{1} (16.65)	6.006×10^{-2} (0.06006)	mmol/d	25.8-43 g/24 h (g/d)	430-716 mmol/d	Alternative quantity: patient (urine), urea (excreted), mole rate. 1 mmol/d = 1.16×10^{-2} μmol/s. The quantity "24-hour urine urea (N), mole rate" yields results having numerical values exactly twice as high.
1.667×10^{-2} (0.01667)	6.000×10^{1} (60)	ml/s	64-99 ml/min	1.07-1.65 ml/s	
3.569×10^{-1} (0.3569)	2.802	mmol/L	7-18 mg/100 ml	2.50-6.41 mmol/L	
3.569×10^{1} (35.69)	2.802×10^{-2} (0.02802)	mmol/d	12.1-20.1 g/d	430-716 mmol/d	

Continued.

CLINICAL TESTS WITH UNITS, NORMAL VALUES, AND CONVERSION FACTORS—cont'd

Test	Sample type	Kind of quantity	Synonyms	Atomic or molecular mass	Current units (A)
Urea nitrogen (N)	Kidneys	Clearance (in, plasma; out, urine; output volume rate > 33 $\mu l/s$ or > 2 ml/min.)	Urea nitrogen clearance		ml/min
Urine	24-hour urine (dU)	Relative density, $\dfrac{dU, 20°C}{H_2O, 20°C}$	Specific gravity		
Urobilin	Urine	Arbitrary molar concentration (Marcussen et al., 1918)			
Urobilinogen	Fasting urine	Arbitrary molar concentration (Ehrlich, 1884; 0-1)	Ehrlich's reaction		

*Numbers without parentheses are in scientific notation; numbers in parentheses are in real numbers.

Conversion factors*		Recommended units (B)	Normal values		Comments
A to B	B to A		Conventional	Recommended SI	
1.667×10^{-2} (0.01667)	6.0×10^{1} (60)	ml/s	64-99 ml/min	1.07-1.65 ml/s	
				Approx. average 1.016	
				10 arbitrary units	Use 0 arbitrary units instead of —; Use 0 or 1 for ±.
				0-1 arbitrary units	Use 0 arbitrary units instead of —; Use 0 or 1 for ±.

Appendix EE
ANSWERS TO PRACTICE PROBLEMS

Chapter 1 Basic mathematics*

1. III	41. +16	h. 6.0
2. XLIII	42. −49	m. 10.25
3. LI	43. +16	d. 12.0
4. XCVI	44. +5	f. 22
5. CLXXIII	45. −26	74. 8
6. DLXVIII	46. −14	75. 32
7. DCCIV	47. +12	76. 18
8. MXX	48. −14	77. 1,360
9. MDCLII	49. +90	78. 3,150
10. L̄MMCCCLXXI	50. −36	79. 7/5, 1.4
11. 1,117	51. −66	80. 15/8, 1.875
12. 45	52. +280	81. 32/24, 1.333
13. 442	53. +18	82. 265/80, 3.3125
14. 6	54. −42	83. 48/9, 5.333
15. 777	55. +80	84. 33/36, 0.9167
16. 65	56. +50	85. 24/4, 6.0
17. 92	57. +5	86. 323/24, 13.4583
18. 43	58. +0.75	87. 131/72, 1.8194
19. 16	59. −5	88. 31/16, 1.9375
20. 1,400	60. −0.2	89. 1/7, 0.1429
21. +16	61. −11	90. −3/15, −0.2
22. +5	62. −0.6	91. 11/12, 0.9167
23. +5	63. +4.0	92. −9/8, −1.125
24. −6	64. +0.1	93. 45/14, 3.2143
25. −8	65. a, d, e, g, i, k, l, n	94. 48/24, 2.0
26. +15	66. g, k, l	95. −14/8, −1.75
27. −30	67. a, d, e, i, n	96. 17/10, 1.7
28. −9	68. f, h	97. 211/88, 2.3977
29. −13	69. b, m	98. 0
30. −59	70. d, l, n	99. 10/49, 0.2041
31. −25	71. c, g, k	100. 24/104, 0.2308
32. +29	72. c, j	101. −196/25, −7.84
33. +18	73. j. 0.09	102. 800/18, 44.4444
34. −8	l. 0.1875	103. −81/16, −5.0625
35. −24	c, g, k. 0.75	104. 27/48, 0.5625
36. −19	a. 1.0	105. −120/18, −6.667
37. +32	n. 1.3125	106. 245/24, 10.2083
38. +12	h. 1.375	107. 174/72, 2.4167
39. +4	i. 1.625	108. 12/35, 0.3429
40. −8	e. 1.8	109. 45/27, 1.6667

*Slightly different answers may be obtained due to rounding off procedures.

Appendix EE   437

110. $-54/36$, -1.5 113. $-9/40$, -0.225 116. $-12/57$, -0.2105
111. $15/30$, 0.5 114. $-12/63$, -0.1905 117. $328/216$, 1.5185
112. $234/120$, 1.95 115. $36/24$, 1.5 118. $49/6$, 8.1667

119. ⓵⁄₃ , ²⁄₄, ②⁄₆ , ⁶⁄₁₀, ⁴⁄₁₅, ⑥⁄₁₈

120. ①¹⁄₃ , 2²⁄₃, 4, ④⁄₃ , ³⁄₄, ①²⁄₉ , 2²⁄₆

121. $2/18$, $4/18$, $6/18$, $7/18$, $9/18$, $10/18$, $13/18$, $15/18$, $20/18$, $25/18$
122. $9/21$, $9/20$, $9/18$, $9/16$, $9/14$, $9/13$, $9/10$, $9/7$, $9/4$, $9/2$

123. 84. 0.9167 124. 95. -1.75 125. 101. -7.84 126. 110. -1.5
     81. 1.333 92. -1.125 105. -6.667 113. -0.225
     79. 1.4 90. -0.2 103. -5.0625 116. -0.210
     87. 1.8194 98. 0 99. 0.2041 114. -0.1905
     80. 1.875 89. 0.1429 100. 0.2308 111. 0.5
     88. 1.9375 91. 0.9167 108. 0.3429 115. 1.5
     82. 3.3125 96. 1.7 104. 0.5625 117. 1.5185
     83. 5.333 94. 2.0 107. 2.4167 109. 1.6667
     85. 6.0 97. 2.3977 106. 10.2083 112. 1.95
     86. 13.4583 93. 3.2143 102. 44.4444 118. 8.1667

127. $\dfrac{42}{100}$, $\dfrac{21}{50}$

128. $\dfrac{39}{10}$, $3\dfrac{9}{10}$

129. $6/1,000$, $3/500$ 153. 1.014
130. $1,145/100$, $229/20$, $11\%_{20}$ 154. -2.814
131. $9,072/10,000$, $567/625$ 155. 1.0914
132. $1,902/100,000$, $951/50,000$ 156. 0.011
133. $10,003/100$, $100³⁄_{100}$ 157. -0.187
134. $2,018/1,000$, $1,009/500$, $2⁹⁄_{500}$ 158. -0.1059
135. 0.1667 159. 0.1059
136. 0.875 160. 0.57
137. 1.25 161. 0.00804
138. 13.2857 162. -6.78
139. 1.2857 163. 1.264
140. 0.6522 164. -0.0356
141. 2.0, ⟨0.2⟩, 0.02, ⟨0.20⟩, ⟨0.2000⟩, 0.002 165. 0.0050
142. ⟨1.5⟩, 1.555, ⟨1.50⟩, 1.505, ⟨1.5000⟩, 1.005 166. 12.4
143. 0.98 167. -7.67
144. -0.82 168. -0.0107
145. 1.84 169. 0.00220
146. 0.273 170. 0.000014
147. 9.702 171. -0.296
148. -6.32 172. -0.0330
149. 13.0547 173. 1.17
150. 0.00858 174. 5.78
151. 1.00 175. -0.856
152. -2.376 176. 1.90

177. 61.1
178. 15.4
179. 0.0323
180. -1.45
181. -0.60
182. 0.0476
183. 2%
184. 0.03%
185. 6.3%
186. 18%
187. 10%
188. 0.15%
189. 4.074%
190. 0.008%
191. 2/100, 1/50
192. 1.006/100, 0.503/50
193. 0.08/100, 0.02/25
194. 32.9/100
195. 0.25/100, 0.01/4
196. $\dfrac{1/10}{100}$, 1/1,000
197. $\dfrac{3\frac{1}{8}}{100}$, $\dfrac{3.125}{100}$, 1/32
198. $\dfrac{25/30}{100}$, $\dfrac{0.833}{100}$, 1/120
199. 0.38
200. 0.0007
201. 0.029
202. 0.0100065
203. 0.00092
204. 0.00125
205. 0.022
206. 0.008
207. 50%
208. 966.67%
209. 30%
210. 80%
211. 712.5%
212. 200%
213. 29%
214. 500%
215. 1620%
216. 1.38%
217. 100.06%
218. 59,298%
219. 13%
220. 6.9%

221. 0.3%
222. $12\frac{1}{8}$%, 12.125%
223. $35\frac{5}{6}$%, 35.833%
224. $\frac{11}{12}$%, 0.917%
225. 20%
226. 2.1%
227. $\frac{5}{16}$%, 0.3125%
228. 0.04%
229. 2.4%
230. $2\frac{17}{18}$%, 12.056%
231. 6.5
232. 0.024
233. 0.004821%
234. 19.8%
235. 200
236. 13.75
237. 520
238. 18.75
239. 66.67%
240. 3,599.71 (or 3,600.0)%
241. $+23.6667$
242. $+37.0$
243. -13.0
244. -50.0
245. $+25.6667$
246. $+10.0$
247. $+61.6328$
248. $+43.6786$
249. $+9.7083$
250. -12.5286
251. $+1.4$
252. $+3.1429$
253. true (11 = 11)
254. true (1.875 = 1.875)
255. true (0.25 = 0.2500)
256. 125
257. 0.8571
258. 24
259. 0.04124
260. 14,400
261. 5,600
262. 0.002344
263. 62.2222
264. 1/2, 0.5
265. $-1/8$, -0.125
266. 5/2, 2.5
267. 7/10, 0.7
268. $-15/8$, -1.875

269. $\dfrac{1}{2\frac{1}{3}}$, $\dfrac{1}{2.33}$, 0.4286, (³⁄₇, 0.4286)

270. $-1/4.5$, -0.2222

271. $-1/0.012$, -83.3333

272. $1/1.19$, 0.8403

273. $1/0.7$, 1.4286

274. 3

275. 1

276. 1

277. 4

278. 3

279. Questionable (see rule 3, p. 26).

280. 7

281. 4

282. 1

283. 2

284. 5

285. 7.6

286. 7.6

287. 7.6

288. 7.6

289. 13.18

290. 44.10

291. 7.12

292. 123.18

293. 33.88

294. 14.5

295. 3.04

296. 7.7

297. 16,777,216

298. 10,000

299. $1/1,000,000$; 0.000001

300. 15,625

301. $1/9$, 0.1111

302. $1/1,000$, 0.001

303. $1/10,000$; 0.0001

304. $1/4,782,969$; 0.000000209

305. 10,000

306. $1/1,000,000$; 0.000001

307. 1,100

308. 0.010001

309. 6^9; 10,077,696

310. 5^2; 25

311. 10^4; 10,000

312. 10^{-6}; 0.000001

313. 9,529,569

314. $216 + 7,776 = 7,992$

315. a^9

316. $b^3 \times c^6$

317. $128 - 4,096 = -3,968$

318. d^3

319. 7^6; 117,649

320. a^4

321. $(a^b)^c$, $a^{b \times c}$

322. $10,000 + 100,000 = 110,000$

323. $0.000003815 + 0.0000000596 =$ $0.0000038746 = 3.8746 \times 10^{-6}$

324. 4^9; 262,144

325. 8^5; 32,768

326. 5^4; 625

327. 13^{-12}; 4.2922×10^{-14}

328. $43,046,721 \times 81 = 3,486,784,401$

329. 9^{-12}; $(531441)^{-2}$; 3.5407×10^{-12}

330. 1×10^3

331. 1×10^5

332. 3.26×10^2

333. 1.59×10^1

334. 3.561×10^3

335. 2.826×10^9

336. 3.3×10^4

337. 1.0101×10^6

338. 1.0×10^{-3}

339. 1.0×10^{-5}

340. 4.21×10^{-2}

341. 3.97×10^{-1}

342. 7.23×10^{-13}

343. 1.01×10^{-1}

344. Should not be done in scientific notation.

345. Should not be done in scientific notation.

346. $(6.42 \times 10^5) \times (3.739 \times 10^6) =$ 2.4004380×10^{12}

347. $(1.5 \times 10^4) \times (1.5 \times 10^5) = 2.25 \times 10^9$

348. $(9.42 \times 10^{-4}) \times (7.84 \times 10^{-3}) =$ 7.38528×10^{-6}

349. $(4.93 \times 10^5) \div (2.5 \times 10^4) =$ 1.972×10^1

350. $(8.0 \times 10^{-8}) \div (3.13 \times 10^{-3}) =$ $2.555910543 \times 10^{-5}$

351. $(4.2 \times 10^2) \div (1.732 \times 10^6) =$ $2.424942263 \times 10^{-4}$

352. $3:9$, $3/9$, $3 \div 9$, 0.3333

353. a. $10:4$ d. $4:14$
     b. $4:10$ e. $14:10$
     c. $14:4$ f. $10:14$

354. a. $x = 9$ c. $x = 8$
     b. $x = 4$ d. $x = 50$

355. a. 3   d. 8
     b. 204   e. 50
     c. 8   f. 2.1

356. 25 g
357. 9 g
358. 0.2 g
359. 6.67 g
360. 3,750 mg
361.

Common fraction	Decimal fraction	Percent (%)	Ratio			
			:	÷	Fraction	Decimal
¾	0.75	75%	3:4	3 ÷ 4	¾	0.75
⁶⁄₁₀₀, ³⁄₅₀	0.06	6%	6:100	6 ÷ 100	⁶⁄₁₀₀	0.06
¹¹⁵⁄₁₀₀	1.15	115%	115:100	115 ÷ 100	¹¹⁵⁄₁₀₀	1.15
¹⁸⁄₁,₀₀₀, ⁹⁄₅₀₀	0.018	1.8%	18:1,000	18 ÷ 1,000	¹⁸⁄₁,₀₀₀	0.018
⁶⁄₇	0.857	85.7%	6:7	6 ÷ 7	⁶⁄₇	0.857
²¹⁄₁₀₀	0.21	21%	21:100	21 ÷ 100	²¹⁄₁₀₀	0.21
¹³⁄₁₀₀	0.13	13%	13:100	13 ÷ 100	¹³⁄₁₀₀	0.13
1⅕, ⁶⁄₅	1.20	120%	6:5	6 ÷ 5	⁶⁄₅	1.20
¹³²⁄₁₀₀, ⁶⁶⁄₅₀, ³³⁄₂₅	1.32	132%	132:100	132 ÷ 100	¹³²⁄₁₀₀	1.32
³⁰⁄₂₀	1.5	150%	3:2	3 ÷ 2	³⁄₂	1.5

Chapter 2 Systems of measure*

1. m milli 10^{-3} n nano 10^{-9}
   a atto 10^{-18} k kilo 10^{3}
   T tera 10^{12} d deci 10^{-1}
   M mega 10^{6} μ micro 10^{-6}
   da deca 10^{1} h hecto 10^{2}
   c centi 10^{-2} f femto 10^{-15}
   p pico 10^{-12} P peta 10^{15}
   G giga 10^{9} E exa 10^{18}
2. μ—micro
   λ—micro
   γ—micro
   millimicro—nano
   micromicro—pico
3. 30,000,000 μg; 3.0×10^{7}
4. 0.30 cg
5. Cannot change grams to liters.
6. 0.016 mm
7. 800 fg
8. 0.4 dl
9. 0.167 μg
10. 1,600 dag
11. 0.00000003265 dl; 3.265×10^{-8} dl
12. 182,900,000,000,000 am; 1.829×10^{14} am
13. 0.01 L
14. 0.560 ml
15. Cannot change grams to meters.
16. 0.32 cg
17. 7,000,000 nl; 7×10^{6} nl
18. 0.09 km
19. Cannot change grams to liters.
20. 5,200 ml
21. 8,000 cl
22. 3,000.970 mm
23. 5,700 mg
24. 0.066 g
25. b
26. d
27. b

*Slightly different answers may be obtained due to rounding off procedures.

28. c
29. c
30. 77
31. 352.7
32. 11.286
33. 1.157
34. 52.49
35. 20.736
36. 104.78
37. 1.215
38. 10.14
39. 28.39

40. 3.43
41. c
42. a
43. d
44. d
45. a
46. 4.23
47. 7,464
48. 128.6
49. 0.78
50. 2,662.4 (approx)
51. approx 59 weeks; cost $113.40

Chapter 3 Temperature conversions*

1. −243°C
2. −284°C
3. −273°C
4. 67°C
5. −353°C
6. 293 K
7. 223 K
8. 273 K
9. 393 K
10. 269 K

11. 104°F
12. −5.8°F
13. 33.8°F
14. 392°F
15. −238.0°F
16. 61.11°C
17. −46.11°C
18. −17.78°C
19. 204.44°C
20. −26.67°C

21. 288.56 K
22. 249.67 K
23. 255.2 K
24. 394.1 K
25. 199.7 K
26. −149.8°F
27. −621.4°F
28. −459.4°F
29. −387.4°F
30. −464.8°F

Chapter 4 Factors*

1. 0.393
2. 0.607
3. 1.648
4. 2.543
5. 2.768
6. 0.361
7. 1.908
8. 0.524
9. 1.739
10. 0.575
11. 1.517
12. 0.659
13. 0.635
14. 1.575
15. 1.288
16. 0.224
17. 0.973
18. Factor = 0.501; 150.3 mg S
19. Factor = 2.513; 52.8 g $CuSO_4$
20. Factor = 1.288; 1,674 mg NaBr; 1.674 g NaBr

21. Factor = 2.496; 1,058.3 mg $CaCO_3$
22. Factor = 0.274; 82.2 mg Na
23. Factor = 1.028; 308.4 mg HCl
24. Factor = 0.776; 77.6 mg Br
25. Factor = 1.435; 502.3 mg KOH
26. Factor = 1.086; 369.2 mg LiBr
27. Factor = 0.326; 6.5 mg P
28. Factor = 0.202; 141.4 mg Mg
29. Factor = 0.947; 38 mg/dl Sulfadiazine
30. Factor = 0.675; 68 mg/dl Sulfanilamide
31. 218 mg/dl Sulfadiazine
32. Factor = 125
33. Factor = 25
34. Factor = 18
35. Factor = 0.926
36. a. Factor = 1.25
    b. Factor = 250
37. 30 mg/dl
38. 88 mEq/L
39. 83 mg/L

*Slightly different answers may be obtained due to rounding off procedures.

Chapter 5 Dilutions*

1. a. 8:2
   b. 8:10
   c. 2:8
   d. 10:2
2. a. 1:14
   b. 2:21
   c. 7:2
   d. 30:15
3. a. 2:28
   b. 6:4
   c. 8:8
4. 3:17, 3/20
5. 4/24 or 1/6, 4:20
6. 2/32 or 1/16
7. 1.0 ml
8. 0.1/5 or 1/50
9. 0.1/4 or 1/40
10. a
11. 10 ml: 20 oz, 10/602 dilution (all parts of a single dilution must be in the same units, 20 oz = approx. 592 ml)
12. 1.8 ml
13. a. 1/15
    b. 1/11.5
    c. 1/1.29
    d. 1/1.5
14. a. 1/15
    b. 1/1.67
    c. 1/2
15. a. 1/5
    b. 1/3.33
    c. 1/7
16. 0.5/80 or 1/160
17. b
18. 50/300 or 1/6 dilution
19. 100 ml
20. 50 ml
21. 120 ml of alcohol diluted up to 300 ml → 300 ml of a 2/5 dilution
22. 5 ml
23. 9 ml
24. 2 ml
25. 29.94 ml
26. c
27. 1/21 dilution
28. 2/25 or 1/12.5 dilution
29. 1 ml of 43% ↑ 5 ml → 5 ml of 8.6%
30. 0.07%

31. 200 ml, 0.1%
32. 60 ml, 20/60 N or 0.33 N
33. 1 ml/100 ml
34. 1,000 mg/500 ml or 200 mg/dl
35. 0.5 mg/ml
36. 0.002 mg/ml
37. Tube #1, 10 ml; #2, 25 ml; #3, 50 ml
38. Before transfer:
    tube #1, 10 ml; #2, 25 ml; #3, 50 ml
    After transfer:
    tube #1, 7 ml; #2, 21 ml; #3, 50 ml
39. Before transfer:
    tube #1, 100 ml; #2, 100 ml; #3, 100 ml
    After transfer:
    tube #1, 88 ml; #2, 92 ml; #3, 100 ml
40. Tube #1, 2/10; tube #2, 3/25; tube #3, 4/50
41. Tube #1, 2/10; tube #2, 3/25; tube #3, 4/50
42. Tube #1, 20/100, 2/10, or 1/5;
    tube #2, 12/100, 3/25, or 1/8.33;
    tube #3, 8/100, 4/50 or 1/12.5
43. Tube #1, 2/10 or 1/5;
    tube #2, 3/25 or 1/8.33;
    tube #3, 4/50 or 1/12.5
44. Tube #1, 2/10 or 1/5;
    tube #2, 6/250 or 1/41.7;
    tube #3, 24/12,500 or 1/520.8
45. Tube #1, 2/10 or 1/5;
    tube #2, 6/250 or 1/41.7;
    tube #3, 24/12,500 or 1/520.8
46. a. Tube #1, 1/6; tube #2, 1/60
    b. Tube #1, 2/5; #2, 2/15;
       #3, 2/120 or 1/60
    c. Tube #1, 1/4; #2, 1/16;
       #3, 1/64
47. Tube #2, 1/5,000 (1/10 is the original concentration)
48. 5/1,000 or 1/200 dilution
49. 1/400% or 0.0025%
50. 4.1/250% or 0.0164%, 25 ml
51. 16/300M or 0.0533M
52. 50 ml, 3/250N or 0.012N
53. 1/250N or 0.004N
54. 5 ml, 1 mg/150 ml or 0.667 mg/dl
55. 45 g/100 liters
56. a. 5 ml, 1/90 dilution
    b. 50 ml, 80 mg/5,000 ml or 1.6 mg/dl
    c. 6 ml, 48/180N or 0.267N
    d. 10 ml, 60 mg/2,000 ml or 3 mg/100 ml

*Slightly different answers may be obtained due to rounding off procedures.

57. a. 9 ml, 48/63M or 0.762M
    b. 9 ml, 20/2,025 dilution or 1/101.25 dilution
    c. 500 ml, 6,000 mg/50,000 ml or 12 mg/dl
58. 0.45 g $CuSO_4$/L
59. None; there is no $CuSO_4$ in NaCl.
60. 1/500 dilution; assuming 50 ml was made, would be 0.1 ml serum present.
61. 0.05 ml
62. a. Dilute 1 ml of 8.5N to 10 ml, dilute 2 ml of this solution to 5 ml, and dilute 4 ml of the second solution to 25 ml.
    b. 25 ml
    c. 34/625N
    d. 0.16 ml
63. a. 1/15% or 0.067%
    b. 6 ml
    c. 0.04 ml
64. 0.1 ml urine
65. a. Dilute 1 ml of 6N to 5 ml, dilute 2 ml of this solution to 3 ml, and dilute 3 ml of the second solution to 15 ml.
    b. 15 ml

c. 4/25N or 0.16N
d. 0.4 ml
66. a. 12 ml
    b. 1/20 dilution
    c. 0.6 ml blood in 12 ml
    d. 0.05 ml blood in 1 ml
67. 0.08 ml
68. 2 ml of 0.5N ↑ 50 ml → 50 ml of 0.02N
69. 12 oz of 10/1,000 ↑ 30 oz → 30 oz of 1/250 solution
70. 1.2 oz of 50/1,000 ↑ 30 oz → 30 oz of 1/500 solution
71. Cannot make a stronger solution from a weaker one.
72. 10 ml of 10% ↑ 200 ml → 200 ml of 0.5%
73. 0.025 ml stock ↑ 50 ml → 50 ml of 0.5 mg/dl
74. There are several solutions possible: 0.1/1, 1/10, 10/100, etc.
75. c
76. Tube 5, 1/32,805 dilution; tube 10, 1/1,937,102,445 dilution
77. Tube 4, 1/1,296 dilution; tube 8, 1/1,679,616 dilution

78.

					Tube Number						
	1	**2**	**3**	**4**	**5**	**6**	**7**	**8**	**9**	**10**	**11**
Tube dilution	1/4	1/2	1/2	1/2	1/2	1/2	1/2	1/2	1/2	1/2	1/2
Solution dilution	1/4	1/8	1/16	1/32	1/64	1/128	1/256	1/512	1/1024	1/2048	1/4096
Substance conc.	1/4	1/8	1/16	1/32	1/64	1/128	1/256	1/512	1/1024	1/2048	1/4096 dilution

79. Tube dilution in tube 4 = 1/2; 0.25 ml urine present before transfer; tube dilution in tube 1 = undiluted.

80.

		Tube Number			
	1	**2**	**3**	**4**	**5**
a.	4 ml	4.5 ml	4.5 ml	4.5 ml	4.5 ml
b.	1/10	1/5.5	1/5.5	1/5.5	1/5.5
c.	1/10	1/55	1/302	1/1,664	1/9,151
d.	0.5 ml	0.1 ml	0.018 ml	3.3×10^{-3} ml	6.01×10^{-4} ml
e.	0.4 ml	0.082 ml	0.0149 ml	2.704×10^{-3} ml	4.917×10^{-4} ml

		Tube Number			
	6	**7**	**8**	**9**	**10**
a.	4.5 ml	4.5 ml	4.5 ml	4.5 ml	4.5 ml
b.	1/5.5	1/5.5	1/5.5	1/5.5	1/5.5
c.	1/50,328	1/276,806	1/1,522,435	1/8,373,394	1/46,053,666
d.	1.09×10^{-4} ml	1.987×10^{-5} ml	3.613×10^{-6} ml	6.568×10^{-7} ml	1.194×10^{-7} ml
e.	8.941×10^{-5} ml	1.626×10^{-5} ml	2.956×10^{-6} ml	5.374×10^{-7} ml	9.771×10^{-8} ml

81.

	Tube Number	
	4	**8**
Serum dilution	1/1,125	1/703,125
Amount of serum present	0.0044 ml	0.0000071 ml

82. a. Tube 1 = 1/10; tube 6 = 1/2
    b. Tube 1 = 1/10; tube 4 = 1/80; tube 7 = 1/640
    c. 0.125 ml
    d. Serum volume = 0.000977 ml; serum concentration = 1/5,120 dilution
83. a. Tube 1 = 1/5; tube 3 = 1/2; tube 5 = 1/2
    b. Tube 1 = 1/5; tube 2 = 1/10; tube 7 = 1/320
    c. Volume = 4 ml; concentration = 1/2,560 dilution
    d. Before transfer = 0.025 ml; after transfer = 0.0125 ml

84.

	Tube Number					
	1	**2**	**3**	**4**	**5**	**6**
a.	1/10	1/2	1/2	1/2	1/2	1/2
b.	1/10	1/20	1/40	1/80	1/160	1/320
c.	0.05 ml	0.025 ml	0.0125 ml	0.00625 ml	0.003125 ml	0.0015625 ml
d.	1/20	1/40	1/80	1/160	1/320	1/640

85. a. 50   d. 60
    b. 45/3 or 15   e. 250/4 or 62.5
    c. 200/2 or 100   f. 3,000
86. 417 mg/dl
87. 3,750 mg/dl
88. 20.5 mg/dl
89. 560 mg/dl
90. 1,600 mg/dl
91. c, Assuming you were not supposed to correct for the 1/20 dilution in the procedure; 250 mg/dl if you need to correct for the 1/20 dilution.
92. 167 mEq/L, same as #91, 1,667 mEq/L if you need to correct for the 1/10 dilution.
93. $1/100 \times 1/100 \times 1/10 = 1/100,000$
94. There are several possible solutions. One is: $0.50/50 \times 1/100 = 1/10,000$
95. There are several possible solutions. One is:
    a. $1/10 \times 1/10 \times 1/100 = 1/10,000$
    b. $3/50 \times 1/10 \times 1/100 = 3/50,000$
    c. $1/100 \times 1/100 \times 1/100 = 1/1,000,000$
    d. $2/60 \times 1/100 \times 1/100 = 2/600,000$

Chapter 6 Solutions*

1. 3,200
2. 26,000
3. 4,520
4. 700
5. 0.016
6. 0.320
7. 200,000
8. 16,200,000
9. 0.0032
10. 0.000063
11. 796
12. 10
13. 1,000
14. 7,000

*Slightly different answers may be obtained due to rounding off procedures.

15. 1,600,000
16. 0.1
17. 155,000
18. 0.0036
19. 2,010,000
20. 0.0000001
21. 2,200,000
22. 0.000979
23. 1.06
24. 0.000001
25. 0.30
26. 0.0555
27. 1.0×10^{10}
28. 1,353,000,000
29. 90,000
30. 193,000
31. d
32. w/w
33. v/v
34. w/v
35. $3\%^{w/w}$
36. $12\%^{v/v}$
37. $6.3\%^{w/v}$
38. $0.00006\%^{w/v}$, 0.06 mg$\%^{w/v}$
39. $0.064\%^{w/v}$, 64 mg$\%^{w/v}$
40. $8.75\%^{w/v}$
41. $12.5\%^{w/w}$
42. $7.89\%^{w/w}$
43. $31.82\%^{w/w}$
44. $0.188\%^{w/v}$
45. 24 gm NaCl ↑ 400 ml
46. 6 ml HCl ↑ 30 ml
47. 60 g HCl ↑ 1200 ml
48. 5.6 g NaOH + 344.4 g H_2O
49. 1,200 g H_2SO_4 ↑ 3,000 ml
50. 0.3 ml HNO_3 ↑ 500 ml
51. $6\%^{w/v}$
52. $3.25\%^{v/v}$
53. $0.065\%^{w/v}$
54. $0.144\%^{w/w}$
55. $0.25\%^{v/v}$
56. $0.064\%^{v/v}$
57. $33.33\%^{w/w}$
58. $0.00105\%^{w/w}$
59. $38\%^{w/v}$
60. $10\%^{w/w}$
61. 160 ml
62. 100 ml
63. 26.4 ml
64. 353.33 ml
65. 80,000 ml
66. 24 g
67. 0.06 g
68. 900 ml
69. 1.25 g
70. 1.62 ml
71. 108 g
72. 9.1% Cl
73. 5 g $(NH_4)_2SO_4$
74. 10.48% K
75. 3.15 g KCl
76. 24 g NaCl
77. 60 ml glacial acetic acid
78. 4.25 g
79. 800 ml HCl ↑ 2,000 ml
80. a. 24.5 ml saline
    b. 16.2 ml saline
81. 15 g NaCl ↑ 300 ml
82. 2.5 g NaCl
83. 124 g HCl ↑ 2,000 ml
84. 20%; 20,000 mg%
85. 100 mg NaCl ↑ 100 ml
86. 130 g NaCl ↑ 650 ml
87. 500 ml
88. 160 g/L
89. 12.5%
90. 38,000 mg/L; 38 g/L
91. 225 ml
92. 3,230 mg/L
93. 50 ml, 20%
94. 6 g
95. 8.1 g NaCl ↑ 135 ml
96. 30 g NaOH
97. 0.45 g NaCl ↑ 50 ml
98. 8.3%
99. 4%
100. 250 ml
101. 4%
102. 49.8 g NaCl
103. 1 g NaOH
104. 600 ml
105. 0.84 %
106. a
107. 75 g NaCl
108. b
109. a. 12 g
     b. 24 g
     c. 1.5 g

110. a. 4%
    b. 45.8%
    c. 0.5%
    d. 46.7%
111. 15 g NaOH
112. 5.3%
113. 7.8 g NaCl
114. Yes
115. 0.2N
116. 0.714N
117. 1.758N
118. 2,970.3 ml
119. 8.25N
120. 9.5 ml
121. b
122. 100 ml
123. 40 ml
124. 4N
125. 125 ml of 1N + 375 ml of 5N
126. 400 ml
127. 333.3 ml
128. 66.7 ml of 0.6N ↑ 1,000 ml → 1,000 ml of 0.04N
129. 0.148N
130. 112.5 ml
131. 100 ml
132. 37.5 ml H_2O
133. Stock solution is 1.008N, 1.76 ml H_2O needed.
134. None; you cannot make NaOH from NaCl.
135. 20,000 ml
136. 40%
137. 28.2 ml H_2O needed
138. 0.05N
139. 4.6N
140. 4,975 ml of remaining 0.6N ↑ 5970 ml → 5970 ml of 0.5N
141. 1.68N
142. Cannot make a stronger solution from a weaker solution.
143. 10%
144. 20 ml 5M
145. 44.4 ml of 9% ↑ 100 ml → 100 ml of 4%
146. 62.1 ml
147. 6%
148. Cannot make a stronger solution from a weaker solution.

149. 112.5 ml
150. 4.5 ml
151. 30 ml
152. 10%
153. 1.25%
154. 5.48%
155. 21.8 ml of 15% + 18.2 ml of 4%
156. Volumes are arbitrary, many combinations possible. One solution: 16.22 ml of 40% + 33.78 ml of 3% → 50 ml of 15%.
157. 0.4 ml 50% ↑ 50 ml → 50 ml of 0.4%; 50 ml
158. a. 159.6
    b. 177.6
159. 42.56 g $CuSO_4 \cdot 10\ H_2O$ ↑ 400 ml → 400 ml of 5% $CuSO_4$
160. 19.8 g Na_2SO_4 ↑ 450 ml → 450 ml of 10% $Na_2SO_4 \cdot 10\ H_2O$
161. 61.06 g $CaCl_2$ ↑ 2,000 ml → 2,000 ml of 8% $CaCl_2 \cdot 10\ H_2O$
162. 15.64 g $CuSO_4 \cdot 5\ H_2O$ ↑ 1,000 ml → 1,000 ml of 1% $CuSO_4$
163. 0.127 g $Co(NO_3)_2 \cdot 6\ H_2O$ ↑ 400 ml → 400 ml of 0.02% $Co(NO_3)_2$
164. 9 g of $CuSO_4 \cdot 5\ H_2O$ ↑ 100 ml
165. a. No
    b. 6% $CuSO_4$
    c. 2.16 g
166. a. 1.2 g $CuSO_4$
    b. 1.2 g $CuSO_4 \cdot 5\ H_2O$
167. 829.7 ml
168. 16.17 g $CH_3COONa \cdot 3\ H_2O$
169. a
170. 300 g
171. 10M
172. 1.71M
173. 0.5M
174. 3.57M
175. 72 g NaOH ↑ 300 ml → 300 ml of 6M
176. 0.67M
177. 11.396M
178. 133.3 ml
179. 58.5
180. 2.67M
181. 98.0
182. 3.125
183. 310.3
184. 22.2 g/L
185. 142.06, 142.06 g

186. 22.4 g
187. 4.0 mol
188. none
189. 35.1 g
190. 444.4 ml
191. 17.55 g
192. 5.85 g
193. 0.878 g
194. 1.314 g
195. 2.0M
196. 142.06 g Na_2SO_4 ↑ 1,000 ml → 1,000 ml of 1M Na_2SO_4
197. a. 39.2 g
    b. 16 g
    c. 44.4 g
    d. 39.24 g
198. 25.2 g $NaHCO_3$ ↑ 500 ml → 500 ml of 0.6M $NaHCO_3$
199. a. 5 M
    b. 0.685M
    c. 0.91M
200. 19.11 g
201. 2.99 g KOH ↑ 800 ml → 800 ml of M/15 KOH
202. 138 g
203. 5.13M
204. 250 ml
205. 46.8 ng
206. 52.05 mmol/L; 13,012.5 μmol/250 ml
207. 129.24 g
208. 117.72 g
209. 0.0183 g
210. 84 g
211. 20.475 μg/350 ml
212. 131.51 mmol/L
213. a. Yes
    b. 6M $CuSO_4$ contains 957.6 g $CuSO_4$; 6M $CuSU_4 \cdot 5\ H_2O$ contains 1497.6 g $CuSO_4 \cdot 5\ H_2O$, of which 957.6 g are $CuSO_4$.
214. a. 127.68 g
    b. 142.08 g
    c. 199.68 g
215. 255 mOsmol/L
216. 18.6 osmol/L
217. 86.02 mOsmol/L
218. 60 mOsmol/L
219. 9 osmol/L
220. 21 mOsmol/L
221. 279.57 mOsmol/L
222. 370.97 mOsmol/L
223. 60 mOsmol/L
224. −0.288°C
225. 430.11 mOsmol/L
226. 370.75 mOsmol NaCl, 0.185M
227. 48 mOsmol/L
228. 376.3 mOsmol/L
229. 255 mOsmol/L
230. 188.2 mOsmol/L
231. 1.8 equivalent weights
232. 65.4 g H_3PO_4 ↑ 500 ml → 500 ml of 4N H_3PO_4
233. 1.3 equivalent weights
234. 399.6 g $CaCl_2$ ↑ 1,000 ml → 1,000 ml of 7.2N $CaCl_2 \cdot 10\ H_2O$
235. c
236. Cannot make a stronger solution from a weaker solution.
237. b
238. 1.58N
239. e
240. 3.1 ml
241. 294.3 g H_3PO_4 ↑ 3,000 ml → 3,000 ml of 3N H_3PO_4
242. 150 ml
243. 0.05N
244. 34.2 g HCl ↑ 7,500 ml → 7,500 ml of N/8 HCl
245. 1.334 g NaOH ↑ 200 ml → 200 ml of N/6 NaOH
246. 4.5N
247. 0.0025N
248. 73.125 g
249. 0.1408N
250. 300.85 g H_3PO_4 ↑ 2,300 ml → 2,300 ml of 4N H_3PO_4
251. 0.04 mEq or 0.8 mg
252. 180 mEq
253. 3
254. 3.126 g $BaCl_2$ ↑ 150 ml → 150 ml of N/5 $BaCl_2$
255. a. 58.5
    b. 58.5
256. 0.05N
257. a. 98.1
    b. 49.05

258. 1.05 g $BaSO_4$ ↑ 300 ml → 300 ml of 0.03N $BaSO_4$
259. a. 98.0
     b. 32.67
260. 360.4 ml
261. 365 g
262. 436.5 g $CaCl_2 \cdot 10\ H_2O$ ↑ 200 ml → 200 ml of 15N $CaCl_2$
263. 132.5 g
264. 1765.8 g H_2SO_4 ↑ 1,800 ml → 1,800 ml of 20N H_2SO_4
265. 4.90 g
266. (To make 20 L): 15 jars or 22.5 lb; $36.00
267. 20.58 g $CaCl_2 \cdot 2\ H_2O$ ↑ 700 ml → 700 ml of 0.4N $CaCl_2$
268. 10N
269. a. 1,036.3 g
     b. 323.3 g
     c. 213.5 g
     d. 199.3 g
270. 1.12 N
271. 4,500 mEq
272. 45 ml
273. 3.998 mEq
274. 7.5N
275. 3,998 mEq
276. 1,250 ml of 1.5N + 1,750 ml of 7.5N → 3,000 ml of 5N
277. 0.00214N
278. 5 ml of 8N ↑ 100 ml → 100 ml of 0.4N
279. 0.08547N
280. 0.0563N
281. 2.5N
282. 0.00282N
283. a. 3
     b. 1
     c. 1
284. 63.01 g
285. 0.15N
286. 0.96N
287. 1.85 g $CaCl_2$ ↑ 200 ml → 200 ml of N/6 $CaCl_2$
288. 0.1N
289. 0.1 molecular weights
290. 2N
291. 5N
292. 216 mEq/L chloride
293. 70.76 g
294. 34.133 g
295. 27.75 g $CaCl_2$ ↑ 100 ml → 100 ml of 5N $CaCl_2 \cdot 10\ H_2O$

296.

	$CuSO_4$	$CuSO_4 \cdot H_2O$	$CuSO_4 \cdot 10\ H_2O$
a.	15 g	15 g	15 g
b.	119.7 g	133.2 g	254.7 g

297. 28 ml conc H_2SO_4 ↑ 200 ml → 200 ml of 25%$^{w/v}$ H_2SO_4
298. 142.75 g
299. 115.76 ml conc HNO_3 ↑ 3,000 ml → 3,000 ml of 0.6N HNO_3
300. 65.66 ml conc H_2SO_4 ↑ 200 ml → 200 ml of 6M H_2SO_4
301. a. 16.67%$^{v/v}$
     b. 28.5%$^{w/v}$
     c. 2.91M
     d. 5.81N
302. 3.75%$^{v/v}$, 6.55%$^{w/v}$
303. 127.21 ml + 272.79 ml H_2O
304. 510.8 ml conc HNO_3 ↑ 1,000 ml → 1,000 ml of 8N HNO_3
305. 17.6M
306. 18.2M
307. 44.1N
308. 14.78 ml of conc H_3PO_4 ↑ 700 ml → 700 ml of 0.3N H_3PO_4
309. 92.26 ml of conc H_2SO_4 ↑ 400 ml → 400 ml of 4M H_2SO_4
310. 363.58 ml of conc HNO_3 ↑ 1,000 ml → 1,000 ml of 6N HNO_3
311. 147.31 ml of conc HCl ↑ 18 L → 18 L 0.1M HCl
312. a. 6%$^{w/v}$
     b. 10.54%$^{v/v}$
     c. 1.075M
     d. 2.15N
313. a. 12.33M
     b. 24.67N
     c. 605 g
314. 0.85
315. 1.55
316. 6,521.7 ml

317. 1.3

318. 10.96M, 10.96N

319. 13.5N

320. 10.8M, 32.45N, 116.6 g

321. 22.3 g

322. 0.84

323. 1.075

324. 9,933.8 ml

325. 6.32

326. 10.77 g

327. 200.8 ml of $4\%^{w/v}$ ↑ 750 ml → 750 ml of $0.6\%^{v/v}$ ($1.071\%^{w/v}$)

328. 0.612N

329. 102.56 mEq Cl/L

330. 3.44 mEq Mg/L

331. 468 mg NaCl/dl

332. 2.41N

333. 28 ml

334. 2.039N

335. 175 ml

336. 119.66 mEq Cl/L

337. $20\%^{w/v}$ = 4.08N; cannot make a stronger solution from a weaker one.

338. 24%

339. $29.2\%^{w/v}$

340. 1.5 ml

341. 11.1N, 11.1M

342. 15 mEq Ca/L

343. a. 5.5 mEq Ca/L
     b. 102.56 mEq NaCl/L
     c. 3.07 mEq K/L

344. 1.71M

345. 0.0256N

346. 0.6M

347. a. 308.2 mg Na/dl
     b. 12 mg Ca/dl
     c. 23.5 mg K/dl

348. 0.1M

349. 16 ml

350. a. 0.6N
     b. 0.6N
     c. 1.8N
     d. 1.2N

351. 83.3 ml

352. a. 0.4M
     b. 0.2M
     c. 0.2M
     d. 0.15M

353. 11.25N

354. 140.4 mEq Na/L

355. a. $6.68\%^{w/v}$
     b. $6.682\%^{v/v}$

356. 3.3 mg Mg/dl

357. 266.67 ml

358. 1.37M, 1.37N

359. 3M

360. 1.84M

361. 21.9N

362. 0.434N

363. 0.154M, 0.154N

364. 0.02N

365. 1.33M

366. 0.045M, 0.090N

367. a. 53.85 mEq NaCl/L
     b. 7.67 mEq K/L
     c. 136.96 mEq Na/L

368. a. 514.75 mg Cl/dl
     b. 3.17 mg Mg/dl

369. 3 ml

370. 14 mg/dl

371. 78.26 mEq NaCl/L

372. $30\%^{w/v}$ = 3.62N; cannot make a stronger solution from a weaker one.

373. 7.5N

374. 526.5 mg NaCl/dl

375. 40 ml

376. $10.95\%^{w/v}$

377. a. 5 mEq Ca/L
     b. 119.66 mEq NaCl/L
     c. 3.58 mEq K/L

378. a. 322 mg Na/dl
     b. 10 mg Ca/dl
     c. 19.55 mg K/dl

379. 2.5M

380. 9N

381. 16.82 ml

382. 10 ml

383. 365.65 mg Cl/dl

384. 15 ml

385. a. $4.62\%^{v/v}$
     b. $2.03\%^{w/v}$
     c. 0.556M
     d. 0.556N

386. 91.18 ml

387. 9.52N, 9.52M

388. a. 0.06M $AgNO_3$
     b. 0.65M $CaCl_2$
     c. 2.5M H_2SO_4
     d. 2.0M NaOH

389. a. 0.02N CaCl$_2$
 b. 4N H$_2$SO$_4$
 c. 0.8N CuSO$_4$
 d. 6N NaOH
390. a. 0.625M
 b. 0.625N
 c. 2.5%$^{w/v}$
 d. 25,000 ppm
391. 288.9 ml
392. a. 1.6%
 b. 0.274N
 c. 0.274M
 d. 16,000 ppm
393. a. 3.5%
 b. 598.3 mEq Na/L
 c. 598.3 mEq Cl/L
 d. 598.3 mEq NaCl/L
 e. 0.598N
 f. 0.598M
 g. 35,000 ppm
394. a. 3,128 mg/dl
 b. 75.05 g/24 hr
 c. 75,072 mg/24 hr
 d. 1,919.6 mmol/d
 e. 31,280 ppm
395. a. 0.154M
 b. 0.154N
 c. 153.85 mEq/L
 d. 900 mg/dl
 e. 9,000 ppm
396. 553.9 ml of conc acid (12.05N) + 196.1 ml H$_2$O
397. 21.42%$^{w/v}$
398. 36.4 ml H$_2$O
399. 5%$^{v/v}$ = 2.2%$^{w/v}$; cannot make a stronger solution from a weaker one.
400. a. 0.5
 b. 0.02
 c. 2.0
 d. 0.282
 e. 0.282
 f. 3.55
 g. 5.85
 h. 0.0585
 i. 0.256
 j. 3.91
 k. 0.0746
 l. 0.435
 m. 0.435
 n. 2.3
 o. 5.85
 p. 0.0585

401. 33.75 mmol/L
402. 29.25 mmol/L
403. 56.54 vol%
404. 23.85 to 34.2 mmol/L
405. a. 0.45
 b. 2.226
406. 5 × 10^5 μg/dl
407. 1.525 × 10^{-11} g/ml
408. 1 × 10^6 mg/ml
409. 5 × 10^5 μg/L
410. 2 × 10^3 ng/μl
411. 46 g/L
412. 36.41 μmol/L
413. 30.78 μmol/L
414. 2.74 mmol/L
415. 2.4 mmol/L
416. 5.33 kPa
417. 84.6 mmol/L
418. 108 mmol/L
419. 3.75 mmol/L
420. 0.0053 mmol/L
421. 34.13 μmol/L
422. 5.51 mmol/L
423. 2.22 mmol/d
424. 20.66 μmol/d
425. 0.54 μmol/L
426. 350 mg/dl
427. 7.78 mg/dl
428. 3.8 mEq/L
429. 3.07 mg/dl
430. 0.62 g/d
431. 1,368.5 mg/d
432. 35 mEq/d
433. 7.0 g/dl
434. 459.8 mg/dl
435. 200 mEq/L
436. 1.68 mg/dl
437. 15.56 mg/dl
438. 7.26 mg/dl
439. 547.6 mm Hg
440. 7.10 pH

Chapter 7 Logarithms*†

1. 0.0128
2. 0.9832
3. 0.4014
4. 0.3010
5. 1.6232
6. 3.5623

*Slightly different answers may be obtained due to rounding off procedures.
†Most of the answers to this chapter were determined using a calculator. Answers derived from a table may vary slightly. In most cases logarithms will be given in calculator form (negative form) and in regular form.

7. $\overline{4}.0$
8. $\overline{6}.0$
9. $\overline{1}.0$
10. $\overline{10}.0$
11. 0
12. 3
13. 1
14. 0
15. 2
16. 4
17. 1
18. −4
19. −1
20. −2
21. −8
22. −1
23. −3
24. −1
25. 11. .1430
   12. .1430
   13. .5798
   14. .6927
   15. .00043
   16. .4724
   17. .1901
   18. .1139
   19. .2938
   20. .1139
   21. .1139
   22. .2866
   23. .002641
   24. .000000035
26. 11. 0.1430
   12. 3.1430
   13. 1.5798
   14. 0.6927
   15. 2.00043
   16. 4.4724
   17. 1.1901
   18. $\overline{4}.1139$, −3.8861
   19. $\overline{1}.2938$, −0.7062
   20. $\overline{2}.1139$, −1.8861
   21. $\overline{8}.1139$, −7.8861
   22. $\overline{1}.2866$, −0.7134
   23. $\overline{3}.002641$, −2.997359
   24. $\overline{1}.000000035$, −0.999999965
27. 1. 1.02991
  2. 9.62055
  3. 2.52000
  4. 1.99986
  5. 41.99523
  6. 3650.05997
  7. 0.0001
  8. 0.09707
  9. 0.45499
  10. 0.00064565
28. 50.0035
29. 5,000.3454
30. 500,034.5350
31. 1,000
32. 5.00035
33. 0.0500035
34. 0.000019999
35. 24,997.6970
36. 44.6992
37. 500,034,535.0
38. 0.00006203
39. 1,000,000,000
40. 34,103.58226
41. −1.0129
42. −0.3420
43. −3.1900
44. −0.0021
45. −2.0160
46. 41. $\overline{2}.9871$
   42. $\overline{1}.6580$
   43. $\overline{4}.8100$
   44. $\overline{1}.9979$
   45. $\overline{3}.9840$
47. 0.000204
48. 1.0000
49. 0.1000
50. 0.00000984
51. a. $\overline{3}.3118$ b. −2.6882 c. 0.00205
52. a. $\overline{2}.9907$ b. −1.0093 c. 0.0979
53. a. $\overline{6}.3879$ b. −5.6121 c. 0.000002442
54. a. $\overline{9}.0207$ b. −8.9793 c. 0.000000001049
55. a. $\overline{1}.0003$ b. −0.9997 c. 0.100069
56. Cannot add and subtract using logarithms.
57. Cannot add and subtract using logarithms.
58. Cannot add and subtract using logarithms.

Problems 59 to 70 were calculated by rounding off the logarithms to four places. The answers using the original figures themselves are presented in parentheses after the answers derived from using logarithms, which are presented in boxes. The more the logarithms are rounded off, the less precise the answer.

59. $1.5185 + 0.3222 + 3.7929 = 5.6336 = \boxed{430,130.2634}$ (430,145.1000)

60. $4.5279 + 6.3012 + 3.5989 = 14.4280 = \boxed{2.679168 \times 10^{14}}$ (2.678949×10^{14})

61. $1.0792 + 0.8573 + 3.7775 = 5.7140 = \boxed{517,606.8319}$ (517,622.4)

62. Cannot be done with logs because of negative number.

63. $1.5046 + (-1.1415) + 1.1139 + (-0.1135) = 1.3635 = \boxed{23.09404}$ (23.09820)

64. $-2.0315 + 4.1358 + 0.7782 + (-4.01773) = -1.13523 = \boxed{0.0732487}$ (0.0732382)

65. $1.6335 - 0.7853 = 0.8482 = \boxed{7.05018}$ (7.04918)

66. $3.6356 - 1.4624 = 2.1732 = \boxed{149.0047}$ (149.000)

67. $2.6021 - (-0.2218) = 2.8239 = \boxed{666.6532}$ (666.667)

68. Cannot be done with logs because of negative number.

69. $0.0374 - 1.6232 = -1.5858 = \boxed{0.0259537}$ (0.0259524)

70. $-1.2147 - (-3.1427) = 1.9280 = \boxed{84.7227}$ (84.72222)

71. $\bar{3}.3292,\ 7.3292 - 10,\ -2.6708$
72. $\bar{1}.97044,\ 9.97044 - 10,\ -0.02956$
73. $\bar{2}.0069,\ 8.0069 - 10,\ -1.9931$
74. $\bar{6}.6006,\ 4.6006 - 10,\ -5.3994$
75. $\bar{4}.8672,\ 6.8672 - 10,\ -3.1328$
76. $\bar{8}.9315,\ 2.9315 - 10,\ -7.0685$
77. $\bar{5}.8403,\ 5.8403 - 10,\ -4.1597$
78. $\bar{7}.6809,\ 3.6809 - 10,\ -6.3191$

Chapter 8 Ionic solutions and pH*

1. a. $[H^+] = 0.021$
   b. $[OH^-] = 4.76 \times 10^{-13}$
   c. pH = 1.678
   d. pOH = 12.322
2. $[H^+] = 0.81$M; pH = 0.0915
3. pH = 3.0
4. $[H^+] = 1 \times 10^{-7}$
5. d
6. b
7. acid
8. pH = 5.0
9. basic
10. pH = 3.0
11. false

12. a. $[H^+] = 0.019$
    b. $[OH^-] = 5.263 \times 10^{-13}$
    c. pH = 1.721
    d. pOH = 12.279
13. 10; acidity
14. 0.001
15. 1×10^{-10}
16. a. $[OH^-] = 5.263 \times 10^{-9}$
    b. $[OH^-] = 3.333 \times 10^{-2}$
    c. $[OH^-] = 1.923 \times 10^{-11}$
17. a. $[H^+] = 9.901 \times 10^{-8}$
    b. $[H^+] = 5.263 \times 10^{-12}$
    c. $[H^+] = 1.555 \times 10^{-5}$

*Slightly different answers may be obtained due to rounding off procedures.

18. a. pOH = 8.25; pH = 5.75
    b. pOH = 1.477; pH = 12.523
    c. pOH = 10.716; pH = 3.284
19. a. pH = 7.004; pOH = 6.996
    b. pH = 11.279; pOH = 2.721
    c. pH = 4.808; pOH = 9.192
20. pH = 9.0
21. $[OH^-] = 1 \times 10^{-6}$
22. pH = 4.0
23. pH = 3.3768
24. pH = 6.3979
25. pH = 2.0315; pOH = 11.9685
26. pH = 5.5086; pOH = 8.4914
27. 1g per 100,000,000 L (1×10^8 L)
28. 1/10,000 g/L (1×10^{-4} g/L)
29. pH = 3.0575; pOH = 10.9425
30. pH = 8.4914; pOH = 5.5086
31. 1.585×10^{-8}
32. 5.4954×10^{-4}
33. 8.5113×10^{-10}
34. 3.0903×10^{-12}
35. 2.3442×10^{-8}
36. 0.0016 g NaOH (1.6×10^{-3} g)
37. 0.0006925 g HCl (6.925×10^{-4} g)
38. pH = 2.0
39. $[H^+] = 3.9811 \times 10^{-9}$; $[OH^-] =$ 2.5119×10^{-6}

40. $[H^+] = 2.5119 \times 10^{-6}$; $[OH^-] =$ 3.9811×10^{-9}
41. 1.3979
42. 1.1749M
43. a. pH = 12.301
    b. pOH = 1.699
    c. $[H^+] = 5.0 \times 10^{-13}$
    d. $[OH^-] = 2 \times 10^{-2}$
44. pH = 12.4771
45. pH = 10.0
46. pH = 6.0
47. pH = 2.5229
48. 8.912×10^{-6}
49. pH = 7.458
50. CO_2 = 17.86
51. pH = 7.416
52. P_{CO_2} = 58.8
53. a. 126 nmol/L
    b. 19.9 nmol/L
54. pH = pK
55. 0.00536 mol/L acid + 0.29464 mol/L salt
56. pK
57. Equal, pK
58. pH = 7.1
59. 0.00343 mol/L acid + 0.59657 mol/L salt

Chapter 9 Colorimetry*

1. 277.8 mg/dl
2. 75 mg/dl
3. 0.071
4. 130.8 µg/dl
5. 255.2 mg/dl
6. 128.6 µg/dl
7. a. 1.0000
   b. 0.456
   c. 0.215
   d. 0.036
8. a. 98%T
   b. 62.2%T
   c. 18.5%T
   d. 12.2%T
9. a
10. a. 1.482×10^{-4} mol/L
    b. 5.091×10^{-5} mol/L
    c. 9.287×10^{-5} mol/L

    d. 5.338×10^{-5} mol/L
    e. 1.787×10^{-4} mol/L
    f. 1.482×10^{-4} mol/L
11. a. 3.789×10^3
    b. 6.188×10^3
    c. 3.33×10^3
12. 1/100,000 dilution should have an *A* of 0.5
13. No, the ϵ is 57,500.
14. ϵ = 78,750
15. *A* = 0.000769
16. a. 6.2×10^{-6} mol/L
    b. 6.2×10^{-6} M
    c. 1.24×10^{-5}N
    d. 0.0868 mg/dl (8.68×10^{-2} mg/dl)
    e. 0.0124 mEq/L (1.24×10^{-2} mEq/L)
    f. 0.868 ppm
    g. 0.0000868%

*Slightly different answers may be obtained due to rounding off procedures.

Chapter 10 Graphs and Standard Curves*

Standard curves

1. 0.006 ml *SS* ↑ 50 ml → 50 ml of a 0.03 mg/dl *WS*
2. 1,000 mg/dl
3. 0.025 ml *SS* ↑ 50 ml → 50 ml of a 0.5 mg/dl *WS*
4. 1 mg/dl
5. 178.3 mg/dl
6. a. 5 mg/dl
   b. 85.5 μmol/L
7. 125 mg/dl
8. 262.3 mg/dl

Establishing a standard curve

9. 0.25 mg/ml; 2.5 ml *SS* ↑ 100 ml → 100 ml of a 0.25 mg/dl *WS*
10. 300 mg/dl; 3,000 μg/ml
11. 22.2 μg/ml
12. a. 400 mg/dl
    b. 0.5 ml
    c. 0.4 mg/ml
    d. 4/10 dilution
    e. Several ways to calculate; picking the concentration wanted is presented below.
       300 mg/dl = 0.375 ml *WS*
       200 mg/dl = 0.25 ml *WS*
       100 mg/dl = 0.125 ml *WS*
    However, these volumes are difficult to measure. Picking the volumes wanted is presented below:
       0.4 ml *WS* = 320 mg/dl
       0.3 ml *WS* = 240 mg/dl
       0.2 ml *WS* = 160 mg/dl
       0.1 ml *WS* = 80 mg/dl
13. 3,000 mg/dl
14. 0.2 mg/ml
15. a. 350 mg/dl
    b. 0.3 ml
    c. 0.35 mg/ml
    d. 7 ml *SS* ↑ 100 ml → 100 ml of 0.35 mg/ml *WS*
    e. Several solutions possible:
       0.1 ml *WS* = 116.7 mg/dl
       0.2 ml *WS* = 233.3 mg/dl
16. 250 mg/dl
17. 15/100 dilution; 0.15 mg/ml
18. 1000 μg/ml
19. a. 600 mg/dl
    b. 1 ml
    c. 0.6 mg/ml
    d. 24/100 dilution of *SS*

*Slightly different answers may be obtained due to rounding off procedures.

  e. Several solutions possible:
     0.75 ml *WS* 450 mg/dl
     0.5 ml *WS* 300 mg/dl
     0.25 ml *WS* 150 mg/dl

Plotting the standard curve

20. b and d

Serum controls

21. 28.32 mg $(NH_4)_2SO_4$ ↑ 100 ml → 100 ml of a 6 mg/dl N standard
22. 20 μg/ml Pb
23. 6.98 mEq K/L; 110.96 mEq Na/L
24. 14.16 mg $(NH_4)_2SO_4$ ↑ 100 ml → 100 ml of a 3 mg/dl N standard
25. 64.2 mg $CO(NH_2)_2$ ↑ 600 ml → 600 ml of a 5 mg/dl N standard
26. 94.4 mg $(NH_4)_2SO_4$ ↑ 500 ml → 500 ml of a 4 mg/dl N standard
27. 2.58 mmol/L
28. 47.2 mg $(NH_4)_2SO_4$ ↑ 100 ml → 100 ml of a 10 mg/dl N standard

Chapter 11 Hematology math*

1. 1/20
2. 1/16.7
3. 1/125
4. 1/33.3
5. 1/100
6. 1/142.8
7. a
8. 1/111.1
9. d
10. c
11. b
12. 62,500 cells/mm³
13. 31 cells/mm³
14. b
15. 0.02 mm³
16. 854,338 cells/mm³
17. 3,029 cells/mm³
18. b
19. a. A = 3 mm
    B = 1 mm
    C = 0.25 mm
    D = 0.2 mm
    E = 0.05 mm
  b. F = 1 mm²
    G = 0.0625 mm²
    H = 0.04 mm²
    I = 0.0025 mm²
20. 1/50 dilution; 50

21. a. 1/25
    b. 10
    c. 0.1
    d. 1.0
    e. 25
22. a. 1/33.3
    b. 33.3
    c. 10
    d. 0.167
    e. 6 mm²
    f. 0.6 mm³
    g. 1.67
    h. 55.5
    i. 5,550 cells/mm³
23. a. 200
    b. 0.056
    c. 111.1
    d. 11.332 platelets/mm³
24. a. 100
    b. 0.0556
    c. 55.6
    d. 2,780 platelets/mm³
25. a. 17,777 WBC/mm³
    b. 22,223 NRBC/mm³
26. a. 69.4
    b. 6,940 cells/mm³
27. 25,000 WBC/mm³
28. a. 33.3

    b. 10
    c. 0.1
    d. 1.0
    e. 33.3
29. a. 40,426 WBC/mm³
    b. 54,574 NRBC/mm³
30. a. 5.0
    b. 2.5
    c. 12.5
    d. 3,125
    e. 3,125,000 cells/mm³
    f. 3.125 × 10⁹ cells/ml
31. 41,720 WBC/mm³
32. 1/25; 25
33. 1/333.3; 333.3
34. a. 10
    b. 500
    c. 1/4; 0.25
    d. 1/0.4; 2.5
35. a. 5.0
    b. 1/12.5
    c. 12.5
    d. 1/.2; 5.0
    e. 1/.04; 25
    f. 312.5
    g. 31,250 cells/mm³
36. a. 200
    b. 0.111

*Slightly different answers may be obtained due to rounding off procedures.

c. 222.2
d. 1.11
e. 50,000 platelets/mm^3

37. a. 10
b. 1/166.7
c. 166.7
d. 1/2; 0.5
e. 1/.2; 5.0
f. 833.5
g. 83,350 cells/mm^3

38. a. 5.0
b. 1/12.5
c. 12.5
d. 1/.6; 1.667
e. 1/.12; 8.333
f. 104.2
g. 5,210 cells/mm^3

39. a. 1/33.3
b. 33.3
c. 10
d. 18 mm^2
e. 0.056
f. 1.8 mm^3
g. 0.556
h. 18.5
i. 925 cells/mm^3
j. 925 $\times$ 10^6/L

40. a. 100
b. 0.2
c. 200
d. 6,800 platelets/mm^3

41. a. 9,709 WBC/mm^3
b. 291 NRBC/mm^3

42. a. 16,667 WBC/mm^3
b. 18,333 NRBC/mm^3

43. a.

	1	2	3	4	5
1.	1/50	1/20	1/16.7	1/14.3	1/12.5
2.	50	20	16.7	14.3	12.5
3.	10	10	10	10	10
4.	0.24 mm^2	0.32 mm^2	18 mm^2	10 mm^2	0.4 mm^2
5.	4.167	3.125	0.056	0.1	2.5
6.	0.024 mm^3	0.032 mm^3	1.8 mm^3	1.0 mm^3	0.04 mm^3
7.	41.67	31.25	0.56	1.0	25.0
8.	2,083.3	625	9.4	14.3	312.5
9.	270,829 cells/mm^3	101,250 cells/mm^3	7,708 cells/mm^3	3,775 cells/mm^3	116,562 cells/mm^3

b.

	1	2	3	4	5
1.	1/333.3	1/250	1/166.7	1/142.8	1/100
2.	333.3	250	166.7	142.8	100
3.	10	10	10	10	10
4.	4 mm^2	0.8 mm^2	0.4 mm^2	0.12 mm^2	2.0 mm^2
5.	0.25	1.25	2.5	8.33	0.5
6.	0.4 mm^3	0.08 mm^3	0.04 mm^3	0.012 mm^3	0.2 mm^3
7.	2.5	12.5	25	83.3	5.0
8.	833.2	3,125	4,167.5	11,895	500
9.	171,639 cells/ mm^3	559,375 cells/ mm^3	1,708,675 cells/ mm^3	4,413,045 cells/ mm^3	25,000 cells/ mm^3

c.

	1	2	3	4	5
1.	1/50	1/20	1/16.7	1/14.3	1/12.5
2.	50	20	16.7	14.3	12.5
3.	5	5	5	5	5
4.	0.24 mm^2	0.32 mm^2	18 mm^2	10 mm^2	0.4 mm^2
5.	4.167	3.125	0.056	0.1	2.5
6.	0.048 mm^3	0.064 mm^3	3.6 mm^3	2.0 mm^3	0.08 mm^3
7.	20.8	15.6	0.278	0.5	12.5
8.	1,041.7	312.5	4.64	7.15	156.2
9.	135,421 cells/ mm^3	50,625 cells/ mm^3	3,805 cells/mm^3	1,888 cells/mm^3	58,263 cells/ mm^3

d.

	1	2	3	4	5
1.	1/333.3	1/250	1/166.7	1/142.8	1/100
2.	333.3	250	166.7	142.8	100
3.	5	5	5	5	5
4.	4 mm^2	0.8 mm^2	0.4 mm^2	0.12 mm^2	2.0 mm^2
5.	0.25	1.25	2.5	8.33	0.5
6.	0.8 mm^3	0.16 mm^3	0.08 mm^3	0.024 mm^3	0.4 mm^3
7.	1.25	6.25	12.5	41.7	2.5
8.	416.6	1,562.5	2,083.8	5,950	250
9.	85,820 cells/ mm^3	279,688 cells/ mm^3	854,358 cells/ mm^3	2,207,450 cells/ mm^3	12,500 cells/ mm^3

44. c
45. d
46. 20,870 WBC/mm^3
47. c
48. a. 91.1 μm^3
    b. 31.1 pg
    c. 34.1%

49. a. 95.9 μm^3
    b. 30.6 pg
    c. 31.9%
50. a. 88.2 μm^3
    b. 30.4 pg
    c. 34.4%

51.

	a	b	c	d	e	f
MCV (μm^3)	75.5	100	80.7	83.0	75.0	100
MCH (pg)	22.9	34.7	29.3	25.5	25.0	42.3
MCHC (%)	30.3	34.7	36.3	30.7	33.3	42.3

52.	a	b	c	d	e	f
MCV (μm^3)	86.5	103.7	95.3	68.9	108.3	114.3
MCH (pg)	29.0	15.9	27.0	23.1	33.8	22.9
MCHC (%)	33.6	15.4	28.3	33.5	31.2	20.0

53. Answers are the same as problem 52.

54. a. 10.3 g%

b.

Standard	+	Diluent	Value
6 ml		0 ml	10.3 g%
5 ml		1 ml	8.6 g%
4 ml		2 ml	6.9 g%
3 ml		3 ml	5.2 g%
2 ml		4 ml	3.4 g%
1 ml		5 ml	1.7 g%
0 ml		6 ml	0 g%

55. a. 8.6 g%

b.

Standard	+	Diluent	Value
5 ml		0 ml	8.6 g%
4 ml		1 ml	6.9 g%
3 ml		2 ml	5.2 g%
2 ml		3 ml	3.4 g%
1 ml		4 ml	1.7 g%
0 ml		5 ml	0 g%

56. a. 9.7 g%

b.

Standard	+	Diluent	Value
6 ml		0 ml	9.7 g%
5 ml		1 ml	8.1 g%
4 ml		2 ml	6.5 g%
3 ml		3 ml	4.8 g%
2 ml		4 ml	3.2 g%
1 ml		5 ml	1.6 g%
0 ml		6 ml	0 g%

57. a. 16.2 g%

b.

Standard	+	Diluent	Value
9 ml		0 ml	16.2 g%
6 ml		3 ml	10.8 g%
3 ml		6 ml	5.4 g%
0 ml		9 ml	0 g%

c. 8.0 g%

Chapter 12 Enzyme calculations*

1. 3.53
2. 5.4
3. 16.7
4. 0.482

*Slightly different answers may be obtained due to rounding off procedures.

Chapter 13 Gastric acidity*

1. e (answer, 106.7°)
2. Free acid = 15°; 15 mmol/L
   Combined acid = 11°; 11 mmol/L
   Total acid = 26°; 26 mmol/L
3. Free acid = 24°; 24 mmol/L
   Combined acid = 16°; 16 mmol/L
   Total acid = 40°; 40 mmol/L
4. 40°
5. 122 mmol/L
6. Free acid = 9.6°; 9.6 mmol/L
   Combined acid = 22.4°; 22.4 mmol/L
   Total acid = 32°; 32 mmol/L

7. BAO
   Fasting = 1.92 mmol/hr
   15 min = 3.4 mmol/hr
   30 min = 5.6 mmol/hr
   45 min = 5.2 mmol/hr
   60 min = 2.3 mmol/hr

   MAO = 4.1 MAO/hr
   PAO = 5.4 PAO/hr

Chapter 14 Renal tests*

Clearance tests

1. 24.1 ml/min; 44.5% of normal
2. a. 2.10 m^2
   b. 0.82
3. 2.8 ml/min; 3.7% of normal
4. 55.6 ml/min
5. a. 1.65 m^2
   b. 1.05
   c. 11.2 ml/min
   d. 11.7 ml/min
   e. 21.7% of normal
   f. 20.7% of normal
6. 8.3 ml/min; 15.4% of normal
7. a. $\dfrac{1.73}{A}$

   b. $C = \dfrac{U}{P} \times V$

   c. $C = \dfrac{U}{P} \times \sqrt{V}$

d. $C = \dfrac{U}{P} \times V \times \dfrac{1.73}{A} \times \dfrac{100}{75}$

e. $C = \dfrac{U}{P} \times \sqrt{V} \times \dfrac{1.73}{A} \times \dfrac{100}{54}$

f. $C = \dfrac{U}{P} \times V \times \dfrac{1.73}{A}$

g. $\log A = (0.425 \times \log W) + (0.725 \times \log H) - 2.144$

8. a. 1.64 m^2
   b. 1.05
   c. 4.4 ml/min
   d. 4.6 ml/min
   e. 8.5% of normal
   f. 8.1% of normal
9. 78.0 ml/min; 104% of normal
10. 32.4 ml/min; 43.2% of normal

General renal test

11. a. 92 mg/dl
    b. 40 mmol/L
    c. 1,334 mg/24 hr
    d. 58 mmol/d
12. 1.5 g/d
13. 0.571%
14. 51 g/d
15. a. 198 mg/150 ml
    b. 1.32 mg/ml

16. a. 267.8 units/2 hr
    b. 1.05 units/ml
    c. 267.8 units/255 ml
17. a. 690 mg/dl
    b. 12.42 g/d
    c. 539.4 mmol/d
    d. 540 mEq/24 hr

*Slightly different answers may be obtained due to rounding off procedures.

Chapter 15 Quality control*

1. d
2.

		WBC	BUN	Hb
a.	s	1,835	1.7	0.14
b.	$\pm 2\,s$	4,208-11,548	19.5-26.3	13.12-13.68
c.	CV	23.3%	7.4%	1.04%

*Slightly different answers may be obtained due to rounding off procedures.

Bibliography

Barnett RN: *Clinical laboratory statistics,* ed 2, Boston, 1979, Little, Brown & Co.

Budavari et al: *The Merck index,* ed 12, Whitehouse Station, N.J., 1996, Merck & Co.

Curtis CA, Ashwood ER, editors: *Teitz textbook of clinical chemistry,* ed 2, Philadelphia, 1994, WB Saunders Co.

Dybkaer R: International Union of Pure and Applied Chemistry and the International Federations of Clinical Chemistry, Expert Panel on Quantities and Units: list of quantities in clinical chemistry (recommendations 1978), *Pure and Applied Chemistry* 51:2481-2502, 1979.

Dybkaer R: International Union of Pure and Applied Chemistry and the International Federations of Clinical Chemistry, Expert Panel on Quantities and Units: quantities and units in clinical chemistry (recommendations 1978), *Pure and Applied Chemistry* 51:2452-2479, 1979.

Dybkaer R, Jørgensen K: *Quantities and units in clinical chemistry, including recommendation 1966 of the Commission on Clinical Chemistry of the International Union of Pure and Applied Chemistry and of the International Federation of Clinical Chemistry,* Baltimore, 1967, Williams & Wilkins Co.

Federal Register Notice: *The metric system of measure (SI),* FR Doc 76-36414, December 10, 1976.

Henry JB: *Todd-Sanford-Davidsohn: clinial diagnosis and management by laboratory methods,* ed 18, Philadelphia, 1990, WB Saunders Co.

IUPAC Commission on Atomic Weights and Isotopic Abundances: Atomic weights of the elements (1993), *Pure and Applied Chemistry* 66:2423, 1994.

Kelly WD: *Basic statistics for laboratories,* New York, 1991, Van Nostrand Reinhold.

Laposata M: *SI unit conversion guide,* Boston, 1992, NEJM Books.

Leigh GJ, editor: *Nomenclature of inorganic chemistry: recommendations 1990,* London, 1990, Blackwell Scientific Publications.

Lide DR: *CRC handbook of chemistry and physics,* ed 76, New York, 1996, CRC Press.

Lippert H, Lehmann HP: *SI units in medicine,* Baltimore, 1978, Urban & Schwarzenberg, Inc.

Martinek RG: Practical mathematics for the medical technologist, *J Am Med Tech* 34: 117-146, 1972.

Mattenheimer H: *The theory of enzyme tests,* New York, Boehringer Mannheim Corp.

McQueen M: *SI unit pocket guide,* 1990, American Society of Clinical Chemistry.

Raphael SS: *Lynch's medical laboratory technology,* ed 4, Philadelphia, 1983, WB Saunders Co.

Robinson JW: *Undergraduate instrumental analysis,* ed 5, New York, 1995, Marcel Dekker, Inc.

Strike PW: *Statistical methods in laboratory medicine,* ed 2, Boston, 1991, Butterworth-Heinemann.

Index